Dentistry: Techniques and Applied Principles

Edited by Edgar Weston

hayle
medical

New York

Hayle Medical,
750 Third Avenue, 9th Floor,
New York, NY 10017, USA

Visit us on the World Wide Web at:
www.haylemedical.com

ISBN: 978-1-63241-476-2

Cataloging-in-Publication Data

Dentistry : techniques and applied principles / edited by Edgar Weston.
    p. cm.
Includes bibliographical references and index.
ISBN 978-1-63241-476-2
1. Dentistry. 2. Dentistry--Practice. I. Weston, Edgar.
RK51.5 .D45 2018
617.6--dc23

Table of Contents

Preface

It is often said that books are a boon to mankind. They document every progress and pass on the knowledge from one generation to the other. They play a crucial role in our lives. Thus I was both excited and nervous while editing this book. I was pleased by the thought of being able to make a mark but I was also nervous to do it right because the future of students depends upon it. Hence, I took a few months to research further into the discipline, revise my knowledge and also explore some more aspects. Post this process, I begun with the editing of this book.

Dentistry is the study and practice of preventing, diagnosing, treating disorders and diseases related to the oral cavity and craniofacial complex. The treatments included in this field are root canal, scaling and root planing, extractions, dental implants, etc. The topics covered in this extensive text deal with the core subjects of dentistry. From theories to research to practical applications, case studies related to all contemporary topics of relevance to the field of dentistry have been included in this book. The text is compiled in such a manner, that it will provide in-depth knowledge about the theory and practice of the subject. It will serve as a reference to a broad spectrum of readers.

I thank my publisher with all my heart for considering me worthy of this unparalleled opportunity and for showing unwavering faith in my skills. I would also like to thank the editorial team who worked closely with me at every step and contributed immensely towards the successful completion of this book. Last but not the least, I wish to thank my friends and colleagues for their support.

Editor

Orthodontic Protocol Using Mini-Implant for Class II Treatment in Patient with Special Needs

Fernando Pedrin Carvalho Ferreira,[1] **Anderson Paulo Barbosa Lima,**[2]
Eliana de Cássia Molina de Paula,[2] **Ana Claudia de Castro Ferreira Conti,**[2]
Danilo Pinelli Valarelli,[2] **and Renata Rodrigues de Almeida-Pedrin**[2]

[1]*CORA Vilhena, Vilhena, RO, Brazil*
[2]*Department of Orthodontics, Universidade do Sagrado Coração, Bauru, SP, Brazil*

Correspondence should be addressed to Anderson Paulo Barbosa Lima; andersonlima@ortodontista.com.br

Academic Editor: Sukumaran Anil

Improving facial and dental appearance and social interaction are the main factors for special needs (SN) patients to seek orthodontic treatment. The cooperation of SN patients and their parents is crucial for treatment success. *Objective.* To show through a case report the satisfactory results, both functional and esthetic, in patients with intellectual disability, congenital nystagmus, and severe scoliosis. *Materials Used.* Pendulum device with mini-implants as anchorage unit. *Results.* Improvement of facial and dental esthetics, correction of Class II malocclusion, and no root resorption shown in the radiographic follow-up. *Conclusion.* Knowing the limitations of SN patients, having a trained team, motivating and counting on the cooperation of parents and patients, and employing quick and low-cost orthodontic therapy have been shown to be the essential factors for treatment success.

1. Introduction

Special needs (SN) patients are the ones who do not engage in normal activities of their age groups. The prevalence of severe malocclusions in these patients is high, which requires orthodontic therapy [1]. The aim of the orthodontic treatment is not only functional but also esthetic improvement [2]. Individuals with SN face a social acceptance barrier, while the improvement of dental esthetics has a positive influence on social interaction, increasing the chances of employment toward self-sufficiency. However, the effectiveness of the orthodontic treatment is limited and not satisfactory for all cases [3].

The concern with facial appearance is what triggers parents to seek orthodontic treatment. Although parents are motivated by the improvement of quality of life of their children, SN patients are less likely to receive treatment. Usually, few SN patients end up being treated, and the main reasons are the fear of parents regarding the cooperation of their children during treatment and finding a trained dental team [4]. The cooperation of SN patients and their parents is essential for the success of orthodontic treatment [1, 4]. The progress over the last years of medical science allowed great developments in the treatment of SN patients in both expectancy and quality of life. The demand for dental treatment from patients with some type of systemic disease and physical or mental disability and elderly and immuno-compromised patients is increasingly high. Acknowledging the pathology and its implications for dental treatment is critical for the success of the therapy applied [5].

Patients with Class II malocclusion are the ones who mostly seek orthodontic treatment [6]. This malocclusion is characterized by maxillary prognathism, mandibular retrognathism, or the association of both [7, 8]. There are several therapeutic possibilities for treatment such as upper molar distalization, which may be performed with extraoral and intraoral appliances [9, 10]. In the case of SN patients, their lack of cooperation during treatment is a determinant factor for selecting the therapy to be applied. The use of intraoral distalizers is an alternative to be considered in these cases.

TABLE 1: Patient information.

Patient demographics	25-year-old Caucasian female 155 cm, 49 kg
Medical history	Nistagmus Scoliosis Visual disability
Allergies	Penicillin
Medications	Topiramate
Social history	Denies
Family history	Mother: none Father: none

Currently, there is a large diversity of intraoral devices in the market, and the pendulum device stands out among them because of the ease of clinical handling and its efficiency in correcting Class II malocclusion [11].

With the appearance of the mini-implant as temporary skeletal anchorage with easy insertion and removal in many areas of the maxilla and mandible, a new outlook was imposed regarding intraoral distalization [9, 12]. Associating the mini-implant as skeletal anchorage for the pendulum device would cancel its negative effects, which has already been described in the literature, improving treatment efficiency and reducing its time.

According to the above, this work aimed to show through a case report the satisfactory results, both functional and esthetic, in patients with intellectual disability, congenital nystagmus, and severe scoliosis. It also aimed to stress the importance of parental and patient cooperation and a trained dental team for treatment success.

2. Case Report

We report the case of a female patient, 1.55 m, 49 kg, 25 years old, with suggestive medical history for congenital nystagmus, severe scoliosis, and visual disability. Further information about the patient, such as past medical history, allergies, medication, and social and family history, is shown in Table 1.

Treatment started with passive lip seal, acceptable facial asymmetry, and closed nasolabial angle. There was prevalence of horizontal growth (Figure 1). The intraoral evaluation revealed the presence of severe crowding in both upper and lower arches, upper canine in buccal-version, and left upper lateral incisor palatal tipped in corssbite position. There are half cusp (1/2) class II malocclusion on the right side and 3/4 cusp class II on the left side and overjet of 2 mm and overbite of 5 mm (Figure 1).

After assessing the panoramic radiography and teleradiography (Figure 2), the patient was diagnosed with maxillary retrusion, thus causing natural compensatory proclination of upper incisors. Mandible was normal with lower incisors well positioned in the symphysis (Table 1).

The options given to the parents of patients were exodontia of third upper molars and first upper premolars (teeth 14 and 24) even with the prevalence of horizontal growth, considering that the amount of crowding would fill the extraction space and the retraction of the anterior quadrant would be small, thus not aggravating the overbite. However, parents refused this option because of the high number of extractions and the potential lack of patient cooperation during surgical therapy. The second option, approved by the parents, was distalization with pendulum supported in mini-implant as skeletal anchorage. As such, the main objectives of the treatment would be achieved: distalization of first upper molars toward Class I position and improvement of dental and facial esthetics.

The treatment had a few steps. First, exodontia of teeth 18 and 28 was requested subsequently under local anesthesia (2% lidocaine hydrochloride with 1 : 50,000 norepinephrine hemitartrate); then, 2 titanium mini screws (SIN, São Paulo, Brazil) of 1.6 cm in diameter and 8 mm in length were installed in the hard palate area, not parallel to each other. After installation, an alginate molding was made and forwarded to the production of the pendulum's anchorage unit, where it would be bonded with photoresin (Figure 3).

After 1 month from the start of distalization of first upper molars, fixed orthodontic appliances were bonded to the upper and lower arches: Roth prescription (Iceram, Orthometric, Marília, SP, Brazil), $0.022'' \times 0.0028''$ slot with $0.014''$ Flexy Super Elastic, Orthometric, wire. A bracket was not bonded to tooth 22 for lack of space in the dental arch (Figure 4). In the fifth month of treatment, the first molars were in Class I, with accentuated buccal torque (Figure 4) and decreasing upper and lower crowding. In this step, the pendulum was removed along with the anchorage unit. Then, space opening for tooth 22 started, with spring (JS) produced with a $0.018''$ steel wire. In the tenth month of treatment, the remaining spaces were closed with chain elastics and with the installation of a $0.019'' \times 0.025''$ steel wire in the upper arch, improving the torque in the first upper molars (Figure 5); a $0.018''$ steel wire was installed in the lower arch. Folds (offset) were applied in the area of teeth 33 and 43, seeking the proper lateral movement (Figure 5).

After 11 months from the start of the treatment, the intercuspation procedure began. By the end of intercuspation and occlusal adjustment, the orthodontic fixed appliance was removed and retainers were produced. A Hawley plate was installed in the upper arch and a 3×3 fixed retainer was installed in the lower arch. Orthodontic therapy lasted 12 months (Figures 6 and 7).

In the first posttreatment control, one month after the removal of the fixed appliance, the upper anterior teeth were rebonded for the repositioning of tooth 22, which presented lingual relapse (Figure 8) due to the lack of patient cooperation in using the upper removable retainer. Releveling lasted 3 months, and after removal a fixed retainer was installed on teeth 21, 22, and 23 (Figure 9).

3. Results

There was an improvement in facial and dental esthetics and retrusion and verticalization of upper incisors, which improved profile and opening of the nasolabial angle, promoting facial balance and harmony (Figure 10). The dental

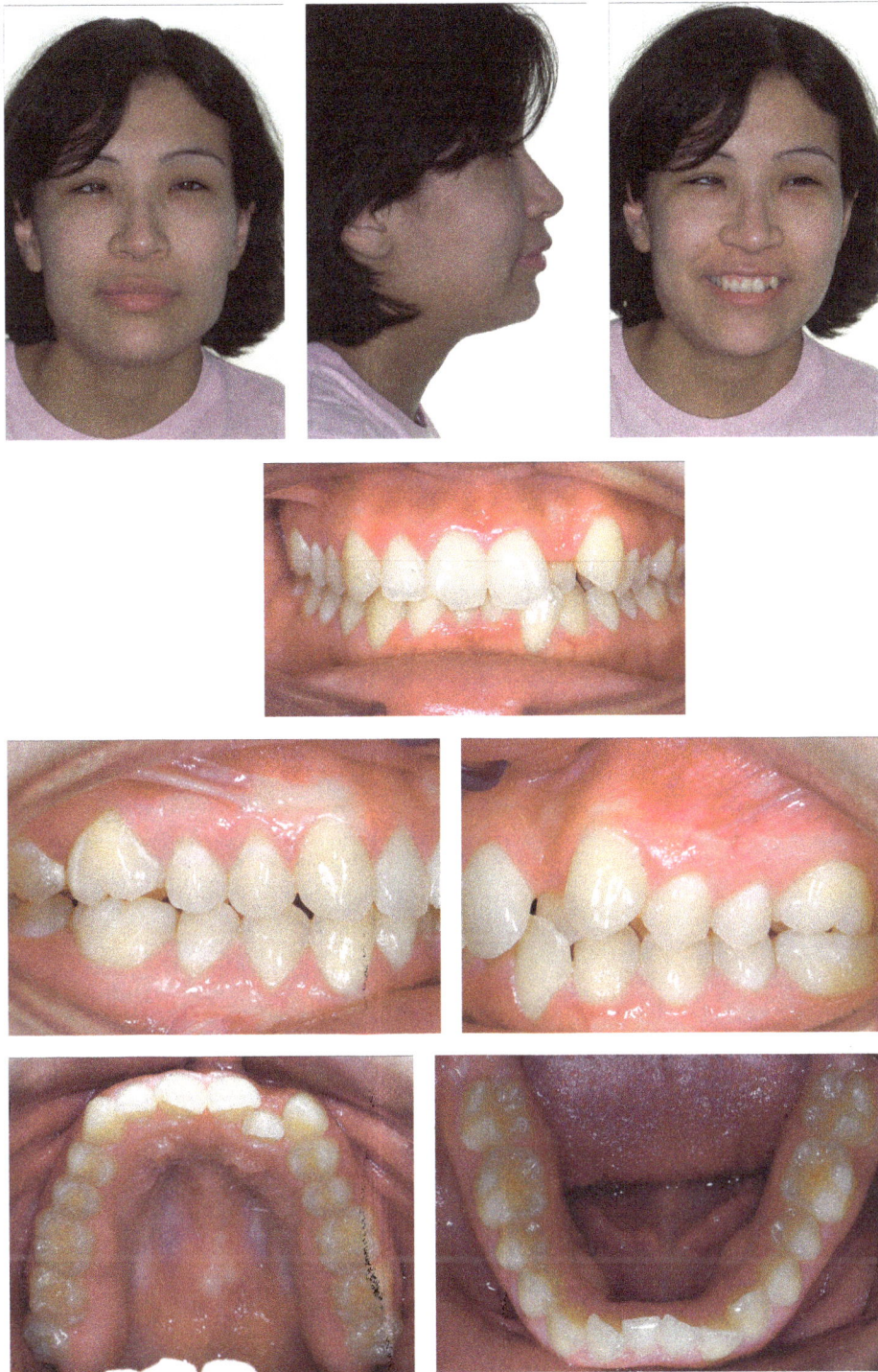

FIGURE 1: Extraoral and intraoral initial photos.

relationship was obtained from an upper tooth with two lower teeth. Overjet and overbite were normal, and maxillary and mandibular median lines coincided. Radiographic follow-up showed no major resorption in teeth roots (Figure 11). Upper molars distalization occurred with the translation movement, which is considered ideal (Figure 11). After 34 months from the end of treatment, the patient was reassessed (Table 2). The results achieved were proven to be stable (Figure 12).

4. Discussion

In Dentistry, the term "special needs patient" includes not only children and adults that take medication for systemic diseases and people with motor impairments and intellectual disabilities but also patients with oral cavity disease, which makes dental treatment more complicated. Therefore, the term "special needs patient" includes every patient that

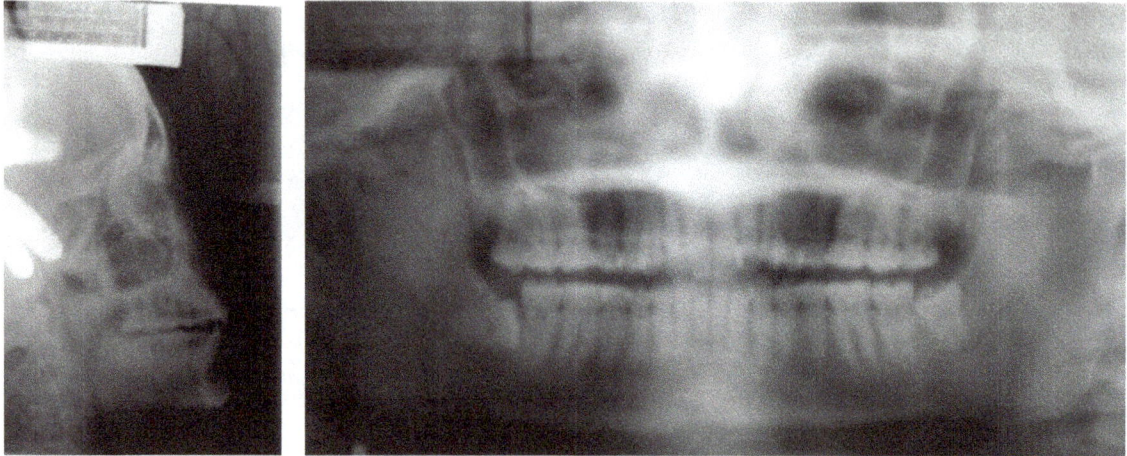

FIGURE 2: Initial panoramic radiography and teleradiography.

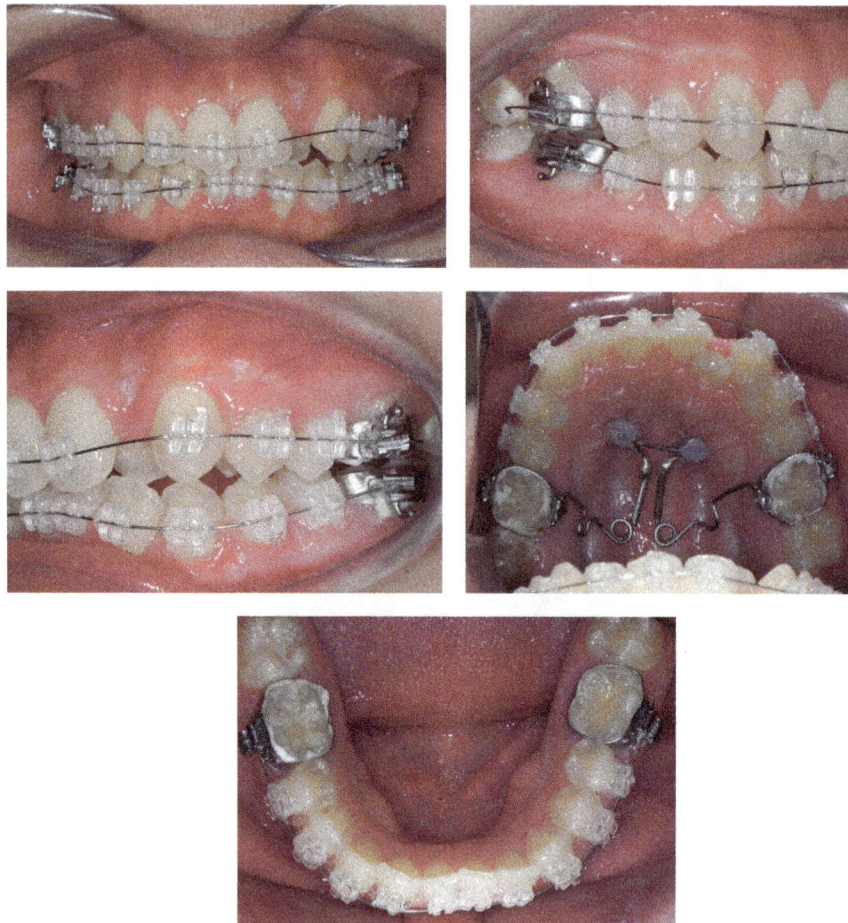

FIGURE 3: Bonding of upper and lower fixed appliances after one month from the start of distalization with pendulum.

requires a broad overview and a thorough physical, psychic, and social assessment in order to provide the correct treatment [5].

Waldman et al. [13] raised the question, "Do disabled people need esthetic and functional considerations to be comparable to 'normal' people?" Improved physical appearance and oral function after orthodontic therapy could increase the quality of life of people with SN and promote better social acceptance [14]. Improved facial appearance and social integration are the major motivators for parents

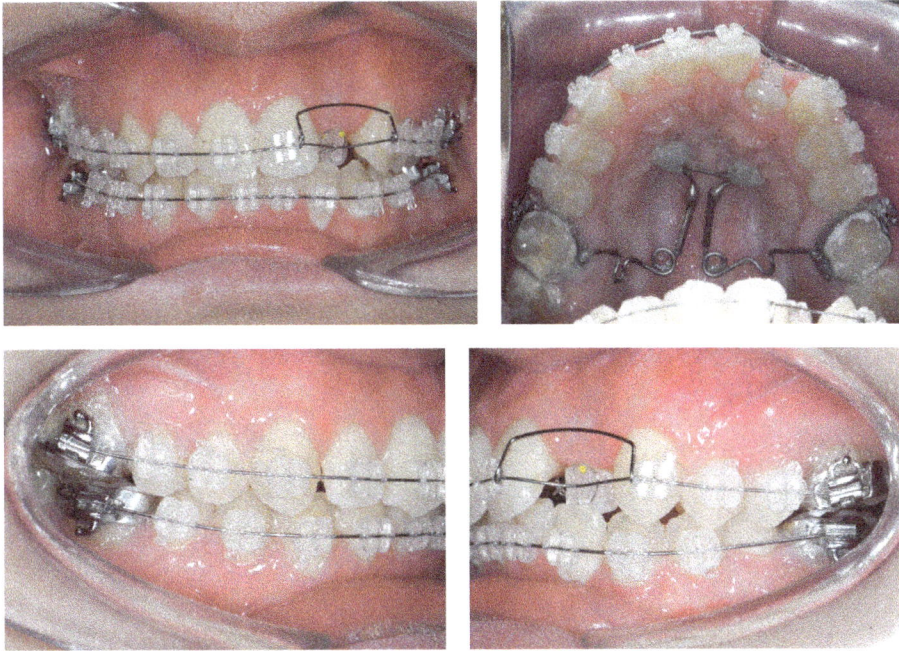

FIGURE 4: Start of tooth 22 alignment. JS spring used for space opening. Buccal torque of first upper molars.

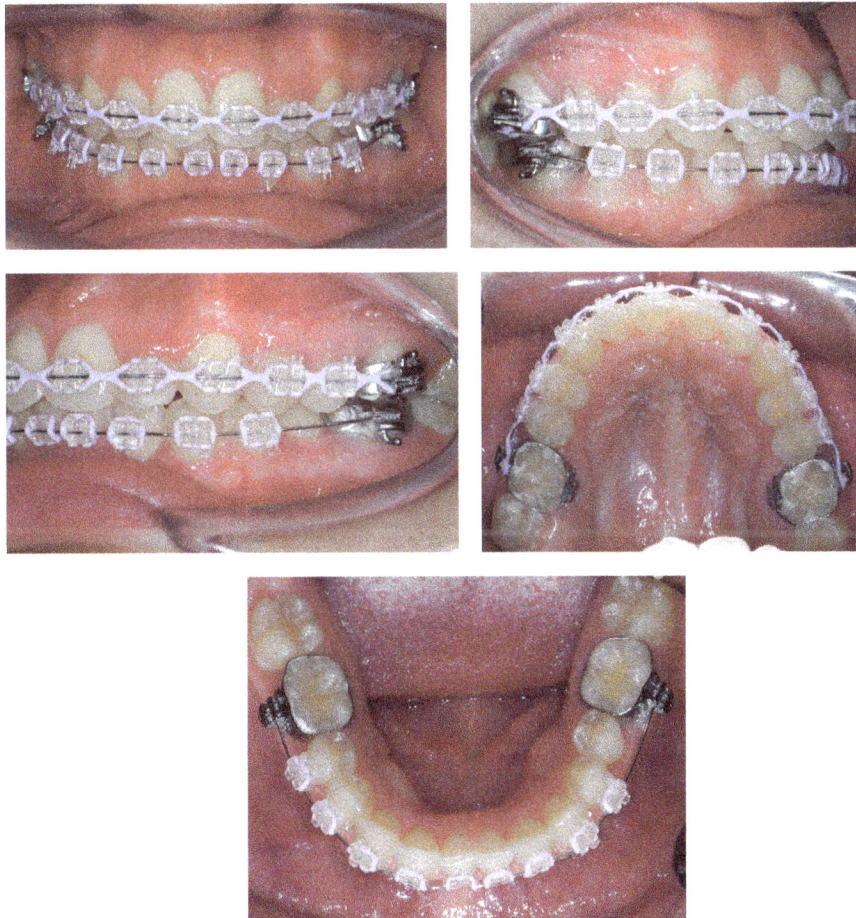

FIGURE 5: Class I upper molars and closing of remaining spaces with chain elastics.

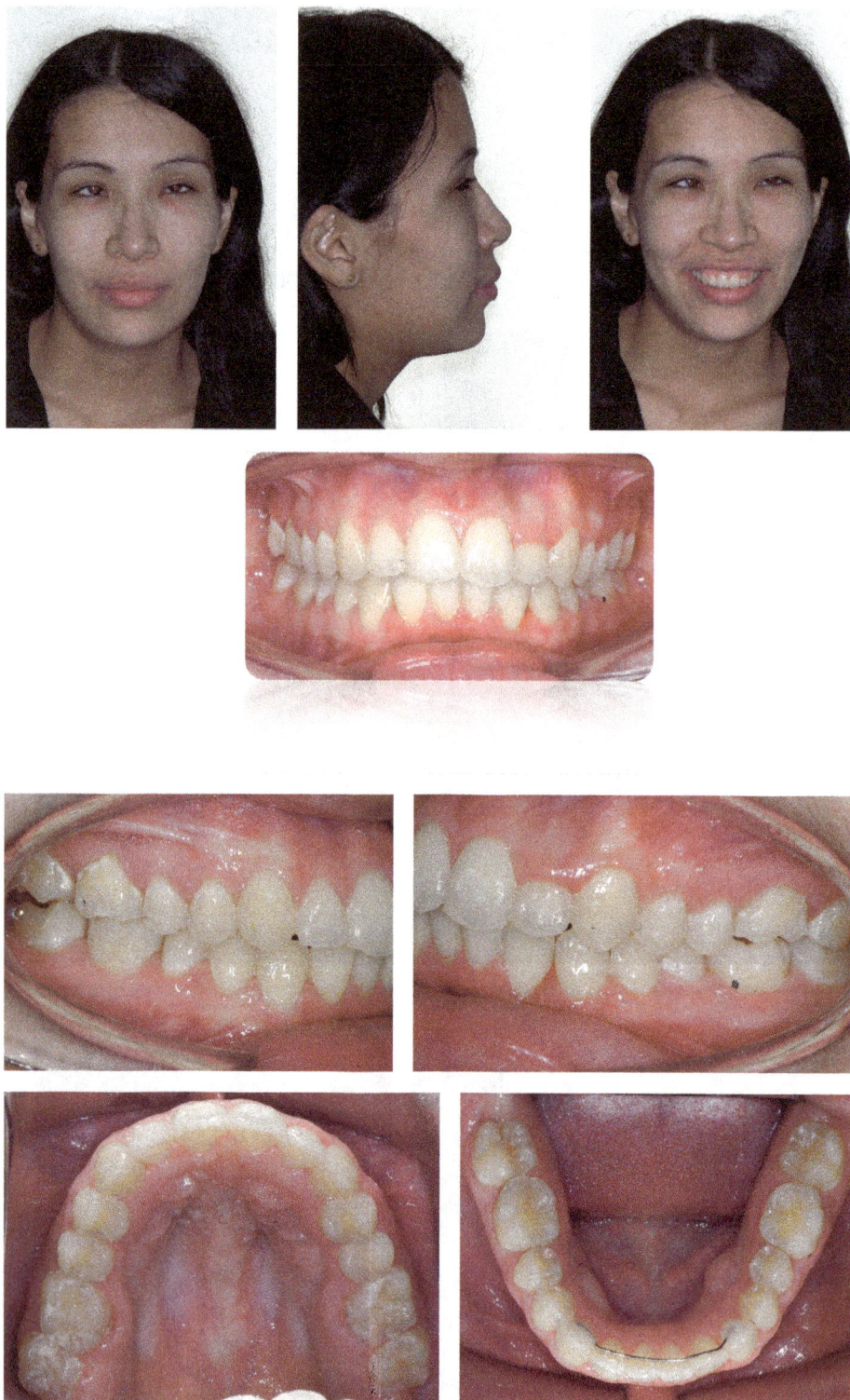

FIGURE 6: Removal of fixed appliance and bonding of 3 × 3 retainer on the lower arch 11 months after treatment started.

to seek orthodontic treatment [14]. Moreover, people with SN are more likely to present periodontal disease, causing severe esthetic malocclusions that hinder social relations and employment opportunities [13].

Children and adolescents with SN present higher prevalence of malocclusions than the normal population due to deleterious habits (thumb sucking, mouth breathing, and tongue interposition), different diet (no intake of solid food

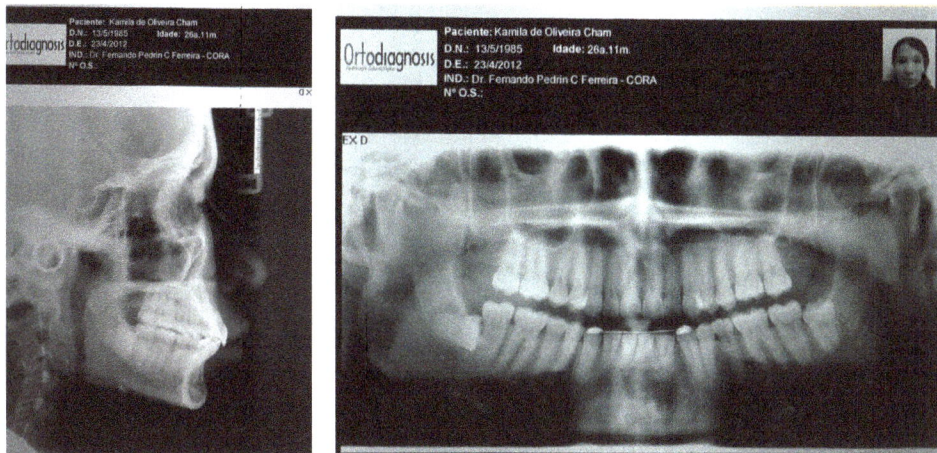

FIGURE 7: Final panoramic radiography and teleradiography.

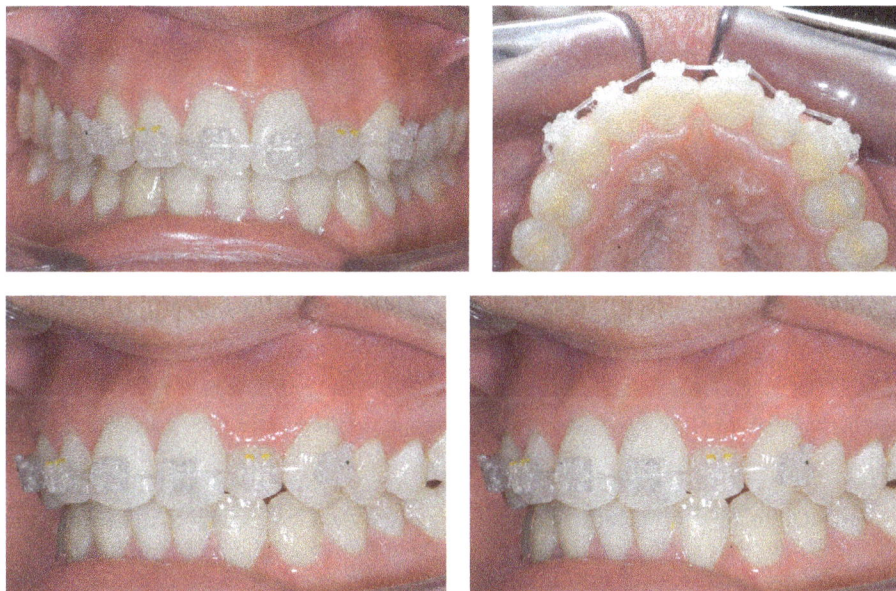

FIGURE 8: Rebonding of fixed appliance to correct relapse.

which requires thorough mastication), increased levels of caries, and early teeth loss. However, malocclusion may have evolved as postpartum trauma, prenatal effects, hereditary factors, or muscle development [13]. Class II malocclusion affects 33.7% of these patients [4].

The treatment for Class II malocclusion varies according to etiology, dentoalveolar involvement, and skeletal discrepancy. Several protocols are described in the literature, including dental extractions, functional orthopedic appliances, distalizers, or orthodontic/surgical treatment [6]. Because of the limitations of the patient reported in this study and the refusal from parents for a high number of extractions, the distalization of molars with pendulum supported in mini-implant was the more likely option to be performed. The mini-implant support eliminated the unwanted effects such as protrusion of anterior teeth (incisors and canines), mesial

movement of premolars, and the increase of overjet, which would extend treatment time [6]. The study by Öncağ et al. [15] on the efficiency of the pendulum device supported in palate mini-implants concluded that there was no protrusion of upper incisors during the distalization process, reducing treatment time and presenting satisfactory esthetics and stable occlusion. The pendulum is a device that presents efficiency in upper molar distalization, eliminating the factor of patient cooperation; it is a low-cost device that is easy to produce and install [11, 16]. The use of extraoral appliances is the best option, but due to esthetic standards imposed by society, it is harder to get patient approval, which consequently leads to treatment failure [6]. The lack of cooperation from the patient exposed was another determinant factor for the selection of the pendulum device supported in mini-implants.

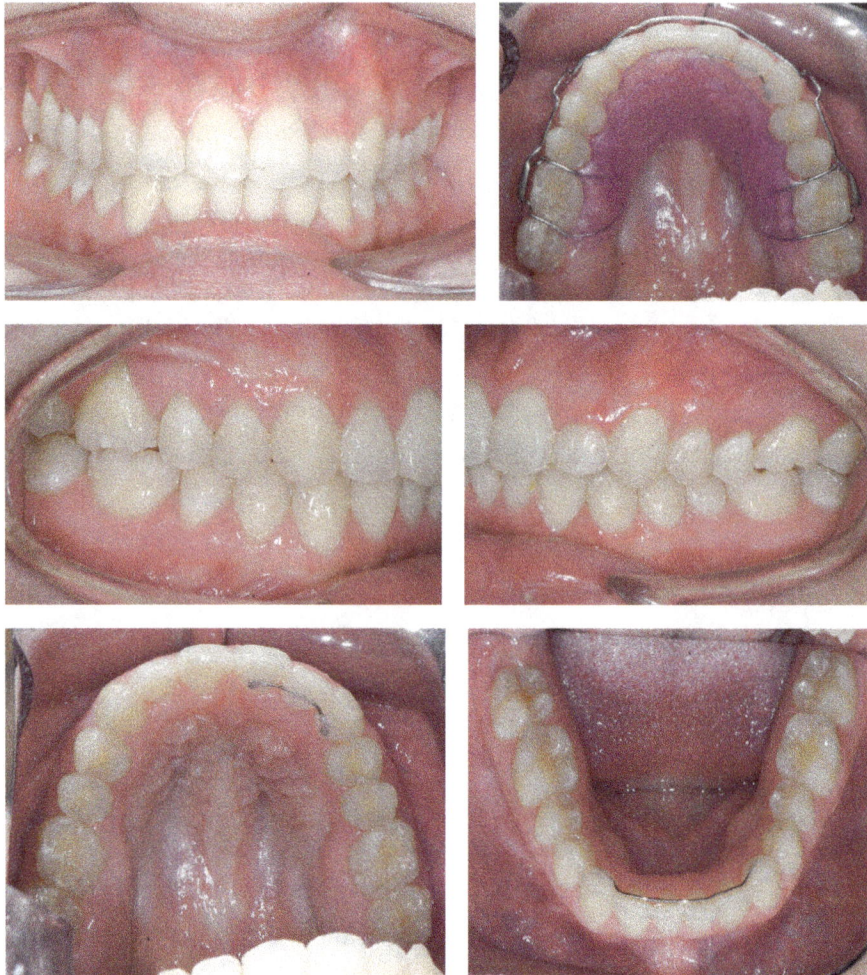

FIGURE 9: After 3 months, the fixed appliance was removed again and an upper fixed retainer was produced from tooth 21 to tooth 23.

With the lack of cooperation of SN patients, parental participation is crucial for the success of orthodontic therapy [17]. Patient motivation does not increase over the different treatment steps, which is influenced by the presence of discomfort and the level of acceptance of the device employed. Parents are significantly more motivated than their children [18].

People with SN are used to receive constant daily attention from their motivated parents who are willing to do everything possible to improve the well-being of their children and are willing to become members of the team [14]. The dental team that receives SN patients and subsequently provides care should assess every aspect of the patient such as communication method, anxiety, and difficulties or challenges concerning behavior in order to maximize the potential for a positive result, which is important for the patient as to make it a successful experience. Some of the precautions to minimize anxiety are online media (websites and blogs) so that patients and parents have access to information about the practice they might experience, brochures showing the patient what might happen during their visit, and accessibility [19].

Usually, SN patients need to be sedated for dental procedures. Currently, propofol and midazolam are the primary

agents used for sedation in dental treatment because of their short half-life and amnesic effects [20, 21]; the most common effect of these drugs is somnolence [22]. Special needs patients often take several drugs and the side effects may affect oral health. Anticonvulsants may cause gingival hyperplasia, and psychotropic and cardiovascular drugs may lead to xerostomia. The high level of sugar in medicines for children may contribute to dental caries [13]. Sedation was not required to install the mini-implants and other orthodontic appliances in the patient treated; only local anesthetic and previous topical anesthetic were needed. Parents were motivated and the patient was conditioned with the procedures to be performed.

Conventional intraoral distalizers take an average of 4–7 months to achieve molar Class I [23], although the literature imposes that the protocol of extraction of two upper premolars is faster than distalization to correct Class II [23]. The use of the pendulum device supported in mini-implants showed efficiency in correcting this malocclusion in a reduced time with satisfactory occlusal results and interesting biological cost, considering the limitations of the patient exposed.

One of the main objectives of the orthodontic treatment is to improve facial esthetics. Nose, lips, and chin should

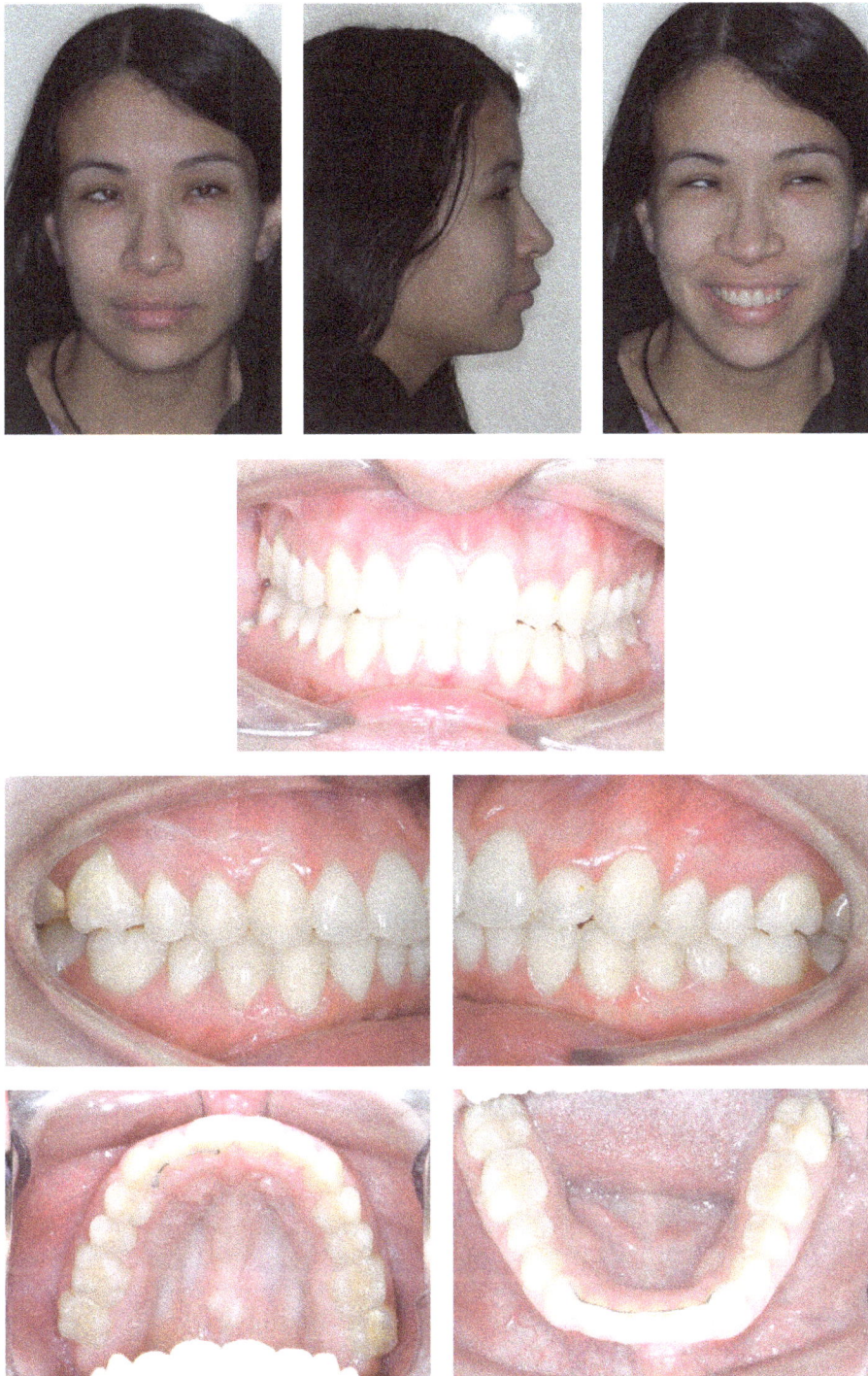

FIGURE 10: Extraoral and intraoral final photos showing improved facial and dental esthetics.

form a gentle outline of the face when seen in profile [24]. It is possible to observe slight retrusion and verticalization of upper incisors and a small opening of the nasolabial angle. Although the cephalometric result was not significant for retrusion and verticalization of upper incisors, the upper lip was posteriorly positioned, making the profile look straighter. Parents noticed the change. In the study by Bowman and Johnston Jr. [25], orthodontists and lay people had the same

perception of the changes in profile after treatment. On the other hand, Cochrane et al. [26] affirm that dentists tend to be more critical than parents and patients regarding the perception of facial esthetics [26]. This corroborates with the study by Pithon et al. [27], where lay people assessed the profile of a female patient with accentuated bimaxillary protrusion. The image was altered to produce a series of photos with different lip positions, and, in conclusion, the

TABLE 2: Cephalometric measurements.

Measurement	Initial (10/10)	Final (4/12)	Follow-up (3/13)
SNA	80.89	80.22	80.22
SNB	77.12	77.32	76.93
ANB	3.77	2.90	3.29
SN-MP	26.93	26.62	27.60
SN.Gn	70.12	70.23	70.50
FMA	17.13	17.84	16.87
1.1	128.17	112.55	119.48
1.NA	28.08	20.66	19.17
1-NA	7.40	6.70	6.27
1.NB	45.64	43.89	38.06
1-NB	7.78	7.63	7.31
IMPA	122.45	119.96	113.53

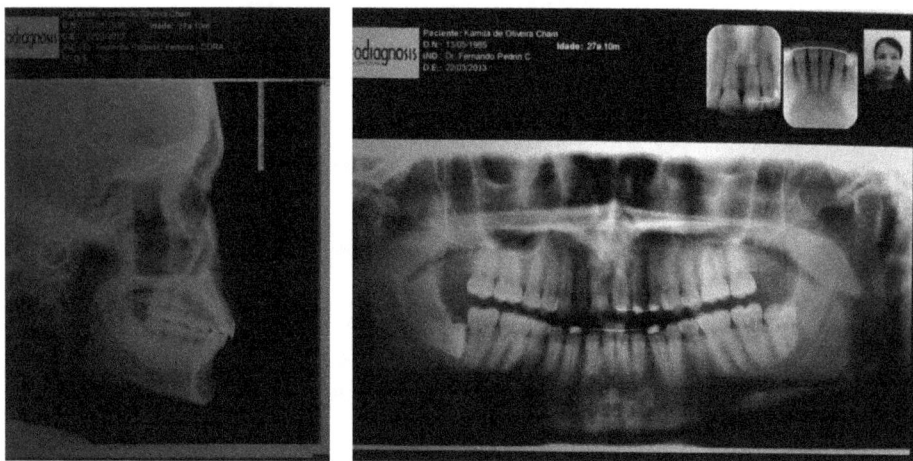

FIGURE 11: Final panoramic radiography and teleradiography. There was no significant root resorption.

straight profile was elected to be the most attractive. The study supports the understanding that people look beyond cephalometric measurements to assess facial appearance [25].

Gingival esthetics in the area of tooth 22 could be improved by finishing folds and arch twists (root buccal torque) [28], the root would be directed toward the buccal side, and root displacement followed by the alveolar bone would make the gingiva thinner, improving smile esthetics. However, parents refused such procedure, considering that the result presented exceeded their expectations. In a study performed in healthy adolescents who received orthodontic treatment, only 34% were completely satisfied with the results, 62% were relatively satisfied, and 4% were dissatisfied [29]. The study by Abeleira et al. [4] with disabled children resulted in 100% of satisfaction from the parents interviewed, and more than 40% affirmed that the results of the orthodontic treatment had exceeded their expectations.

Inadequate oral hygiene may be the greatest obstacle for orthodontic treatment success. People with SN may not understand the need for oral hygiene or present physical limitations [13]. The patient treated presented good oral hygiene, no dental caries, and low level of biofilm. The hygiene routine proposed by the parents was effective.

The "ghost" of dental treatment in SN patients is a label given by dental professionals. The lack of training of professionals and their teams may be the greatest aggravating factor. Knowing the limitations of these patients, providing a friendly environment, and motivating parents were the key factors for a satisfactory orthodontic treatment for both.

5. Conclusion

The treatment of a disabled patient requires special care. Patient motivation and conditioning added by parent cooperation are essential factors for treatment success. The selection of adequate orthodontic mechanics and the presence of a trained team are determinant factors for a more favorable prognosis.

Competing Interests

The authors declare that they do not have a significant financial or professional interest in any company, product, or service mentioned in the article.

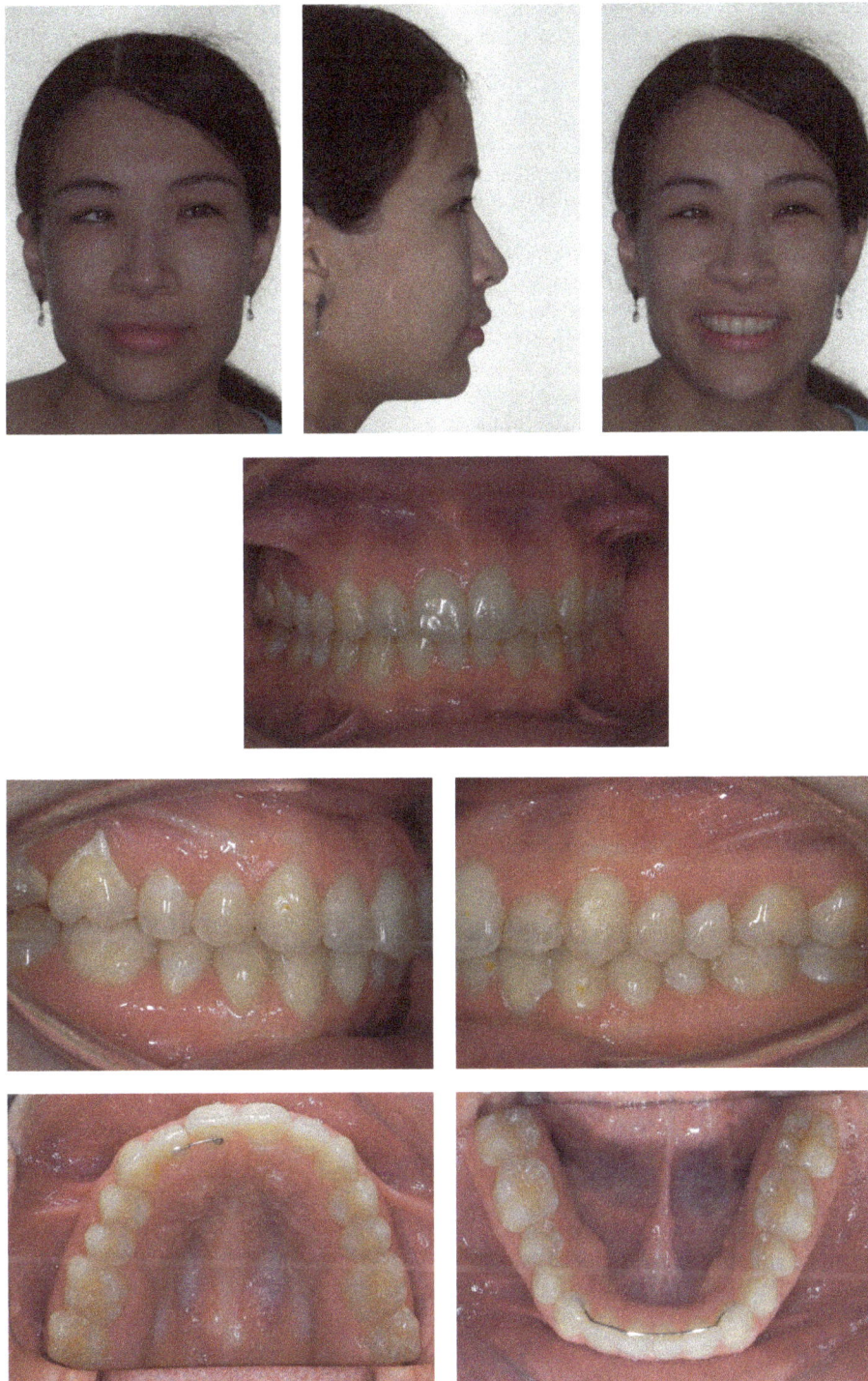

FIGURE 12: Extraoral and intraoral photos 34 months after the end of treatment.

References

[1] A. Becker, S. Chaushu, and J. Shapira, "Orthodontic treatment for the special needs child," *Seminars in Orthodontics*, vol. 10, no. 4, pp. 281–292, 2004.

[2] S. Chaushu and A. Becker, "Behaviour management needs for orthodontic treatment of children with disabilities," *European Journal of Orthodontics*, vol. 22, pp. 143–149, 2000.

[3] A. Becker and J. Shapira, "Orthodontics for the handicapped child," *European Journal of Orthodontics*, vol. 18, no. 1, pp. 55–67, 1996.

[4] M. T. Abeleira, E. Pazos, I. Ramos et al., "Orthodontic treatment for disabled children: a survey of parents' attitudes and overall satisfaction," *BMC Oral Health*, vol. 14, no. 1, article 98, 2014.

[5] M. M. Matesanz, G. E. Gómez, B. G. Chías, C. G. García, and R. C. Lapiedra, "Descriptive study of the patients treated at

the clinic 'Integrated Dentistry for patients with special needs' at Complutense University of Madrid (2003–2012)," *Medicina Oral, Patología Oral y Cirugía Bucal*, vol. 20, no. 2, pp. e211–e217, 2015.

[6] T. E. V. Mendes Jr., A. B. A. Lima, T. E. V. Mendes, C. V. A. T. Mendes, H. D. A. Rosário, and L. R. E. Paranhos, "Distalization controlled with the use of lip-bumper and mini-screw as anchorage: a new approach," *International Journal of Orthodontics*, vol. 26, no. 1, pp. 29–32, 2015.

[7] K. Nagayama, H. Tomonari, F. Kitashima, and S. Miyawaki, "Extraction treatment of a Class II division 2 malocclusion with mandibular posterior discrepancy and changes in stomatognathic function," *Angle Orthodontist*, vol. 85, no. 2, pp. 314–321, 2015.

[8] L. Z. Saikoski, R. H. Cançado, F. P. Valarelli, and K. M. S. de Freitas, "Dentoskeletal effects of Class II malocclusion treatment with the Twin Block appliance in a Brazilian sample: a prospective study," *Dental Press Journal of Orthodontics*, vol. 19, no. 1, pp. 36–45, 2014.

[9] R. H. Shimizu, A. R. Ambrosio, I. A. Shimizu, J. Godoy-Bezerra, J. S. RIbeiro, and K. R. Staszak, "Biomechanic principles of the headgear appliance," *R Dental Press Ortodon Ortop Facial*, vol. 9, pp. 122–156, 2004.

[10] T. Bussick and J. McNamara, "Dentoalveolar and skeletal changes associated with the pendulum appliance," *American Journal of Orthodontics and Dentofacial Orthopedics*, vol. 7, pp. 333–343, 2000.

[11] R. R. Almeida, M. R. Almeida, A. Fuziy, and J. F. C. Henriques, "Modificação do aparelho Pendulum/Pend-X. Descrição do aparelho e técnica de construção," *Revista Dental Press de Ortodontia e Ortopedia Facial*, vol. 4, no. 6, pp. 12–19, 1999.

[12] I. E. Gelgör, T. Büyükyilmaz, A. I. Ý. Karaman, D. Dolanmaz, and A. Kalayci, "Intraosseous screw-supported upper molar distalization," *Angle Orthodontist*, vol. 74, no. 6, pp. 838–850, 2004.

[13] H. B. Waldman, S. P. Perlman, and M. Swerdloff, "Orthodontics and the population with special needs," *American Journal of Orthodontics and Dentofacial Orthopedics*, vol. 118, no. 1, pp. 14–17, 2000.

[14] A. Becker, J. Shapira, and S. Chaushu, "Orthodontic treatment for disabled children: motivation, expectation, and satisfaction," *European Journal of Orthodontics*, vol. 22, no. 2, pp. 151–158, 2000.

[15] G. Öncağ, S. Akyalçın, and F. Arıkan, "The effectiveness of a single osteointegrated implant combined with pendulum springs for molar distalization," *American Journal of Orthodontics & Dentofacial Orthopedics*, vol. 131, no. 2, pp. 277–284, 2007.

[16] J. Ghosh and R. S. Nanda, "Evaluation of an intraoral maxillary molar distalization technique," *American Journal of Orthodontics and Dentofacial Orthopedics*, vol. 110, no. 6, pp. 639–646, 1996.

[17] K. Winter, L. Baccaglini, and S. Tomar, "A review of malocclusion among individuals with mental and physical disabilities," *Special Care in Dentistry*, vol. 28, no. 1, pp. 19–26, 2008.

[18] A. S. Daniels, J. D. Seacat, and M. R. Inglehart, "Orthodontic treatment motivation and cooperation: a cross-sectional analysis of adolescent patients' and parents' responses," *American Journal of Orthodontics and Dentofacial Orthopedics*, vol. 136, no. 6, pp. 780–787, 2009.

[19] R. Valle-Jones and D. Chandler, "Special care dentistry: two sides of a coin," *British Dental Journal*, vol. 218, no. 5, pp. 313–314, 2015.

[20] U. Padmanabhan, K. Leslie, A. S. Eer, P. Maruff, and B. S. Silbert, "Early cognitive impairment after sedation for colonoscopy: the effect of adding midazolam and/or fentanyl to propofol," *Anesthesia & Analgesia*, vol. 109, no. 5, pp. 1448–1455, 2009.

[21] M. M. Wahidi, P. Jain, M. Jantz et al., "American College of Chest Physicians consensus statement on the use of topical anesthesia, analgesia, and sedation during flexible bronchoscopy in adult patients," *Chest*, vol. 140, no. 5, pp. 1342–1350, 2011.

[22] S. Maeda, Y. Tomayasu, H. Higuchi et al., "Independent factors affecting recovery time after sedation in patients with intellectual disabilities," *The Open Dentistry Journal*, vol. 9, pp. 146–149, 2015.

[23] C. R. Pinzan-Vercelino, A. Pinzan, G. Janson, R. R. Almeida, J. F. Henriques, and M. R. Freitas, "Comparação entre os resultados oclusais e os tempos de tratamento da má oclusão de Classe II por meio da utilização do aparelho Pendulum e das extrações de dois pré-molares superiores," *Dental Press Journal of Orthodontics*, vol. 15, no. 1, pp. 89–100, 2010.

[24] K. O'Neill, M. Harkness, and R. Knight, "Ratings of profile attractiveness after functional appliance treatment," *American Journal of Orthodontics & Dentofacial Orthopedics*, vol. 118, no. 4, pp. 371–376, 2000.

[25] S. J. Bowman and L. E. Johnston Jr., "The esthetic impact of extraction and nonextraction treatments on caucasian patients," *Angle Orthodontist*, vol. 70, no. 1, pp. 3–10, 2000.

[26] S. M. Cochrane, S. J. Cunningham, and N. P. Hunt, "Perceptions of facial appearance by orthodontists and the general public," *Journal of Clinical Orthodontics*, vol. 31, no. 3, pp. 164–168, 1997.

[27] M. M. Pithon, I. S. N. Silva, I. O. Almeida et al., "Photos vs silhouettes for evaluation of profile esthetics between white and black evaluators," *The Angle Orthodontist*, vol. 84, no. 2, pp. 231–238, 2014.

[28] G. Janson, D. P. Valarelli, F. P. Valarelli, M. R. de Freitas, and A. Pinzan, "Atypical extraction of maxillary central incisors," *American Journal of Orthodontics & Dentofacial Orthopedics*, vol. 138, no. 4, pp. 510–517, 2010.

[29] L. E. Anderson, A. Arruda, and M. R. Inglehart, "Adolescent patients' treatment motivation and satisfaction with orthodontic treatment," *Angle Orthodontist*, vol. 79, no. 5, pp. 821–827, 2009.

2

Congenital Unilateral Agenesis of the Parotid Gland

Afshin Teymoortash and Stephan Hoch

Department of Otolaryngology, Head and Neck Surgery, Philipp University, Marburg, Germany

Correspondence should be addressed to Stephan Hoch; hochs@med.uni-marburg.de

Academic Editor: Anastasios Markopoulos

Congenital unilateral agenesis of the parotid gland is a rare condition with only few cases reported in the literature. A review of 21 cases in the available literature is presented in this article. We report on a further case of a 34-year-old woman with agenesis of the left parotid gland and lipoma of the right cheek. Clinicopathological characteristics of described cases in the literature were discussed.

1. Introduction

The major salivary glands start to develop between the sixth and seventh week of gestation beginning with the parotid gland which arises from ectodermal lining of the stomatodeum [1]. The submandibular and sublingual glands develop later and arise from the endodermal layer of the floor of the stomatodeum. Congenital absence of major salivary glands is a rare condition of unclear etiology. It is usually bilateral and sometimes associated with other development anomalies of the head and neck area. Unilateral agenesis of the parotid gland, especially, is an extremely rare condition with only few cases reported in the literature. The first report of a salivary gland agenesis was mentioned in 1885 by Gruber [2]. Since then, few cases of the unilateral submandibular gland agenesis have been reported in the literature [3].

Agenesis of parotid glands may occur alone or in association with anomalies of the submandibular or lacrimal gland, first brachial arch developmental disturbances, or other congenital anomalies [4–7]. The true incidence of agenesis of the parotid gland is difficult to ascertain because the condition is often asymptomatic [8]. Because saliva is mostly produced by other major and minor salivary glands, xerostomia does not occur and the absence of parotid gland is not noticed by the patient in the majority of cases [4].

We present a case of unilateral agenesis of the parotid gland in combination with a lipoma of the cheek on the opposite site. The clinical and radiological findings in this patient are described. A review of the unilateral parotid gland agenesis in the literature is also presented considering a summary of the data regarding gender, age, defect site, and combined manifestations.

2. Case Report

A 34-year-old woman was referred to our department for evaluation of painless swelling of the right cheek over the last seven months. In addition, she often bit her right cheek. The swelling did not vary in size during eating and the patient had no other clinical symptoms and no history of recurrent parotitis. Xerostomia was not noted. There was no other relevant medical history and no family history of similar problems was reported. On clinical examination the oral mucosa was moistened by saliva. Bilateral hemifacial contour was normal, and there were no depressions in either preauricular region. Physical examination of the head and neck was without pathological findings, except for the absence of the left parotid gland papilla (Figure 1).

Ultrasonographic examination of the head and neck area showed that the parotid gland on the left side was totally absent. The other major salivary glands were present without any pathology. A tumor in the right cheek ventral to parotid gland was observed with characteristic sonographic appearance of lipoma. For further evaluation of the tumor in the right cheek and assessment of the function of the other salivary glands magnetic resonance imaging (MRI) and

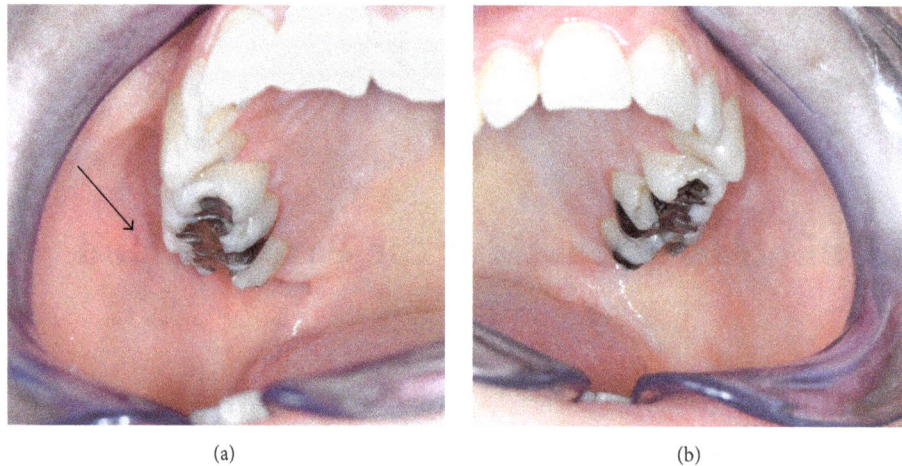

(a)   (b)

FIGURE 1: (a) Intraoral view of the right buccal mucosa shows the papilla of Stensen's duct. (b) Intraoral view of the left buccal mucosa. The papilla of Stensen's duct is absent.

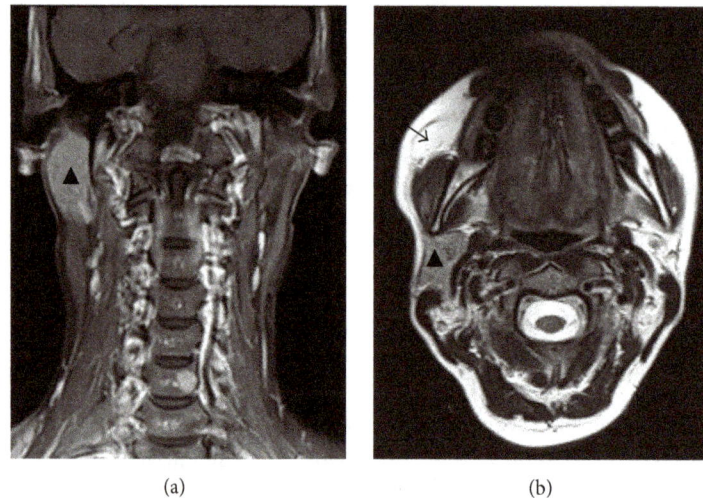

(a)   (b)

FIGURE 2: MRI scan of the parotid gland shows the unilateral agenesis of the parotid gland. (a) Coronary scan and (b) axial scan. The arrow points to the lipoma of the cheek and the triangle points to the right parotid gland.

scintigraphy with Technetium (Tc-99m) sodium pertechnetate were performed. MRI confirmed a lipoma of the cheek on the right side and a unilateral absence of the left parotid gland (Figure 2). Other pathological findings in the head and neck area could not be found. Salivary gland scintigraphy showed no activity in the area of the left parotid gland with normal function of the other major salivary glands (Figure 3). The patient had no clinical symptoms associated with the absence of the parotid gland. The buccal tumor was removed via parotidectomy incision and exposition of the facial nerve. Histological examination of the specimen confirmed the clinical suspicion of lipoma (Figure 4). The postoperative recovery proceeded without complications. There was no further follow-up after wound healing was accomplished.

3. Discussion

Congenital absence of the salivary glands is a rare condition which has been described to affect the parotid or submandibular glands [26]. Agenesis of salivary glands may be unilateral or bilateral and multiple major salivary glands can be involved [27–29].

The true incidence of unilateral agenesis of the parotid gland is difficult to ascertain because it is often asymptomatic [10]. Congenital unilateral absence of the parotid gland is uncommon with only few cases reported. The absence of bilateral parotid glands has been observed in lacrimoauriculodentodigital (LADD) syndrome [30], in hypoplasia of the lacrimal glands or absence of lacrimal puncta [31], in hemifacial microstomia, and in ectodermal dysplasia. The resulting disturbances affect primarily the lacrimal glands, the inner and outer ear, the salivary glands, and the osseous frame work [24, 30]. Aplasia of the major salivary glands may be associated with aplasia/hypoplasia of the lacrimal glands. This condition is confirmed as autosomal dominant disorder [32]. Single cases of bilateral parotid gland agenesis associated with cleft lip and palate, Down syndrome, or Klinefelter

TABLE 1: Reported cases of unilateral parotid gland agenesis in the literature ($n = 22$).

Number	Authors	Year	Age	Sex	Site	Combined manifestations	Papilla of Stensen's duct
1	Kelly et al. [9]	1990	28	m	Right	Sialosis of contralateral parotid gland	Absent
2	Almadori et al. [10]	1997	38	m	Left	Hypertrophy of contralateral parotid gland	Absent
3	Bhide and Warshawsky [11]	1998	16	m	Right	Ipsilateral accessory of parotid tissue	Unknown
4	Sichel et al. [12]	1998	4.5	f	Right	First branchial cleft cyst type II	Unknown
5	Hyang et al. [13]	1999	22	f	Left	Hypertrophy of contralateral parotid gland	Unknown
6	Martínez Subías et al. [14]	2000	21	f	Right	Hypertrophy of contralateral parotid gland	Unknown
7	Daniel et al. [15]	2003	5	m	Right	Hypertrophy of contralateral parotid gland	Unknown
8	Salvinelli et al. [16]	2004	53	m	Right	Ipsilateral angioma of the cheek	Absent
9	Martín-Granizo and García-González [17]	2004	58	m	Right	Hypertrophy of contralateral parotid gland	Absent
10	Karakoc et al. [18]	2005	35	f	Left	Pleomorphic adenoma of contralateral parotid gland	Absent
11	D'Ascanio et al. [8]	2006	53	f	Right	Hypoplasia of the thyroid's right lobe and homolateral angioma of the cheek	Absent
12	Lee [19]	2010	65	f	Right	Pleomorphic adenoma in the ipsilateral buccal space	Unknown
13	Chen et al. [20]	2011	75	m	Right	Contralateral compensation hypermetabolism of FDG	Unknown
14	Udall and Cho [21]	2011	0.8	m	Right	Metastases from left craniocervical neuroblastoma	Unknown
15	Capaccio et al. [22]	2012	44	m	Right	Recurrent inflammation of accessory parotid tissue	Present
16	Seith et al. [23]	2013	41	m	Left	Pleomorphic adenoma of ipsilateral accessory parotid gland	Absent
17	Sun et al. [24]	2013	15	w	Left	Partial duplication of the mandible facial cleft, accessory parotid gland	Unknown
18	Günbey et al. [25]	2014	45	w	Right	Hypertrophy of contralateral parotid gland	Absent
19			52	w	Left		Absent
20			63	m	Left		Absent
21	Özçelik et al. [7]	2014	0.1	w	Right	Ipsilateral facial cleft, accessory mandible, facial weakness	Absent
22	Present case	2016	30	w	Left	Contralateral cheek lipoma	Absent

m = masculine; f = feminine; FDG = fluorodeoxyglucose.

syndrome have been reported [1, 33–35]. Some cases of familial salivary gland agenesis have also been documented [31]. Bilateral forms of agenesis could be responsible for a severe lack of saliva causing dental caries, periodontal disease, and candidosis [8].

In the available literature, only 22 cases of unilateral agenesis of the parotid gland have been described including the present case (Table 1). Among the 22 cases, 11 (50%) of the patients were male and 11 (50%) were female. At the time of diagnosis the youngest patient was 50 days old and the oldest was 75 years old with an average age of 34.7 years. The unilateral absence of the right parotid gland was nearly twice as frequent as the left side (14/8 cases). The papilla of

Stensen's duct was present in only one case. In the other cases the parotid papilla was absent ($n = 12$) or the presence of the parotid papilla was not documented ($n = 9$).

In most reported cases the unilateral agenesis of the parotid gland was associated with a painless swelling of the contralateral parotid gland or facial asymmetry without any other significant clinical symptoms [9, 10, 13–15, 17, 20, 25]. According to the authors the swelling of the contralateral parotid gland was as a compensatory functional hypertrophy of the parotid gland [14, 15, 17, 25]. Association with other pathologies of the head and neck area could not be found in those cases. Sialosis of the contralateral parotid gland was found in one case; the diagnosis was confirmed by

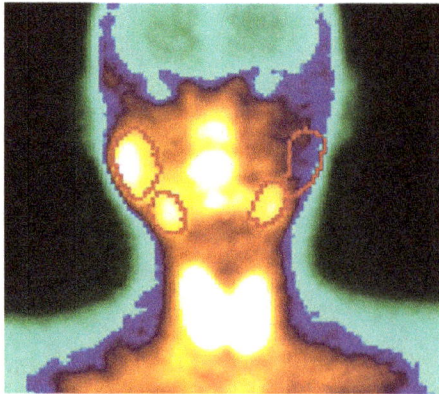

FIGURE 3: Technetium-99m pertechnetate scintiscan showing no activity in the left parotid gland and a normal activity in the other major salivary glands.

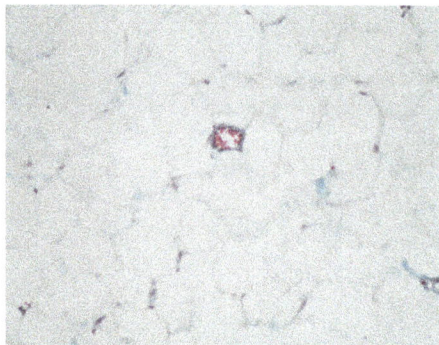

FIGURE 4: Histological examination of the buccal lipoma on the right side by Goldner's Trichrome staining.

an open biopsy of the parotid gland [9]. One case showed ipsilateral agenesis of the parotid gland in association with first branchial cleft cysts [12]. Another two patients suffered from lateral facial cleft associated with accessory mandible [7, 24]. Pleomorphic adenoma of the contralateral parotid gland, the ipsilateral accessory parotid gland, or buccal space was reported in each case [18, 19, 23]. In another case agenesis of parotid gland was masqueraded in I-123 metaiodobenzylguanidine scan with SPECT/CT by a metastasis of a left craniocervical neuroblastoma [21]. In other cases agenesis of the parotid gland was associated with ipsilateral angioma of the cheek and ipsilateral accessory parotid tissue [8, 11, 16, 22]. The present case described a patient with agenesis of the left parotid gland and a lipoma of the right cheek.

The unilateral agenesis of the parotid gland may be clinically silent. Clinical suspicion should arise in cases of asymmetrical parotid areas and a painless unilateral swelling of the parotid gland. Clinical examination, especially the absence of the papilla of Stensen's duct, could be helpful for diagnosis. Mostly the unilateral agenesis of the parotid gland seems to be a coincident finding. We were able to confirm the diagnosis of parotid gland agenesis by using a combination of MRI and salivary gland scintigraphy.

Competing Interests

The authors declare that there is no conflict of interests regarding the publication of this paper.

References

[1] C. Matsuda, Y. Matsui, K. Ohno, and K.-I. Michi, "Salivary gland aplasia with cleft lip and palate," *Oral Surgery, Oral Medicine, Oral Pathology, Oral Radiology, and Endodontics*, vol. 87, no. 5, pp. 594–599, 1999.

[2] W. Gruber, "Congenitaler Mangel beider Glandulae submaxillares bei einem wohlgebildeten, erwachsenen Subjecte," *Archiv für Pathologische Anatomie und Physiologie und für Klinische Medicin*, vol. 102, no. 1, pp. 9–11, 1885.

[3] M. YIlmaz, A. Yücel, S. Dereköy, and A. Altuntaş, "Unilateral aplasia of the submandibular gland," *European Archives of Oto-Rhino-Laryngology*, vol. 259, no. 10, pp. 554–556, 2002.

[4] N. Al-Talabani, I. S. Gataa, and S. A. Latteef, "Bilateral agenesis of parotid salivary glands, an extremely rare condition: report of a case and review of literature," *Oral Surgery, Oral Medicine, Oral Pathology, Oral Radiology and Endodontology*, vol. 105, no. 3, pp. e73–e75, 2008.

[5] D. Z. Antoniades, A. K. Markopoulos, E. Deligianni, and D. Andreadis, "Bilateral aplasia of parotid glands correlated with accessory parotid tissue," *Journal of Laryngology and Otology*, vol. 120, no. 4, pp. 327–329, 2006.

[6] M. J. Higley, T. W. Walkiewicz, J. H. Miller, J. G. Curran, and R. B. Towbin, "Aplasia of the parotid glands with accessory parotid tissue," *Pediatric Radiology*, vol. 40, no. 3, pp. 345–347, 2010.

[7] D. Özçelik, G. Toplu, A. Türkseven, D. A. Şenses, and B. Yiğit, "Lateral facial cleft associated with accessory mandible having teeth, absent parotid gland and peripheral facial weakness," *Journal of Cranio-Maxillofacial Surgery*, vol. 42, no. 5, pp. e239–e244, 2014.

[8] L. D'Ascanio, C. Cavuto, M. Martinelli, and F. Salvinelli, "Radiological evaluation of major salivary glands agenesis. A case report," *Minerva Stomatologica*, vol. 55, no. 4, pp. 223–228, 2006.

[9] S. A. Kelly, M. J. M. Black, and J. V. Soames, "Unilateral enlargement of the parotid gland in a patient with sialosis and contralateral parotid aplasia," *British Journal of Oral and Maxillofacial Surgery*, vol. 28, no. 6, pp. 409–412, 1990.

[10] G. Almadori, F. Ottaviani, M. Del Ninno, G. Cadoni, G. De Rossi, and G. Paludetti, "Monolateral aplasia of the parotid gland," *Annals of Otology, Rhinology & Laryngology*, vol. 106, no. 6, pp. 522–525, 1997.

[11] V. N. Bhide and R. J. Warshawsky, "Agenesis of the parotid gland: association with ipsilateral accessory parotid tissue," *American Journal of Roentgenology*, vol. 170, no. 6, pp. 1670–1671, 1998.

[12] J.-Y. Sichel, D. Halperin, I. Dano, and E. Dangoor, "Clinical update on type II first branchial cleft cysts," *Laryngoscope*, vol. 108, no. 10, pp. 1524–1527, 1998.

[13] S. J. Hyang, J. K. Gyo, C. K. Yu, and K. K. Soo, "Unilateral parotid glandular aplasia and ductal atresia," *Korean Journal of Otorhinolaryngology*, vol. 42, no. 3, pp. 377–379, 1999.

[14] J. Martínez Subías, J. Royo López, and H. Vallés Varela, "Congenital absence of major salivary glands," *Acta Otorrinolaringologica Espanola*, vol. 51, no. 3, pp. 276–278, 2000.

[15] S. J. Daniel, S. Blaser, and V. Forte, "Unilateral agenesis of the parotid gland: an unusual entity," *International Journal of Pediatric Otorhinolaryngology*, vol. 67, no. 4, pp. 395–397, 2003.

[16] F. Salvinelli, C. Marte, L. D'Ascanio et al., "Congenital aplasia of the parotid gland with omolateral cheek angioma: case report and review of the literature," *Acta Oto-Laryngologica*, vol. 124, no. 3, pp. 328–330, 2004.

[17] R. Martín-Granizo and D. García-González, "Unilateral agenesis of the parotid gland: a case report," *Oral Surgery, Oral Medicine, Oral Pathology, Oral Radiology and Endodontology*, vol. 98, no. 6, pp. 712–714, 2004.

[18] O. Karakoc, T. Akcam, M. Kocaoglu, and S. Yetiser, "Agenesis of the unilateral parotid gland associated with pleomorphic adenoma of the contralateral parotid gland," *Journal of Laryngology and Otology*, vol. 119, no. 5, pp. 409–411, 2005.

[19] B. H. Lee, "Unilateral agenesis of the parotid gland associated with a pleomorphic adenoma in the ipsilateral buccal space," *Japanese Journal of Radiology*, vol. 28, no. 3, pp. 224–226, 2010.

[20] Y.-K. Chen, C.-J. Kuo, and C.-L. Yeh, "Unilateral agenesis of the parotid gland with contralateral compensation hypermetabolism of FDG," *Clinical Nuclear Medicine*, vol. 36, no. 8, pp. 710–711, 2011.

[21] D. Udall and S. Y. Cho, "Congenital agenesis of right parotid gland confounds MIBG scan interpretation in craniocervical neuroblastoma," *Clinical Nuclear Medicine*, vol. 36, no. 11, pp. e162–164, 2011.

[22] P. Capaccio, N. Luca, P. E. Sigismund, and L. Pignataro, "Recurrent inflammation of accessory parotid tissue associated with unilateral parotid gland aplasia: diagnostic and therapeutic implications," *European Archives of Oto-Rhino-Laryngology*, vol. 269, no. 5, pp. 1551–1554, 2012.

[23] A. B. Seith, A. Gadodia, R. Sharma, and R. Parshad, "Unilateral parotid agenesis associated with pleomorphic adenoma of ipsilateral accessory parotid gland," *Ear, Nose and Throat Journal*, vol. 92, no. 1, pp. E13–E15, 2013.

[24] L. Sun, Z. Sun, and X. Ma, "Partial duplication of the mandible, parotid aplasia and facial cleft: a rare developmental disorder," *Oral Surgery, Oral Medicine, Oral Pathology and Oral Radiology*, vol. 116, no. 3, pp. e202–e209, 2013.

[25] H. P. Günbey, E. Günbey, F. Tayfun, and S. K. Kaytez, "A rare cause of unilateral parotid gland swelling: compensatory hypertrophy due to the aplasia of the contralateral parotid gland," *Journal of Craniofacial Surgery*, vol. 25, no. 3, pp. e265–e267, 2014.

[26] A. Srinivasan, J. S. Moyer, and S. K. Mukherji, "Unilateral submandibular gland aplasia associated with ipsilateral sublingual gland hypertrophy," *American Journal of Neuroradiology*, vol. 27, no. 10, pp. 2214–2216, 2006.

[27] F. G. McDonald, J. Mantas, C. G. McEwen, and M. M. Ferguson, "Salivary gland aplasia: an ectodermal disorder?" *Journal of Oral Pathology*, vol. 15, no. 2, pp. 115–117, 1986.

[28] E. Berta, G. Bettega, P. S. Jouk, G. Billy, F. Nugues, and B. Morand, "Complete agenesis of major salivary glands," *International Journal of Pediatric Otorhinolaryngology*, vol. 77, no. 10, pp. 1782–1785, 2013.

[29] R. P. S. Mohan, S. Verma, V. R. Chawa, and K. Tyagi, "Non-syndromic non-familial agenesis of major salivary glands: a report of two cases with review of literature," *Journal of Clinical Imaging Science*, vol. 3, article 2, 2013.

[30] M. Lehotay, M. Kunkel, and H. Wehrbein, "Lacrimo-auriculo-dento-digital syndrome. Case, report of the literature, and clinical spectrum," *Journal of Orofacial Orthopedics*, vol. 65, no. 5, pp. 425–432, 2004.

[31] A. P. S. Ferreira, R. S. Gomez, W. H. Castro, N. S. Calixto, R. A. P. Silva, and M. J. B. Aguiar, "Congenital absence of lacrimal puncta and salivary glands: report of a brazilian family and review," *American Journal of Medical Genetics*, vol. 94, no. 1, pp. 32–34, 2000.

[32] D. B. Chapman, V. Shashi, and D. J. Kirse, "Case report: aplasia of the lacrimal and major salivary glands (ALSG)," *International Journal of Pediatric Otorhinolaryngology*, vol. 73, no. 6, pp. 899–901, 2009.

[33] M. M. Ferguson and Y. Ponnambalam, "Aplasia of the parotid gland in Down syndrome," *British Journal of Oral and Maxillofacial Surgery*, vol. 43, no. 2, pp. 113–117, 2005.

[34] M. Odeh, M. Hershkovits, J. Bornstein, N. Loberant, M. Blumenthal, and E. Ophir, "Congenital absence of salivary glands in Down syndrome," *Archives of Disease in Childhood*, vol. 98, no. 10, pp. 781–783, 2013.

[35] Y. F. Yilmaz, A. Titiz, N. Yurur-Kutlay, M. Ozcan, and A. Unal, "Congenital bilateral parotid gland agenesis in Klinefelter syndrome," *Journal of Cranio-Maxillofacial Surgery*, vol. 38, no. 4, pp. 248–250, 2010.

3

Treatment of an Erratic Extraction Socket for Implant Therapy in a Patient with Chronic Periodontitis

Yusuke Hamada, Srividya Prabhu, and Vanchit John

Department of Periodontics and Allied Dental Program, Indiana University School of Dentistry, Indianapolis, IN 46204, USA

Correspondence should be addressed to Yusuke Hamada; yuhamada@iupui.edu

Academic Editor: Sukumaran Anil

As implant therapy becomes more commonplace in daily practice, preservation and preparation of edentulous sites are key. Many times, however, implant therapy may not be considered at the time of tooth extraction and additional measures are not taken to conserve the edentulous site. While the healing process in extraction sockets has been well investigated and bone fill can be expected, there are cases where even when clinicians perform thorough debridement of the sockets, connective tissue infiltration into the socket can occur. This phenomenon, known as "erratic healing," may be associated with factors that lead to peri-implant disease and should be appropriately managed and treated prior to surgical implant placement. This case report describes the successful management of an erratic healing extraction socket in a 62-year-old Caucasian male patient with chronic periodontitis and the outcomes of an evidence-based treatment protocol performed prior to implant therapy. Careful preoperative analysis and cone beam computed tomography imaging can help detect signs of impaired healing in future implant sites and prevent surgical complications.

1. Introduction

Over the past decade, the oral rehabilitation of fully or partially edentulous patients with dental implants has become routine in everyday clinical practice. Implants are placed either in sockets following the extraction of teeth, in sockets following grafting and healing, or in fully healed native bone. The characteristics and progression of healing in extraction sockets have been extensively investigated in animal models and in human clinical trials [1–3]. These studies have included clinical and radiographic dimensional changes, as well as histological analyses [4]. A systematic review of the existing literature assessed the magnitude of dimensional changes for hard and soft tissues of the alveolar ridge up to 12 months after tooth extraction in humans. The results from human reentry studies show that 29–63% horizontal bone loss and 11–22% vertical bone loss occur 6 months following tooth extraction [5]. Current evidence indicates that alveolar ridge preservation treatment at the time of extraction can minimize the degree of ridge dimension shrinkage [6, 7]. Not all patients consider or plan on future implant therapy at the time of

their extractions, so they may go without the alveolar ridge preservation procedure. This ultimately can have an effect on ridge dimensional change and the healing process following extraction.

The sequence of cellular and tissue healing following tooth extraction in humans starts with blood clot formation within the socket; the clot is then replaced by granulation tissue, and, subsequently, osteoid formation occurs [1]. Histologic evaluation of extraction sites has primarily been investigated with teeth devoid of pathological features. In daily practice, many extracted teeth are periodontally or endodontically involved or are extracted from medically compromised individuals. In some cases, even when surgeons perform thorough debridement of the sockets, connective tissue infiltration into the socket can occur [8]. Some reports showed that bacterial contamination during implant insertion and premature loading, bone microfractures, and the presence of a preexisting inflammation (bacteria, inflammatory cells, and/or remaining cells from a cyst or granuloma) are the etiologic factors of retrograde peri-implantitis. Retrograde peri-implantitis is often accompanied by symptoms of pain, tenderness, swelling, and/or the presence of a sinus tract. The appropriate treatment methods for retrograde peri-implantitis are still unclear [9, 10]. Kim et al. defined "erratic healing" as healing where fibrous scar tissue is found occupying the extraction site rather than bone after 12 or more weeks of healing. Erratic healing is a not a rare complication. In their retrospective study, the authors showed that, in 5.71% of subjects receiving extractions, 4.24% of extraction sites demonstrated some degree of erratic healing sites [11]. Appropriate treatment for extraction sites with erratic healing is needed prior to or at the same time of implant surgical therapy to maintain long-term stability of the implant. The purpose of this paper is to illustrate a clinical case and suggest an evidence-based treatment protocol for sockets with erratic healing prior to implant placement.

2. Case Presentation

A 62-year-old Caucasian male was referred to the Graduate Periodontics Clinic at Indiana University School of Dentistry, Indianapolis, Indiana, USA, from a general dentist's office for periodontal treatment. The patient reported a history of hypertension, coronary artery blockage with stent replacement in 2006, osteoarthritis, and hyperlipidemia. The clinical examination demonstrated increased periodontal probing depths, up to 6 mm, on the posterior teeth. Tooth #30 had previously been extracted due to a combined periodontic-endodontic lesion (Figure 1). The radiographic examination revealed horizontal bone loss on the posterior teeth. The periodontal diagnosis was generalized mild chronic periodontitis with localized moderate chronic periodontitis associated with teeth #2, 3, 14, 15, 18, and 19 [12]. The patient's oral hygiene was considered to be acceptable. An O'Leary plaque score of 29% was recorded at the initial appointment. The possible treatment interventions for the periodontitis and edentulous ridge #30 were explained to the patient. These included (1) oral hygiene instructions, (2) nonsurgical periodontal therapy, (3) surgical intervention (resective osseous treatment) around posterior teeth, and, following good control of the patient's periodontal condition, (4) replacement of #30 with a dental implant-supported restoration. The goal of the anti-infective therapy (nonsurgical therapy) was to reduce the bacterial load and inflammation. The patient underwent a periodontal maintenance session and received individualized oral hygiene instructions. His oral hygiene improved, and an O'Leary plaque score of 9% was noted. Shortly after the periodontal maintenance appointment, osseous resective surgery on UL, LL, and UR quadrants was rendered to achieve shallower probing depth and a better periodontal environment for the posterior teeth prior to implant surgery on #30. The patient elected to follow through with implant therapy for #30 with a single implant-supported crown (Figure 2).

On the day of implant placement on #30, infiltration of 2% lidocaine with 1 : 100,000 epinephrine was administered. Following a crestal incision over the edentulous ridge of #30 and intrasulcular incisions along the distal surface of #29 and mesial surface of #31, a full-thickness flap was reflected. After flap reflection, granulation tissue was noted filling the crestal area of the #30 extraction socket. The buccal and lingual

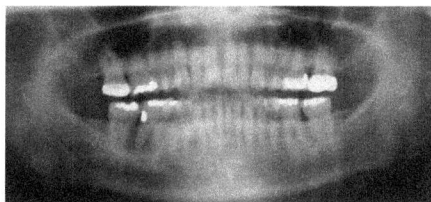

FIGURE 1: Panoramic radiograph at the initial appointment (#30 was extracted by the referring dentist).

walls of the socket were intact. Thorough debridement was attempted. Gaining access to the bottom of the defect was challenging due to the complexity of the defect shape. A small amount of crestal bone was removed with a high-speed handpiece and round burs to allow the surgeon access to the apex of the bony defect. Granulation tissue was removed from the socket and submitted for pathological examination to obtain a formal diagnosis. Following thorough irrigation with saline, hydrated freeze-dried bone allograft (FDBA: particle size $250 \mu m$–$1000 \mu m$, Sunstar) was grafted into the socket and covered with Bio-Gide (non-cross-linked porcine collagen membrane, Geistlich). Primary closure of the site was obtained with single interrupted and horizontal mattress sutures, using 4-0 Cytoplast suture material (Figure 3). Postoperative instructions were given, and the patient was prescribed 500 mg amoxicillin, to be taken three times daily for 1 week. He was instructed to rinse for 30 seconds twice daily with 0.12% chlorhexidine gluconate for 2 weeks. Sutures were removed at 2 weeks after the surgical procedure. The site healed uneventfully, and the pathology report revealed that the tissue sample presented with edema along with intense lymphoplasmacytic infiltrate. The bulk of the specimen consisted of dense, hyalinized mineralized debris. The diagnosis given was residual chronically inflamed granulation tissue with fibrous connective scar tissue (Figure 4).

Five months after the graft procedure, implant placement was planned. Preoperative periapical radiograph showed increased bone density in the #30 site. Following a crestal incision and full-thickness flap elevation, a surgical guide was mounted intraorally, and an osteotomy was created as per the manufacturer's instructions. No soft tissue or granulation tissue was found within the osteotomy site. A Zimmer implant $4.7 \times 11.5 \, (D \times H)$ was placed with insertion torque of 35 N/cm (Figure 5). An Osstell device was used to measure the stability, and an ISQ (Implant Stability Quotient) of 76 was measured from buccal and lingual positions. No adverse events were noted during the osteointegration phase. A custom abutment and a gold cast crown were delivered by a restorative dentist. Radiograph and clinical features showed soft and hard tissue stability at one year following crown delivery, without any symptoms or radiographic evidence of retrograde peri-implantitis (Figure 6).

3. Discussion

Observations of radiolucencies and the presence of fibrous scar tissue occupying an extraction socket rather than bone

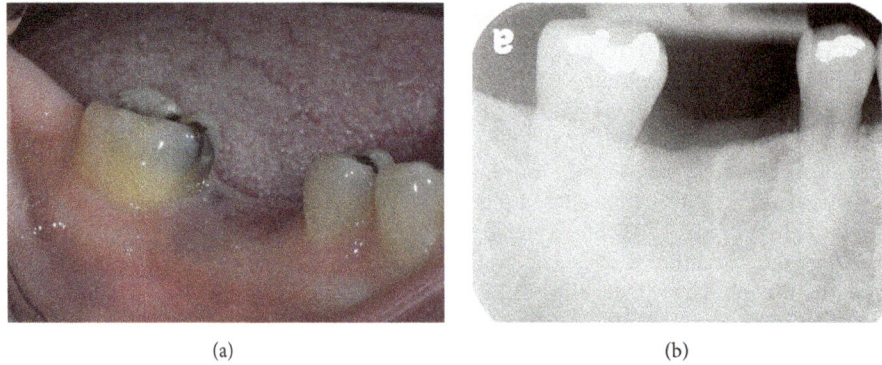

(a)   (b)

FIGURE 2: Preoperative views: (a) intraoral; (b) periapical radiograph.

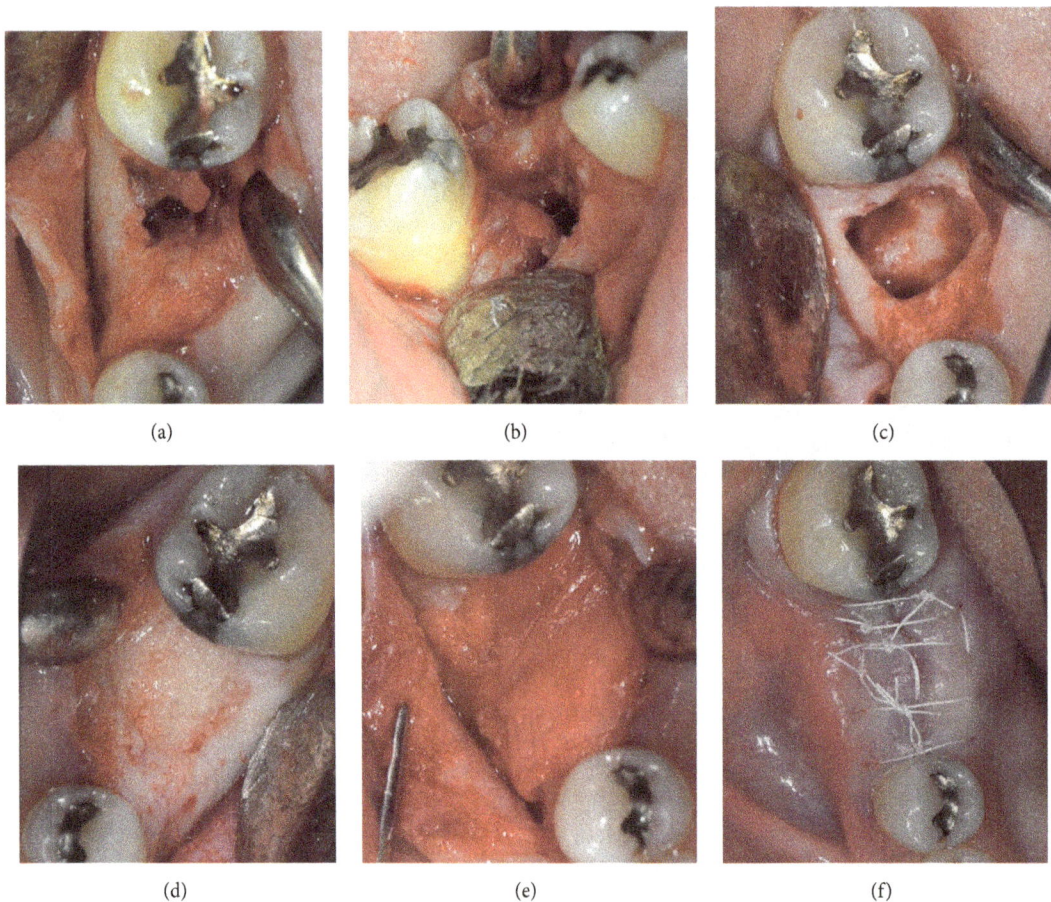

(a)   (b)   (c)

(d)   (e)   (f)

FIGURE 3: Guided bone regeneration procedure was performed on the erratic extraction site (a–f). After a full-thickness flap was elevated, granulation tissue was noted filling the previously extracted site (a and b). Following thorough debridement and irrigation, the site was determined to be a containable defect (c). FDBA was gently packed in the socket and covered with non-cross-linked collagen membrane (d and e). Complete primary closure was achieved with a combination of horizontal mattress and single interrupted sutures (f).

precluded the placement of a dental implant in that site. A retrospective study elucidated factors potentially impeding healing in post-extraction sites with computerized tomography. This study revealed that maxillary incisor/canine sites showed the lowest prevalence of erratic healing, whereas mandibular molar sites had the highest prevalence. The results of the multivariable analysis indicated that erratic healing was more likely to occur in subjects who are <60 years old (OR = 2.23), subjects with hypertension (OR = 2.37), molar sites (OR = 4.91), and single tooth extraction sites (OR = 2.98). This case report fits into all of these conditions except age [11].

In this case report, the buccal and lingual bone of the patient's extraction site was intact, and there was more than 2 mm of thickness on both sides. Additionally, the edentulous

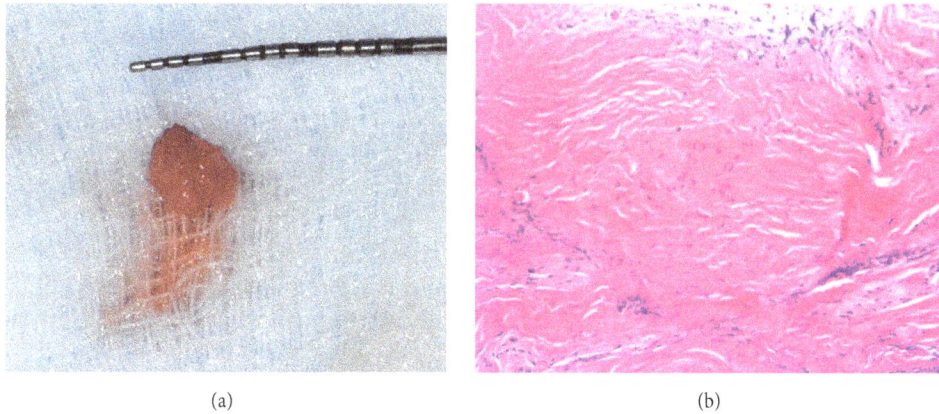

FIGURE 4: The removed specimen and histopathological picture (H&E stain). Approximate $5 \times 5 \times 3$ mm elastic hard granulation tissue was removed from the erratic extraction site (a). Fibrous connective tissue with inflammatory cells infiltration (b).

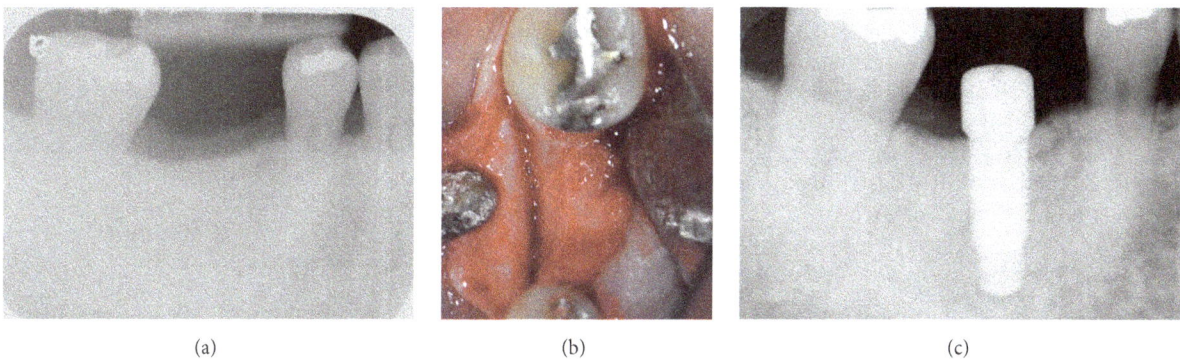

FIGURE 5: Implant placement five months after the graft procedure. The erratic healing extraction site showed increased radioopacity five months after the bone graft surgery (a). Bone fill was found on the crestal portion of the site (b). Implant was placed at a restoratively driven position (c).

site was free of inflammation, which allowed the surgeon to obtain primary closure. Primary closure is one of the keys that allows for optimal results with guided bone regeneration. Wang and Boyapati [13] described those major biologic principles as "PASS" for predictable bone regeneration: "Primary wound closure" to ensure undisturbed and uninterrupted wound healing, "Angiogenesis" to provide necessary blood supply and undifferentiated mesenchymal cells, "Space maintenance" to facilitate adequate space for bone ingrowth, and "Stability of wound" to induce blood clot formation and an uneventful healing process. This case satisfied those four factors at the time of the graft procedure since the defect shape was containable and healthy soft tissue was available to cover the defect. However, almost 85% of erratic healing extraction sites presented with loss of either or both of the buccal and lingual walls [11]. If a defect is not containable, it is difficult to stabilize the wound, and a more rigid membrane or space maintainer, such as titanium-reinforced membrane or titanium mesh, may be needed to prevent tissue collapse [14]. Moreover, if a defect is noncontainable and large amount of bone augmentation is required to develop the implant site, placement of a bone graft material with a slow resorption rate (Deproteinized Bovine Bone Minerals, DBBM, etc.) and

application of growth factors are suggested. Nevins et al. utilized recombinant human platelet-derived growth factor BB (rh-PDGF-BB) to regenerate large alveolar extraction sites with tenting screws, DBBM, and collagen membranes [15]. In this case series, eight sites were treated, and all sites healed successfully with evidence of bone-like hard tissue that was confirmed histologically as vital bone around the remaining graft particulate.

Since the erratic healing extraction site in this case report showed enough buccal-lingual ridge dimension to accommodate an implant fixture, the authors planned the implant surgery using cast models and periapical radiographs. The surgical plan changed unexpectedly during the first surgery. The clinical discovery of granulation and scar tissue in extraction socket was explained to the patient during the surgery, and the surgical plan was changed. However, a more careful presurgical examination, including cone beam computed tomography (CBCT), should be performed to minimize the risk of altering the surgical plan. The detection of erratic healing extraction lesions prior to surgery is beneficial for both patients and surgeons in order to discuss and create a comprehensive treatment plan that includes the duration and cost of the treatment needed. The American Academy of Oral and

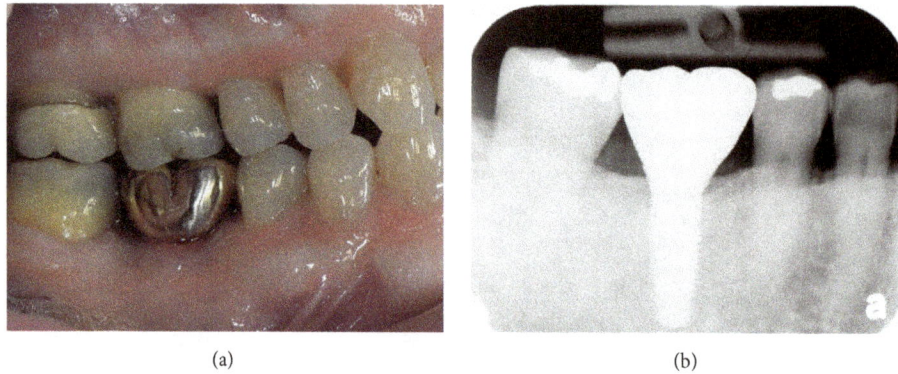

FIGURE 6: One-year follow-up after crown delivery. There is no evidence of inflammation or symptoms (a). Crestal bone loss or typical retrograde peri-implantitis was not noted on the periapical radiograph (b).

Maxillofacial Radiology (AAOMR) published a position statement regarding CBCT for dental implantology. The AAOMR recommends that cross-sectional imaging be used for the assessment of all dental implant sites and that CBCT be the imaging method of choice for gaining this information [16]. The decision to perform a CBCT examination must be clinically justified and conducted based on professional judgment (i.e., the judgment of the clinician that a CBCT image will potentially provide information needed for prosthetic treatment planning, implant selection, and/or surgical placement).

4. Conclusions and Practical Implication

This case report demonstrates successful treatment of erratic healing of an extraction site with guided bone regeneration. This therapy resulted in oral rehabilitation of edentulous site with a dental implant-supported restoration without any complications for one year after the prosthesis was delivered. Impaired extraction sites can be treated adequately if basic principles of biology, such as "PASS" principles, are followed. However, additional radiographic analysis with CBCT to detect a lesion prior to opening a surgical flap is highly useful for diagnosis and treatment planning.

Competing Interests

The authors declare no competing interests related to this study.

Acknowledgments

The authors would like to thank Dr. Susan Zunt (Professor and Chair, Oral Pathology, Medicine & Radiology at Indiana University School of Dentistry) for providing an oral pathology diagnosis and photos of histopathologic images.

References

[1] M. H. Amler, "The time sequence of tissue regeneration in human extraction wounds," Oral Surgery, Oral Medicine, Oral Pathology, vol. 27, no. 3, pp. 309–318, 1969.

[2] C. I. Evian, E. S. Rosenberg, J. G. Coslet, and H. Corn, "The osteogenic activity of bone removed from healing extraction sockets in humans," Journal of Periodontology, vol. 53, no. 2, pp. 81–85, 1982.

[3] J. Pietrokovski and M. Massler, "Alveolar ridge resorption following tooth extraction," The Journal of Prosthetic Dentistry, vol. 17, no. 1, pp. 21–27, 1967.

[4] M. G. Araújo and J. Lindhe, "Dimensional ridge alterations following tooth extraction. An experimental study in the dog," Journal of Clinical Periodontology, vol. 32, no. 2, pp. 212–218, 2005.

[5] W. L. Tan, T. L. T. Wong, M. C. M. Wong, and N. P. Lang, "A systematic review of post-extractional alveolar hard and soft tissue dimensional changes in humans," Clinical Oral Implants Research, vol. 23, supplement 5, pp. 1–21, 2012.

[6] R. Horowitz, D. Holtzclaw, and P. S. Rosen, "A review on alveolar ridge preservation following tooth extraction," Journal of Evidence-Based Dental Practice, vol. 12, no. 3, pp. 149–160, 2012.

[7] A. Horváth, N. Mardas, L. A. Mezzomo, I. G. Needleman, and N. Donos, "Alveolar ridge preservation. A systematic review," Clinical Oral Investigations, vol. 17, no. 2, pp. 341–363, 2013.

[8] C. H. F. Hämmerle, S. T. Chen, and T. G. Wilson Jr., "Consensus statements and recommended clinical procedures regarding the placement of implants in extraction sockets," International Journal of Oral and Maxillofacial Implants, vol. 19, supplement, pp. 26–28, 2004.

[9] G. E. Romanos, S. Froum, S. Costa-Martins, S. Meitner, and D. P. Tarnow, "Implant periapical lesions: etiology and treatment options," Journal of Oral Implantology, vol. 37, no. 1, pp. 53–63, 2011.

[10] M. Quirynen, R. Vogels, G. Alsaadi, I. Naert, R. Jacobs, and D. V. Steenberghe, "Predisposing conditions for retrograde peri-implantitis, and treatment suggestions," Clinical Oral Implants Research, vol. 16, no. 5, pp. 599–608, 2005.

[11] J.-H. Kim, C. Susin, J.-H. Min et al., "Extraction sockets: erratic healing impeding factors," Journal of Clinical Periodontology, vol. 41, no. 1, pp. 80–85, 2014.

[12] G. C. Armitage, "Development of a classification system for periodontal diseases and conditions," Annals of Periodontology, vol. 4, no. 1, pp. 1–6, 1999.

[13] H.-L. Wang and L. Boyapati, "'PASS' principles for predictable bone regeneration," Implant Dentistry, vol. 15, no. 1, pp. 8–17, 2006.

[14] I. A. Urban, J. L. Lozada, S. A. Jovanovic, H. Nagursky, and K. Nagy, "Vertical ridge augmentation with titanium-reinforced, dense-PTFE membranes and a combination of particulated autogenous bone and anorganic bovine bone-derived mineral: a prospective case series in 19 patients," *International Journal of Oral & Maxillofacial Implants*, vol. 29, no. 1, pp. 185–193, 2014.

[15] M. L. Nevins, M. A. Reynolds, M. Camelo, D. M. Kim, and M. Nevins, "Recombinant human platelet-derived growth factor BB for reconstruction of human large extraction site defects," *The International Journal of Periodontics & Restorative Dentistry*, vol. 34, no. 2, pp. 157–163, 2014.

[16] D. A. Tyndall, J. B. Price, S. Tetradis, S. D. Ganz, C. Hildebolt, and W. C. Scarfe, "Position statement of the American Academy of Oral and Maxillofacial Radiology on selection criteria for the use of radiology in dental implantology with emphasis on cone beam computed tomography," *Oral Surgery, Oral Medicine, Oral Pathology and Oral Radiology*, vol. 113, no. 6, pp. 817–826, 2012.

4

Pernicious Effects of Toe Sucking Habit in Children

Deepika Pai,[1] Saurabh Kumar,[1] Abhay T. Kamath,[2] and Vipin Bhaskar[3]

[1]*Department of Pedodontics & Preventive Dentistry, Manipal College of Dental Sciences, Manipal, Manipal University, Manipal, India*
[2]*Department of Oral and Maxillofacial Surgery, Manipal College of Dental Sciences, Manipal, Manipal University, Manipal, India*
[3]*Department of Pedodontics & Preventive Dentistry, Mahe Institute of Dental Sciences, Mahe, Kerala, India*

Correspondence should be addressed to Deepika Pai; deepikapai0479@gmail.com

Academic Editor: Hüsamettin Oktay

Digit sucking is common nonnutritive sucking habit in childhood. However it is unusual to find toe sucking habit in children. We report a case of a seven-year-old child sucking great toe of the left foot. The child was referred by her paediatrician for dental evaluation due to her complaint of recurrent episodes of pyrexia. A dental evaluation was warranted as no particular system contributed to such recurrent episodes of fever in this child. Although dental examination did not reveal any cause for recurrent episodes of pyrexia, as a part of routine history taking we discovered that this child indulges frequently in sucking the great toe of her left foot since infancy. Any nonnutritive sucking habit is considered deleterious; this habit also caused significant effect on the child's dentofacial structures, sucked toe, and her general health. Hence the treatment plan was formulated for immediate cessation of habit. Appropriate interception of habit and timely orthodontic intervention led to not only early interception of cross-bite but also decrease in pyrexial episodes. This case report describes the pernicious effects of toe sucking habit and its relevance to recurrent pyrexia in children.

1. Introduction

Digit sucking habit is characterized by the placement of one or more digits to varying depths in the mouth. This habit develops in uterine life and continuation of habit after age of four-five years can cause deleterious effects on dentofacial structures and sucked digit [1, 2]. The reported incidence of digit sucking habit ranges from 13 to 100% in infancy and up to 61–90% in early childhood [3, 4].

Several unusual cases of nonnutritive sucking habits have been reported in literature. Inclusive of such reports are sucking of forearm resulting in dentofacial deformities and keloid formation of sucked area [5]. A case report on digit sucking habit in a child with cleft lip and palate reported splaying of nasal and alveolar segments of clefts under the influence of aberrant pressure created by sucking habit which significantly affected their treatment planning for rehabilitation of cleft lip and palate [6]. Some authors have reported development of onychophagia resulting from transference of earlier existing thumb sucking habit [7]. It was also found that prolonged intense parafunctional habit like digit sucking habit caused gingival recession and pathologic migration of teeth [8]. Also,

there have been reports of correlation of chronic parasitic infections due to prevalence of digit sucking habit affecting the general wellbeing of the children [9]. These unusual case reports have widen the arena of identifying unusual parafunctional habit as etiological factors for unusual or at times common dental problems and associated with general health of a child. We hereby report one such unusual case of pernicious effects of toe sucking habit and its relevance to recurrent pyrexia.

2. Case Report

A seven-year-old girl was referred by her paediatrician with complaint of recurrent pyrexia of untraceable origin. Since low grade chronic dental infections can cause repeated episodes of fever, the paediatrician desired for a dental evaluation. During history taking the patient's mother revealed recurrent episodes of fever ranging from 101 to 102 degrees Fahrenheit with two episodes in a month for the past one year. The fever subsided on taking medication. Adding further she also gave a history of occasional abdominal pain. Upon systemic review with her paediatrician we learnt that she

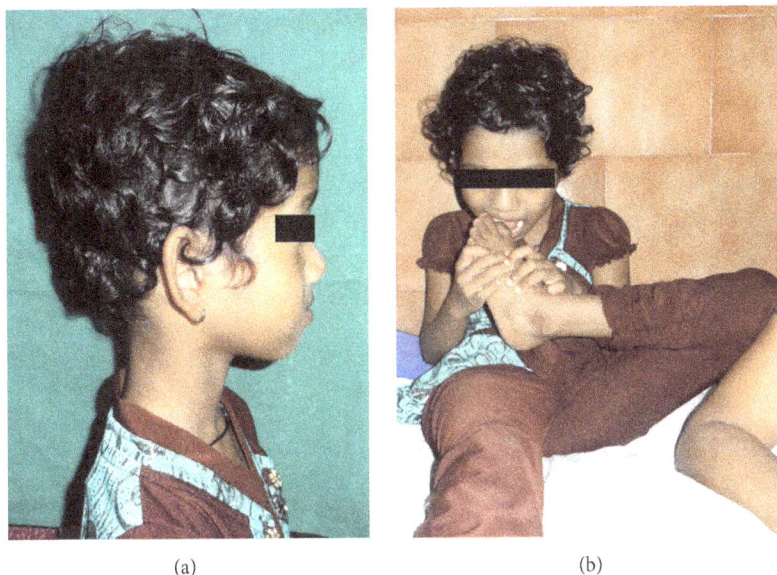

FIGURE 1: (a) Picture showing convex facial profile. (b) Picture showing child sucking the great toe of the left feet.

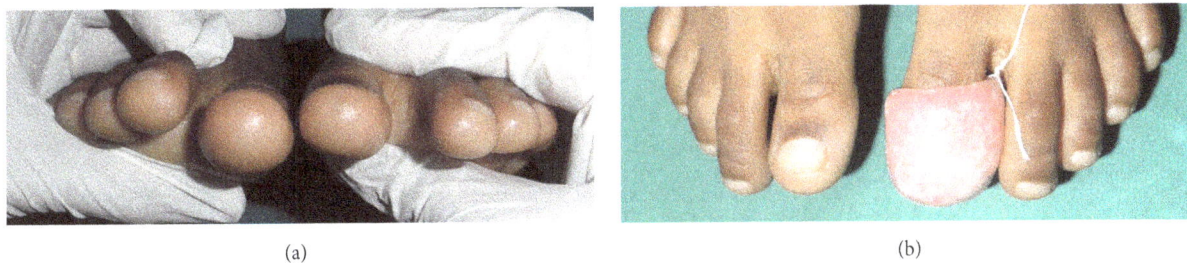

FIGURE 2: (a) Picture showing deformed great toe of left feet. (b) Picture showing acrylic toe guard fitted onto the great toe of left feet.

had no history of shortness of breath, chest pain, diarrhoea, rashes, sore throat, ear ache, or urinary symptoms that could indicate the system responsible for such recurrent episodes of pyrexia. The paediatrician also revealed that her chest X-ray and blood profile were normal. There were no abnormalities detected in her urine and stool analysis as well.

On examination her facial profile was convex (Figure 1(a)) with normal overjet and overbite. Intraoral examination did not reveal any deep carious lesions or any soft tissue abnormalities or palpable lymph nodes that could have been responsible for recurrent episodes of fever. On taking history for oral habits, the mother stated that the child sucks the great toe of her left feet since infancy (Figure 1(b)). On examination, the great toe of her left foot was deformed compared to that of the right foot (Figure 2(a)) which led to the diagnosis of toe sucking habit and its possible implication on recurrent episodes of fever. Since the mother and child were supportive to drop the habit, the detailed treatment plan was formulated.

On the next visit the parent and the patient were counselled for stopping the habit and they were educated on how it could be deleterious for the developing orofacial structures and on general health of the child. As a reminder

therapy, the child was instructed to cover her foot with socks. In the subsequent visit upon finding the patient was reluctant to wear the socks, we implemented the method of negative reinforcement and reminder therapy which was accomplished with a toe guard fabricated with acrylic which fitted the great toe involved in sucking habit (Figure 2(b)).

By three weeks the patient reported reduced frequency of toe sucking habit and episodes of fever. By now the upper incisor showed abnormal pathway of eruption (Figure 3) probably due to abnormal pressure exerted by the toe during sucking event that led to deflection of the developing tooth to an abnormal path. This developing cross-bite was intervened by tongue blade therapy. In the subsequent follow-up visit we noticed that the upper incisors showed distoangular rotation as they erupted into occlusion (Figure 4). The patient is currently using a preorthodontic trainer (T4K® Phase I, Preorthodontic Trainer for Kids, MRC, Australia) (Figure 5). The preorthodontic trainer was advocated to realign the incisors as well for myofunctional retraining of the oral musculature.

As of now the mother and the child did not report any secondary or substitutional habit after the cessation of toe sucking habit. Also no episodes of fever have been reported.

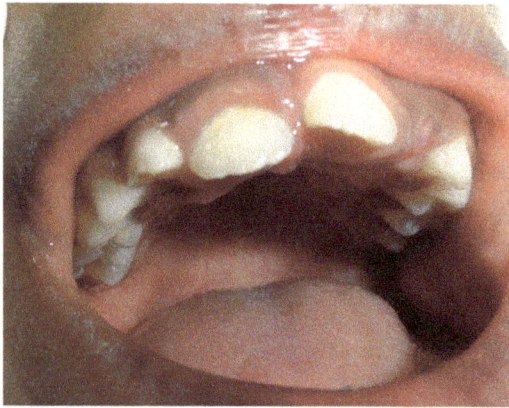

FIGURE 3: Picture showing right central incisor erupting in an abnormal pathway.

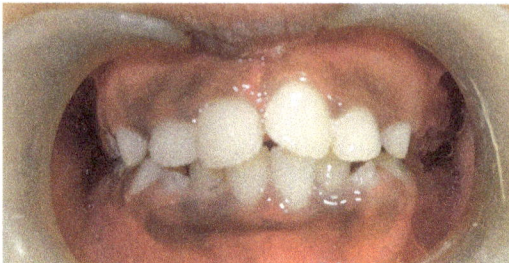

FIGURE 4: Picture showing right central incisor not in cross-bite and distoangular rotation of upper central incisors.

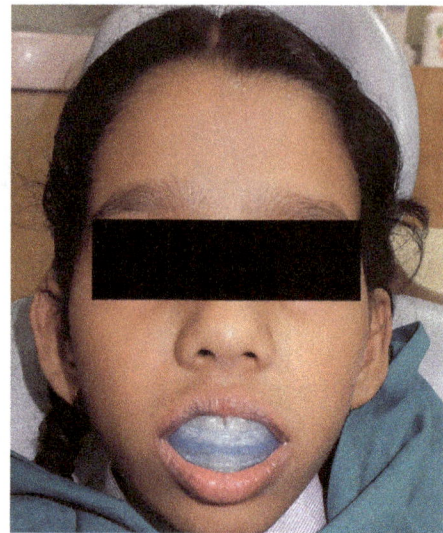

FIGURE 5: Picture showing patient wearing preorthodontic trainer for correction of distoangular rotation.

3. Discussion

The sucking habit develops as a result of rooting reflex in a neonate, which is an inherent biologic drive for sucking. The development of hand to mouth movements is described as a result of complex neurological development as well as muscular development stimulated by proprioceptive and rooting reflexes [10]. In early fetal life fore and hind limbs do not have distinguished functions; therefore it is not uncommon to find infants sucking the toe. As in our case also, the mother gave the history of toe sucking since infancy. It is when the child learns to stand and walk; the risk brought about by sucking of hand or toe may vary. Along with its deleterious effects on dentofacial structures, systemic wellbeing of the child can also be affected by the toe sucking habit [9].

Recurrent pyrexia can usually be triggered by environmental causes, with definite source of exposure. It is commonly seen in preschooler children attending day care centres [11, 12]. Since the children are exposed to outdoor activities the digit and the toe might act as a carrier for different microorganisms which may affect the general health of the patient.

In our case no definitive diagnosis could have been established for the recurrent episodes of fever since investigations like blood culture, chest X-ray, and USG abdomen were not conclusive.

According to few reported cases, allergic rhinitis and parasitic infections are attributed to be caused by digit sucking habit [9]. Analogously we can hypothesise that toe sucking habit as in our case could have led to recurrent pyrexia. The sucking of toe leads to contaminated source through establishment of a possible oropedal route leading to a wide range of parasitic, bacterial, and other agents to cause involvement of different systems like sometimes respiratory, sometimes gastrointestinal, and so on causing recurrent episodes of fever.

Digits of the hand establish a stronger influence on the dentoalveolar and orofacial structures than the digit of the feet, due to its proximity to the oral cavity. This explains why the toe sucking habit in our case did not cause severe malocclusion like presence of anterior open bites, posterior cross-bites, and so forth which are generally associated with finger sucking habits [13, 14]. However it caused deflection of the erupting permanent incisor and deformity of the great toe owing to the duration of the practiced habit.

The identification and intervention of this habit at the right time as in our case have helped in limiting the extent of malocclusion and also relieved the child from complaints of recurrent fever, which has restored the normal living in this child.

4. Conclusion

The aim of this paper is to report the influence of toe sucking habit on general health and dentofacial structures of the children.

Competing Interests

The authors declare that they do not have any conflict of interests regarding the publication of this paper.

References

[1] J. J. Warren, R. L. Slayton, T. Yonezu, S. E. Bishara, S. M. Levy, and M. J. Kanellis, "Effects of nonnutritive sucking habits on occlusal characteristics in the mixed dentition," *Pediatric Dentistry*, vol. 27, no. 6, pp. 445–450, 2005.

[2] J. Srinivasan, J. W. Hutchinson, and F. D. Burke, "Finger sucking digital deformities," *Journal of Hand Surgery*, vol. 26, no. 6, pp. 584–588, 2001.

[3] K. Duncan, C. McNamara, A. J. Ireland, and J. R. Sandy, "Sucking habits in childhood and the effects on the primary dentition: findings of the Avon Longitudinal Study of Pregnancy and Childhood," *International Journal of Paediatric Dentistry*, vol. 18, no. 3, pp. 178–188, 2008.

[4] S. E. Bishara, J. J. Warren, B. Broffitt, and S. M. Levy, "Changes in the prevalence of nonnutritive sucking patterns in the first 8 years of life," *American Journal of Orthodontics and Dentofacial Orthopedics*, vol. 130, no. 1, pp. 31–36, 2006.

[5] N. Chowdhary, H. Gaffur, Sandeep, and R. Chowdhary, "An unusual sucking habit in a child," *Contemporary Clinical Dentistry*, vol. 4, no. 1, pp. 249–250, 2010.

[6] S. Satyaprasad, "An unusual type of sucking habit in a patient with cleft lip and palate," *Journal of Indian Society of Pedodontics and Preventive Dentistry*, vol. 27, no. 4, pp. 260–262, 2009.

[7] O. M. Tanaka, R. W. F. Vitral, G. Y. Tanaka, A. P. Guerrero, and E. S. Camargo, "Nailbiting, or onychophagia: a special habit," *American Journal of Orthodontics and Dentofacial Orthopedics*, vol. 134, no. 2, pp. 305–308, 2008.

[8] A. R. Pradeep and D. C. G. Sharma, "Gingival recession and pathologic migration due to an unusual habit," *Journal of the International Academy of Periodontology*, vol. 8, no. 3, pp. 74–77, 2006.

[9] O. A. Idowu, O. Babatunde, T. Soniran, and A. Adediran, "Parasitic infections in finger-sucking school age children," *Pediatric Infectious Disease Journal*, vol. 30, no. 9, pp. 791–792, 2011.

[10] B. Medoff-Cooper and W. Ray, "Neonatal sucking behaviors," *Image*, vol. 27, no. 3, pp. 195–200, 1995.

[11] S. S. Long, "Distinguishing among prolonged, recurrent, and periodic fever syndromes: approach of a pediatric infectious diseases subspecialist," *Pediatric Clinics of North America*, vol. 52, no. 3, pp. 811–835, 2005.

[12] N. B. Tripathi and S. N. Patil, "Treatment of class II division 1 malocclusion with myofunctional trainer system in early mixed dentition period," *Journal of Contemporary Dental Practice*, vol. 12, no. 6, pp. 497–500, 2011.

[13] T. A. Yemitan, O. O. daCosta, O. O. Sanu, and M. C. Isiekwe, "Effects of digit sucking on dental arch dimensions in the primary dentition," *African Journal of Medicine and Medical Sciences*, vol. 39, no. 1, pp. 55–61, 2010.

[14] E. N. Gale and W. A. Ayer, "Thumb-sucking revisited," *American Journal of Orthodontics*, vol. 55, no. 2, pp. 167–170, 1969.

5

Diastema Closure in Anterior Teeth Using a Posterior Matrix

Ayush Goyal,[1] Vineeta Nikhil,[1] and Ritu Singh[2]

[1]Department of Conservative Dentistry & Endodontics, Subharti Dental College, Meerut, Uttar Pradesh, India
[2]Department of Paediatric and Preventive Dentistry, Subharti Dental College, Meerut, Uttar Pradesh, India

Correspondence should be addressed to Ayush Goyal; ayush2106.goyal@gmail.com

Academic Editor: Tatiana Pereira-Cenci

Presence of diastema between anterior teeth is often considered an onerous esthetic problem. Various treatment modalities are available for diastema closure. However, not all diastemas can be treated the same in terms of modality or timing. The extent and the etiology of the diastema must be properly evaluated. Proper case selection is of paramount importance for a successful treatment. In this case report, diastema closure was performed with direct composite restorations. One bottle etch-and-rinse adhesive was used and a single shade was used to close the diastemas. Contoured sectional posterior matrix was used to achieve anatomic contouring of the proximal surfaces of the teeth. This was followed by finishing and polishing using polishing discs. Patient was kept on recall every 6 months. *Conclusion.* Diastema closure with correct anatomic contouring is easy to perform using the contoured sectional matrices. At 14-month recall, no clinical signs of failure like discoloration or fracture were evident. Also, patient did not complain of any sensitivity. Thus, direct composite restorations serve as durable and highly esthetic restorations leading to complete patient satisfaction.

1. Introduction

Midline diastema is defined as anterior midline spacing greater than 0.5 mm between the proximal surfaces of central incisors [1]. Midline diastema or spacing in anterior teeth is a common condition that can present itself anytime to the dental office. It has been reported that maxilla has a higher prevalence of midline diastema than mandible [2]. Midline diastema is multifactorial in etiology. Some of the causes include maxillary incisor proclination, labial frenum, incomplete coalescence of the interdental septum, pseudo-microdontia, presence of a mesiodens, peg-shaped lateral incisors, congenital absence of lateral incisors, pathologies (e.g., cysts in the midline region), habits such as finger sucking, tongue thrusting, and/or lip sucking, discrepancy in the dental and skeletal parameters, and probably genetics [3].

Once the etiology is known, a decision must then be taken whether to utilize a multidisciplinary approach or to simply close the spaces by means of direct and/or indirect restorative treatment. If the teeth are correctly aligned and positioned, but the tooth size is the culprit, the clinician is left with the task of selecting the best restorative procedure [4].

The development of composite resins with superior mechanical properties and excellent polishability allows the clinician to mimic the natural dentition and render a long-lasting restoration to the patient. Also, composite resins permit conservative treatment and at the same time offer quicker results [5].

Recent aesthetic composite resin materials have similar physical and mechanical properties to that of the natural tooth and possess an appearance like natural dentin and enamel. They offer a diverse range of shades and varying opacities designed specifically for layering technique [6, 7].

Creating an anatomic contour without "black triangles" is an arduous task when closing diastemas using resin-based composites. This case report describes diastema closure in the maxillary anterior region using resin-based composite material with the help of stainless steel precontoured matrices.

2. Case Report

A 52-year-old male patient reported to the department of Conservative Dentistry and Endodontics, Subharti Dental College, with a chief complaint of spacing in his upper

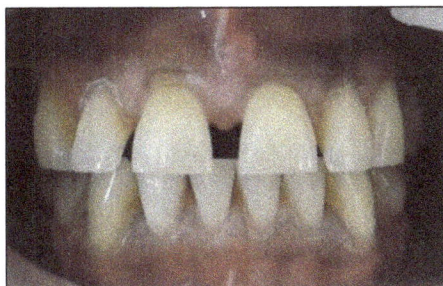

FIGURE 1: Preoperative intraoral view of the patient shows interdental spacing in maxillary anterior regions.

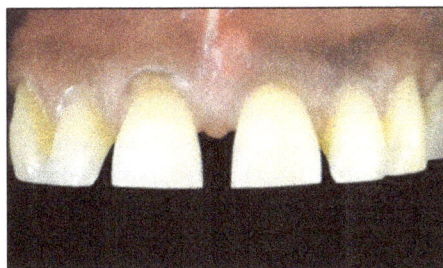

FIGURE 2: Preoperative intraoral view of maxillary anterior regions.

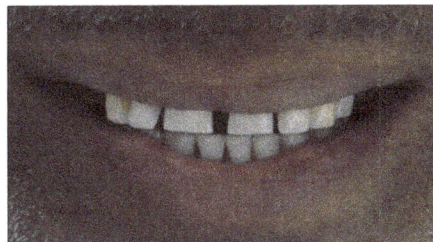

FIGURE 3: Preoperative extraoral view of the patient.

front teeth region. Patient's medical history was noncontributory and intraoral examination using a Vernier Caliper (Aerospace Digital Vernier Caliper, India) revealed interdental spacing between maxillary central incisors (~4 mm) and maxillary central and lateral incisors (~1.5 mm) (Figures 1–3). No dental caries were observed upon both clinical and radiographic examinations.

The patient was satisfied with the color of his teeth. He had a thick gingival biotype and a fairly symmetrical gingival architecture. Patient demonstrated good periodontal health upon clinical examination. Plaque Index [8] was used for periodontal evaluation. The score obtained was 0.57 which signifies good oral hygiene.

Among the different treatment options for this case, we selected the most conservative because of patient's desire for quick results and his financial constraints. Also, though not a regular visitor to the dentist, the patient demonstrated good oral health.

Before starting the treatment, preoperative photographs (Nikon® Coolpix L810) were taken. Following oral prophylaxis, shade selection was done using the VITAPAN® Classical Shade guide (A2) and an intraoral mock-up was done with A2B shade of Filtek™ Supreme XT (3 M/ESPE, St. Paul, MN, USA) but without etching and bonding. Two bulk increments of the composite were placed on the mesial surfaces of 11 and 21 and gross contouring was done with a composite instrument. Then, the composite was cured only for 20 seconds and the outcome was shown to the patient. Since etching and bonding procedures were not done, the bulk of composite restorative material could be easily removed using a sharp instrument. Once the patient was satisfied, it was decided that only a single shade (A2B) would

be used to close all the diastemas. The midline diastema was closed by building up the mesial surfaces of central incisors one by one. It was decided to restore 21 first. No tooth preparation is necessary prior to adhesive procedures. Roughening of the enamel is recommended only when self-etch adhesives are to be used. 37% phosphoric acid (Etching Gel, Kerr, USA) was applied on the mesial surface for 15 seconds, rinsed for 20 seconds, and slightly air-dried. It is advisable to etch a little more surface area (labial) as the exact location of final restoration margin is uncertain [9]. Then, two coats of a single bottle bonding agent (Adper Single Bond, 3M ESPE, USA) were applied using applicator tips and polymerized for 20 seconds with an LED light (Elipar™ 2500, 3M ESPE Dental products, US). Care was taken to apply uniform coats of the bonding agent especially near the gingival area. Since pooling of the bonding agent compromises solvent evaporation, after careful application of the bonding agent near the sulcus, it was air-thinned using oil-free syringe.

Following this, a small increment was placed near the "future" contact area and manually contoured over the mesial surface using a long bladed titanium instrument (Figures 4(a) and 4(b)). The composite was then sculpted beneath the free gingival margin and shaped to ideal contours. A brush was then used to thin the material to obtain an imperceptible margin (Figure 4(c)). The increment was cured with LED light for 40 seconds, both from labial and palatal aspects. Then, a contoured sectional matrix (Palodent® System, DENTSPLY Caulk, Milford, Delaware, US) was placed on the mesial surface of 21 with one end slightly into the sulcus (Figure 5). This is to assure the progressive emergence profile of the resin composite. This contoured matrix was then stabilized by holding it from the palatal side and resin composite was then added incrementally to complete the build-up of 21. These contoured matrices are much rigid (unlike mylar strip) which confers them some degree of self-stability. A mylar strip can be placed on the palatal aspect to act as a frame against which to pack composite (Figure 5). Although, some clinicians prefer a gloved finger for this purpose. Each increment was cured for 40 seconds from both labial and palatal aspects. An ET 9 bur (Brasseler, USA) was used to contour and finish the restoration margins. It is recommended to slightly overbuild the first tooth, so that, after finishing and polishing, the tooth achieves the correct mesiodistal dimension.

The same procedure was repeated for 11 (Figures 6 and 7). Care should be taken to place the matrix slightly into the sulcus (Figure 6). Placing and stabilizing sectional matrix

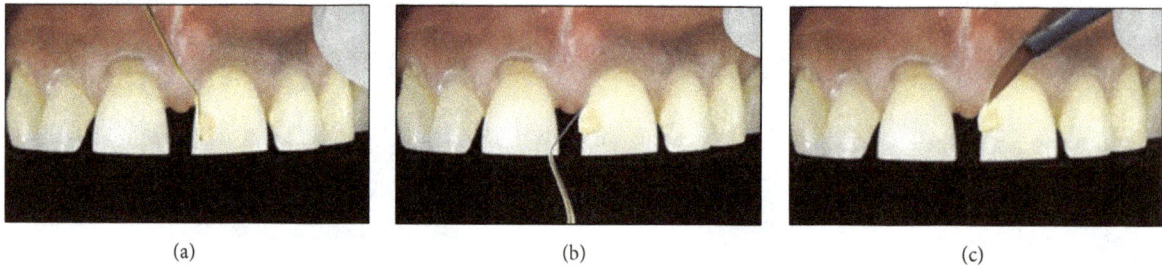

FIGURE 4: (a) A small increment of composite is taken. (b) This increment is flattened with the instrument and is sculpted towards free gingival margin. (c) Composite is then thinned with a brush to achieve an imperceptible margin.

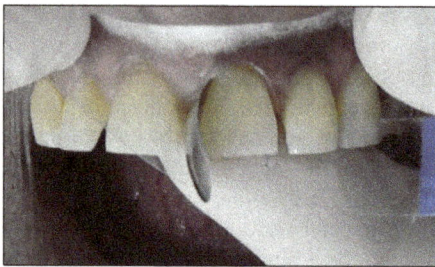

FIGURE 5: Palodent matrix and mylar strip were applied for restoration of 21.

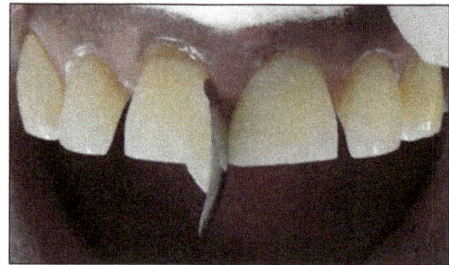

FIGURE 7: Anatomic contours can be easily achieved using the contoured matrix.

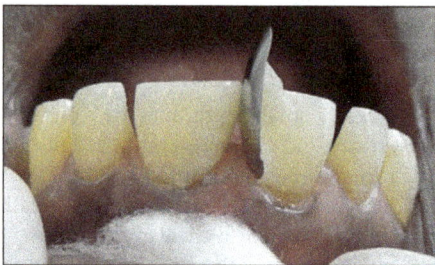

FIGURE 6: Restoration of 11-matrix should be inserted slightly into the sulcus for correct emergence profile of the composite.

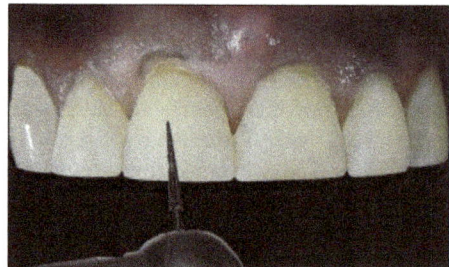

FIGURE 8: Finishing is done with an ET 9 bur.

in 11 would be much simpler as the mesial surface of 21 would provide it with a "positive stop." Once the midline diastema was restored, the diastema between central and lateral incisors was closed in the same manner. Once the diastema closure was accomplished in all the teeth, an ET 9 bur was used again for finishing procedure (Figure 8). Final finishing and polishing were accomplished with Sof-Lex discs (3M ESPE Dental Products. St. Paul, MN, USA). The incisal embrasures were kept small and general anatomic forms of teeth were kept flat and broad which best suited his face and body type (see flat canines of the patient). No or minimal characterization was given on the labial aspects of the teeth. Final outcome of the restorative procedure can be seen in Figures 9–11.

Once all the restorations were placed, the occlusion was verified in both centric and eccentric relations using an articulating paper.

The patient was motivated for oral hygiene and informed for recalls. After 6 months, the restorations were only polished using Sof-Lex discs. The patient was recalled after another 6 months. However, he could not return until 8 months. At 14-month recall (Figure 12), the restorations were evaluated according to modified United States Public Health Service (USPHS) criteria [10]. The scores for all the test procedures were found to be A (Alpha).

3. Discussion

Resin-based composite restorations are single-visit procedures and bypass laboratory work which reduces cost of the treatment. They usually do not require wax-ups and preliminary models. In addition to this, some added advantages that these restorations have over other common treatment modalities are that (a) they are gentle towards the opposing dentition, unlike ceramic materials and (b) they are easy to repair in case of fracture. With porcelain restorations,

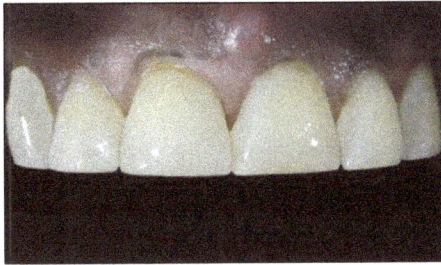

FIGURE 9: Labial view of upper anterior regions after diastema closure.

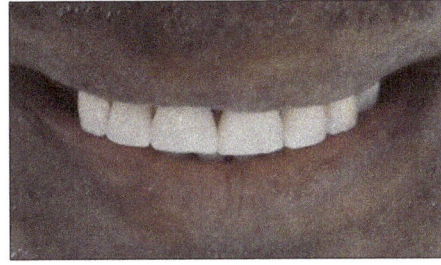

FIGURE 11: Postoperative extraoral view of the patient.

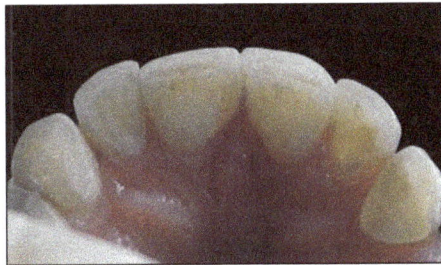

FIGURE 10: Occlusal view after diastema closure.

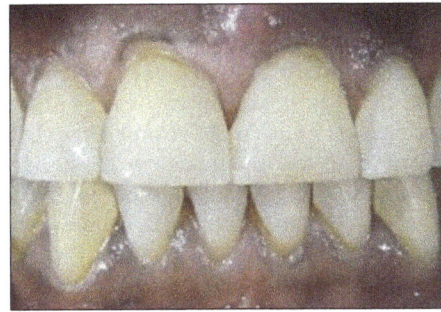

FIGURE 12: View of the restorations at 14-month recall.

any modification means a return-trip to the laboratory for correction [11, 12].

However, there are some distinct disadvantages that these restorations possess which makes case selection critical. Composite restorations possess less color stability compared to ceramics. This of course is related to the degree and quality of polishing but also depends on the patient maintenance [13]. Our patient demonstrated good oral hygiene and was given further instructions regarding the same. Secondly, they possess less fracture toughness and compressive and shear strength and hence are not suited for high-stress bearing areas [14].

In spite of these disadvantages, the clinicians have been offered the best quality resin materials today which allow them to yield esthetic, functional, economical, and durable restorations. We chose to close the diastema using composite restorative material because it was the most conservative treatment possible, the patient exhibited good periodontal health, and also the patient was not willing for an expensive treatment. Excellent outcomes have been reported by numerous authors who have used resin composites for diastema closures [4, 15, 16]. Willhite [17] proposed three criteria for successful diastema closure: an increased emergence profile with natural contours at the interface between the gingiva and tooth; a completely closed gingival embrasure (i.e., no black triangle); and a smooth subgingival margin that does not catch on or shred dental floss.

A common technique of restoring diastemas is to make impression of the wax-up model and fabricating a silicon putty-index [18, 19]. However, in this case using another technique using contoured sectional matrices was decided. The mesial surfaces of teeth were restored one by one; that is, the first tooth was finished and polished to completion

prior to initiation of the second tooth. This allowed us to precisely duplicate the centrals, resulting in two teeth which were mirror images of each other. Most importantly, mesial anatomic contouring could be easily achieved because of the inherent shape of the matrices. One of the biggest challenges that the clinicians face is the failure to avoid "black triangles" when closing diastemas. The restorative technique described here can be applied with relative ease to avoid the "black triangles." A similar technique by Gresnigt et al. has been previously used in literature for direct laminate veneers [20].

These matrices are especially useful in cases where large diastemas (3-4 mm) have to be closed using direct composite resin restorations. The matrices used in this case are polished stainless steel matrices intended for single use only. Since they are polished and made of "soft" metal, there is no risk of epithelial damage when passively inserted into the sulcus. The manufactures recommend steam autoclaving the matrices at 134°C for 3 minutes prior to clinical use. Unlike the BiTine® rings which can be autoclaved 700 times, the matrices can be autoclaved only once [21].

The composite resins used for anterior restorations must demonstrate good handling (nonsticky and nonslumping) and aesthetic (polishability) characteristics. Few commercially available resin composites (e.g., Estelite Sigma, Tokuyama [Tokyo, Japan]; Filtek Supreme Ultra, 3M ESPE [St. Paul, MN]; Premise, Kerr [Orange, CA]; Renamel Microfill, Cosmedent [Chicago, IL]) are well suited for this purpose [22]. Also, they should contain a high filler content by volume (>65%) and particle size smaller than 5 μm [23]. In the present case, we used Filtek Supreme XT which has a filler loading of 78.5% by weight and an average filler particle size of 0.6–1.4 μm [24].

Though the technique mentioned in this report is easy to perform, but the creation of correct midline and optimal contact area requires experience and skill. The dentist should be well experienced with both the technique and the restorative material to perform the procedure correctly. Although use of rubber dam is said to be of paramount importance in placing composite restorations, using cotton-roll isolation in this case was decided. This is primarily because of two reasons. Ideally, the midline of teeth should coincide with midline of face and while restoring midline diastema, it becomes difficult to visualize the midline of face with the rubber dam in place [25]. Secondly, if the midline is shifted by 4 mm or less it is hardly perceptible to the naked eye, but if it is tilted mesiodistally by even 1° (i.e., canted midline), it is discernible. In the authors' opinion, without rubber dam, it is easy to circumvent both the above problems. On the other hand, this step in no way should compromise the longevity of the restoration. A follow-up after 14 months shows no evidence of discolorations, fractures, debonding, or sensitivities (Figure 12). Although a 14-month follow-up might not seem long enough, the abovementioned restoration related failures generally manifest within 6 months after treatment [5]. Diastema closure only under cotton-roll isolation has been demonstrated previously as well [9].

Apart from silicon putty-index technique and common indirect restorative therapy like ceramic veneers, an indirect ceramic restoration called the "ceramic fragment" is also a treatment option for these cases. However, being an indirect procedure, it requires at least two appointments [6].

Recent studies have concluded that direct composite restorations can be considered aesthetic, functional, and stable restorations in patients with favorable occlusion. Prabhu et al. [26] conducted a study in which midline diastema closure was done in maxillary and mandibular central incisors in a total of 45 patients. Recall visits were made every 6 months for a period of 60 months. The authors stated that composite restorations exhibited satisfactory survival rates. Similarly, Demirci et al. [27] evaluated direct composite build-ups for space closure after orthodontic treatment for 4 years and concluded that survival rates for the restorations were favorable for the specified period. Taking into account that failures such as discoloration, marginal leakage, fracture, and debonding usually occur within 6 months of the placement of the restoration, these long-term studies seem to be predictable indicators of long- life of composite restorations.

By taking the past and current literature into consideration, an experienced clinician with the required skill, proper technique, and case selection can create aesthetic and long-lasting direct resin composite restorations much to the satisfaction of his patients as with the case presented in this report.

Competing Interests

The authors of this manuscript declare that there is no conflict of interests regarding the publication of this manuscript.

References

[1] H. J. Keene, "Distribution of diastemas in the dentition of man," *American Journal of Physical Anthropology*, vol. 21, no. 4, pp. 437–441, 1963.

[2] J. T. Kaimenyi, "Occurrence of midline diastema and frenum attachments amongst school children in Nairobi, Kenya," *Indian Journal of Dental Research*, vol. 9, no. 2, pp. 67–71, 1998.

[3] W. J. Huang and C. J. Creath, "The midline diastema: a review of its etiology and treatment," *Pediatric Dentistry*, vol. 17, no. 3, pp. 171–179, 1995.

[4] S. Ardu and I. Krejci, "Biomimetic direct composite stratification technique for the restoration of anterior teeth," *Quintessence International*, vol. 37, no. 3, pp. 167–174, 2006.

[5] B. Korkut, F. Yanikoglu, and D. Tagtekin, "Direct midline diastema closure with composite layering technique: a one-year follow-up," *Case Reports in Dentistry*, vol. 2016, Article ID 6810984, 5 pages, 2016.

[6] B. Bağış and H. Y. Bağış, "Porselen laminate veneerlerin klinik uygulama aşmaları: klinik bir olgu sunumu," *Ankara Üniversitesi Diş Hekimliği Fakültesi Dergisi*, vol. 33, no. 1, pp. 49–57, 2006.

[7] R. Hickel, D. Heidemann, H. J. Staehle, P. Minnig, and N. H. Wilson, "Direct composite restorations: extended use in anterior and posterior situations," *Clinical Oral Investigations*, vol. 8, no. 2, pp. 43–44, 2004.

[8] J. Silness and H. Löe, "Correlation between oral hygiene and periodontal condition," *Acta Odontologica Scandinavica*, vol. 22, no. 1, pp. 121–135, 1964.

[9] B. Margeas, "Free Hand Diastema Closure," Oral Health (April issue), 2014.

[10] G. Ryge, "Clinical criteria," *International Dental Journal*, vol. 30, no. 4, pp. 347–358, 1980.

[11] P. Magne and U. C. Belser, "Porcelain versus composite inlays/onlays: effects of mechanical loads on stress distribution, adhesion, and crown flexure," *International Journal of Periodontics and Restorative Dentistry*, vol. 23, no. 6, pp. 543–555, 2003.

[12] S. Berksun, P. S. Kedici, and S. Saglam, "Repair of fractured porcelain restorations with composite bonded porcelain laminate contours," *The Journal of Prosthetic Dentistry*, vol. 69, no. 5, pp. 457–458, 1993.

[13] D. A. Garber, R. E. Goldstein, and R. A. Feinman, *Porcelain Laminate Veneers*, Quintessence Publishing, Chicago, Ill, USA, 1988.

[14] R. E. Jordan, *Esthetic Composite Bonding Techniques and Materials*, Mosby-Year Book, St. Louis, Mo, USA, 2nd edition, 1993.

[15] M. Lenhard, "Closing diastemas with resin composite restorations," *The European Journal of Esthetic Dentistry*, vol. 3, no. 3, pp. 258–268, 2008.

[16] E. M. De Araujo Jr., S. Fortkamp, and L. N. Baratieri, "Closure of diastema and gingival recontouring using direct adhesive restorations: a case report," *Journal of Esthetic and Restorative Dentistry*, vol. 21, no. 4, pp. 229–240, 2009.

[17] C. Willhite, "Diastema closure with freehand composite: controlling emergence contour," *Quintessence International*, vol. 36, no. 2, pp. 138–140, 2005.

[18] M. J. Koczarski, "Achieving natural aesthetics with direct resin composites: predictable clinical protocol," *Practical Procedures & Aesthetic Dentistry*, vol. 17, no. 8, pp. 523–525, 2005.

[19] B. W. Small, "Repair of central incisors on a child with diastema using a novel matrix," *General Dentistry*, vol. 55, no. 5, pp. 390–391, 2007.

[20] M. M. M. Gresnigt, W. Kalk, and M. Özcan, "Randomized controlled split-mouth clinical trial of direct laminate veneers with two micro-hybrid resin composites," *Journal of Dentistry*, vol. 40, no. 9, pp. 766–775, 2012.

[21] The Palodent® System. Instruction manual (Dentsply), https://www.dentsply.com/content/dam/dentsply/pim/manufacturer/Restorative/Accessories/Matrix_Systems/Sectional_Systems/Palodent_Sectional_Matrix_System/Palodent-zv2lpax-en–1402.

[22] M. Vargas, "A step-by-step approach to a diastema closure," *Journal of Cosmetic Dentistry*, vol. 26, no. 3, pp. 40–45, 2010.

[23] C. H. Chu, C. F. Zhang, and L. J. Jin, "Treating a maxillary mid-line diastema in adult patients. A general dentist's perspective," *The Journal of the American Dental Association*, vol. 142, no. 11, pp. 1258–1264, 2011.

[24] V. L. Schmitt, R. M. Puppin-Rontani, F. S. Naufel, F. P. Nahsan, M. A. C. Sinhoreti, and W. Baseggio, "Effect of the polishing procedures on color stability and surface roughness of composite resins," *ISRN Dentistry*, vol. 2011, Article ID 617672, 6 pages, 2011.

[25] A. S. Brisman, "Esthetics: a comparison of dentists' and patients' concepts," *The Journal of the American Dental Association*, vol. 100, no. 3, pp. 345–352, 1980.

[26] R. Prabhu, S. Bhaskaran, K. R. G. Prabhu, M. A. Eswaran, G. Phanikrishna, and B. Deepthi, "Clinical evaluation of direct composite restoration done for midline diastema closure—long-term study," *Journal of Pharmacy and Bioallied Sciences*, vol. 7, no. 6, pp. S559–S562, 2015.

[27] M. Demirci, S. Tuncer, E. Öztaş, N. Tekçe, and Ö. Uysal, "A 4-year clinical evaluation of direct composite build-ups for space closure after orthodontic treatment," *Clinical Oral Investigations*, vol. 19, no. 9, pp. 2187–2199, 2015.

6

Total CAD/CAM Supported Method for Manufacturing Removable Complete Dentures

Arthur Furtado de Mendonça,[1] Mario Furtado de Mendonça,[1] George Shelby White,[2] Georges Sara,[2] and Darren Littlefair[3]

[1]*Department of Prosthodontics, Fluminense Federal University, Niterói, RJ, Brazil*
[2]*Department of Prosthodontics, Columbia University College of Dental Medicine, New York, NY, USA*
[3]*University of Manchester (Formerly UMIST), Manchester, UK*

Correspondence should be addressed to Arthur Furtado de Mendonça; arthurgsfm@gmail.com

Academic Editor: Maria Beatriz Duarte Gavião

The incorporation of computer-aided design/computer-aided manufacturing (CAD/CAM) technology into complete denture fabrication brings about several advantages to the fabrication process, providing better predictability of the desired outcomes and high accuracy of denture fit, mainly because the milling of prepolymerized acrylic resin eliminates the shrinkage of the acrylic base. Also, there is a decrease in the porosity when compared to a conventionally processed denture, and consequently there is a decrease in the retention of *Candida albicans* on the denture base. The presented workflow for complete denture fabrication presents a totally wax-free manufacturing process, combining rapid prototyping (RP) and rapid milling. With the presented technique, the maxillomandibular relation (MMR) and the ideal setup of the tooth arrangement are developed by using occlusion rims and trial setup made with RP. For the definitive final denture, the denture base and the basal surfaces of the conventional denture teeth were milled according to the individual clinical situation. Posteriorly, the teeth were adapted and bonded into the milled sockets of the milled base.

1. Introduction

Since the introduction of computer-aided design/computer-aided manufacturing (CAD/CAM) techniques, considerable changes have taken place in dentistry; fixed dental prostheses have been extensively reported, while clinical reports of total CAD/CAM workflow for complete removable dentures are scarce. Some systems are available for the fabrication of removable dentures, including milling and rapid prototyping, but still some limitations and disadvantages can be found, such as manufacturing challenges caused by making impression, establishing occlusal vertical dimension (OVD), maxillomandibular relation (MMR) transfer, inability to define the mandibular occlusal plane, expensive materials, and increased laboratory costs compared with those for conventional methods [1]. Also, some systems do not provide a trial denture, which is considered an important step in validating

comfort, function aesthetics, and patient acceptance before the final fabrication is issued to the patient.

Current innovations and developments in dental technology address these limitations and allow the fabrication of removable dentures by using CAD/CAM from start to finish, achieving a less traumatic experience for the patients for better fitting dentures. The first step for manufacturing the digital dentures is to prepare the casts using conventional impression techniques or intraoral digital impression; therefore, casts are scanned and the MMR is registered using occlusion rims manufactured using RP. Stereolithography (STL) files with the appropriate OVD and MMR are generated with the scans of the occlusion rims after the interocclusal records, tooth selection, and arrangement. Subsequently, the trial denture is 3D printed using RP and the clinical parameters are evaluated, so the final denture can be milled.

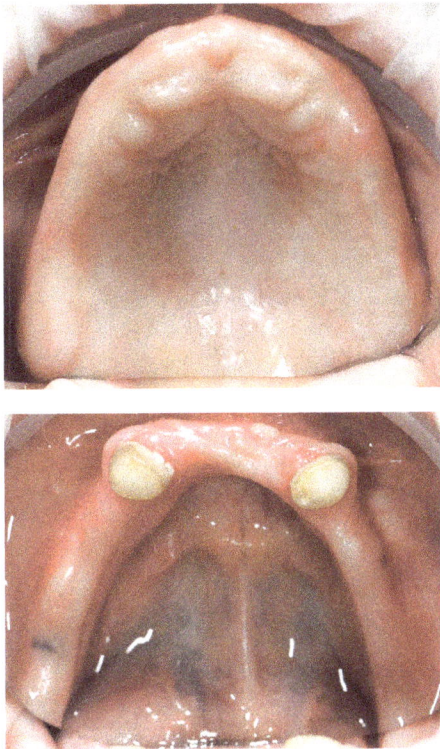

FIGURE 1: Clinical condition.

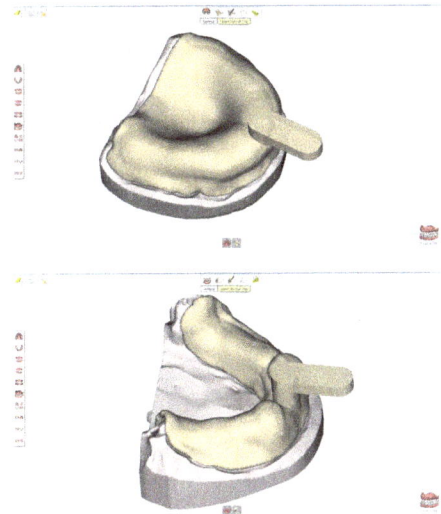

FIGURE 2: Design of special trays.

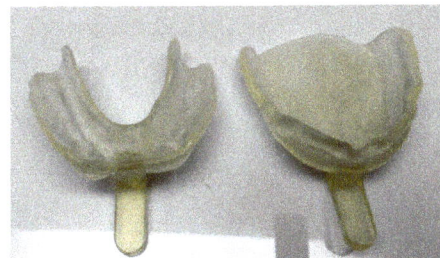

FIGURE 3: Special trays manufactured by rapid prototyping.

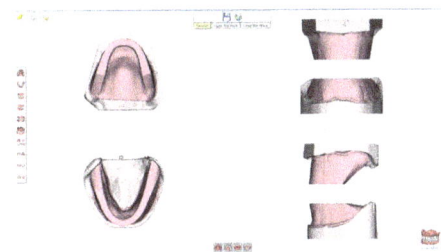

FIGURE 4: Digital design of the occlusal rims.

The presented report of a clinical study provides a detailed description of a total CAD/CAM supported method for manufacturing removable complete dentures. The workflow is managed using the Prosthetic Design Centre software (PDC, Stoneglass Industries).

2. Case Presentation

A 63-year-old woman presented without any significant medical problems to replace her current removable denture. On the mandibular arch, the prepared teeth 33 and 34 were presented (Figure 1). For the primary casts, conventional impressions using alginate (Alginoplast, regular set; Heraeus Kulzer GmbH) were made for subsequent scanning and digital designed special trays (first clinical appointment). The correct path of insertion and the extension and width of the trays were designed and managed within the PDC software. The trays were manufactured with rapid prototyping process (ProJet MP 3500, 3D Systems Inc., USA) (Figures 2 and 3). Once the definitive impressions (Impregum Penta; 3M ESPE) of the maxilla and mandible were completed with the 3D printed special trays (second clinical appointment), the secondary casts were fabricated, which then are scanned for the digital design of the occlusal rims (Figure 4).

The third clinical appointment is dedicated to adjusting the occlusion rims and recording the clinical data following the basic protocol for removable dentures, like the vertical dimension of occlusion, smile line, the position of the canines, and the midline. When the occlusion rims were articulated properly, the MMR was registered with a bite registration material (Blu-Mousse, Parkell Inc., USA) (Figure 5) and scanned for the digital design of teeth and gingival tissues. The scan of the MMR was made in two steps: first, the casts were mounted on an articulator (Artex, Amann Girrbach, USA) and then the casts were scanned separately with an optical scanner (IScan d104i, Imetric 3D Scanning Systems, Switzerland), and with a precalibrated device the MMR was transferred to a STL file.

Following the PDC workflow, tooth selection and arrangement can be accomplished by using the data on the adjusted occlusion rims for appropriate lip support and optimal aesthetics (Figures 6 and 7). The first prototype is then 3D printed (ProJet MP 3500, 3D Systems Inc., USA) for the patient's trial setup. After making proper adjustments to the RP clinical setup, occlusal landmarks can be validated

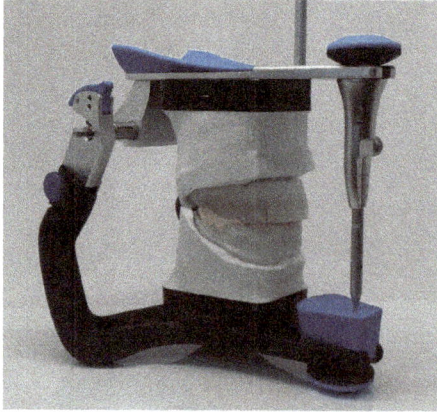

FIGURE 5: Record of the maxillomandibular relation.

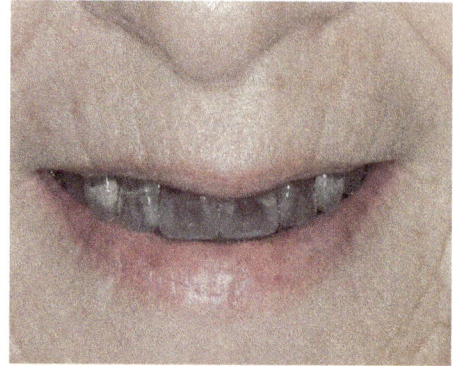

FIGURE 6: Digital design of the teeth.

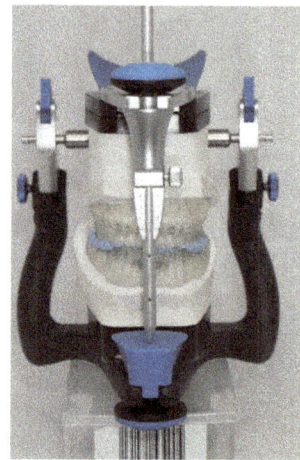

FIGURE 7: First prototype.

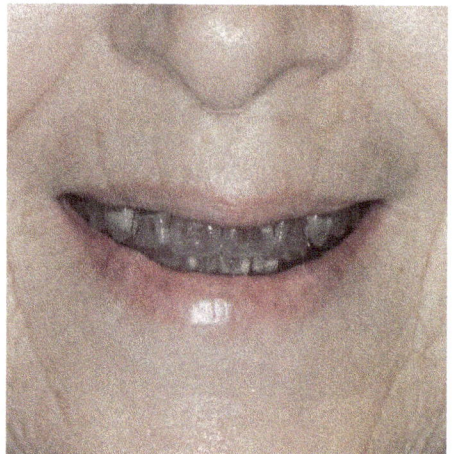

FIGURE 8: Clinical evaluation of the first prototype.

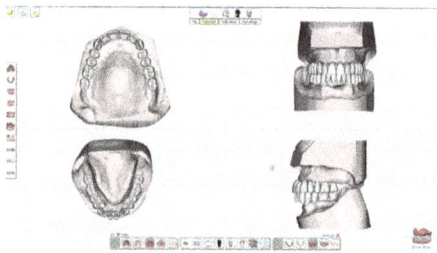

FIGURE 9: Bite record after the primary changes on the occlusion plane.

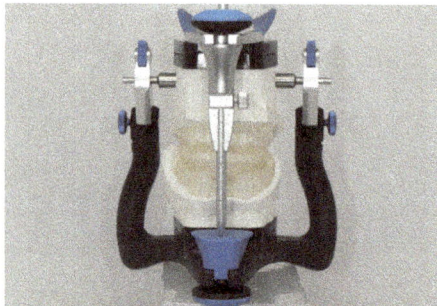

FIGURE 10: Second prototype.

(fourth clinical appointment). Adjustments were necessary on the plane of occlusion and the MMR. Final adjustments can be made if necessary (Figures 8 and 9). After the clinician has verified the occlusal data and patient acceptance has been established (Figure 10), the final prosthesis can be sent for milling and are ready to be issued.

The base of the denture is ready to be manufactured by milling a poly(methyl methacrylate) (PMMA) block with the information provided by the CAD software. Milling will provide individual sockets for each tooth (Figure 11). The conventional denture teeth (Heraeus Kulzer GmbH, Germany) were modified according to the individual clinical situation. For that purpose, they were mounted in a special device and had their basal surfaces milled according to prior computation. The teeth were bonded in the milled sockets of the denture base by mechanic retention done in the milling of the denture tooth (each tooth was milled according to its respective socket

on the denture base with additional physical retention), and also chemical bonding was obtained by acrylic and monomer activation (Heraeus Kulzer GmbH, Germany). Denture base was stained with Heraeus Kulzer Pala cre-active Stains. The complete denture was polished and delivered (Figures 12 and 13). No adjustments were made in the delivery of the denture,

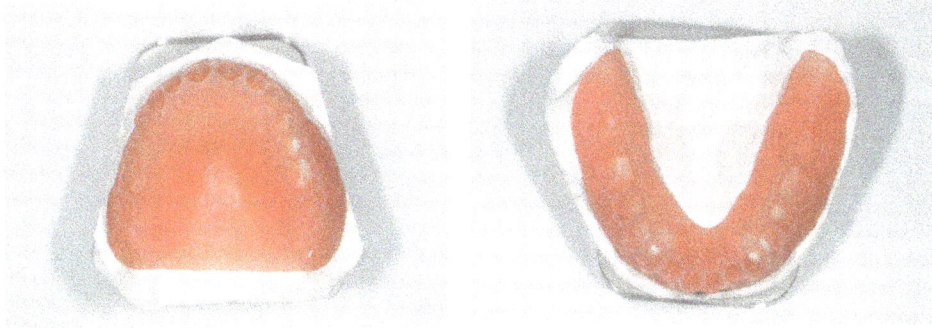

FIGURE 11: Denture bases.

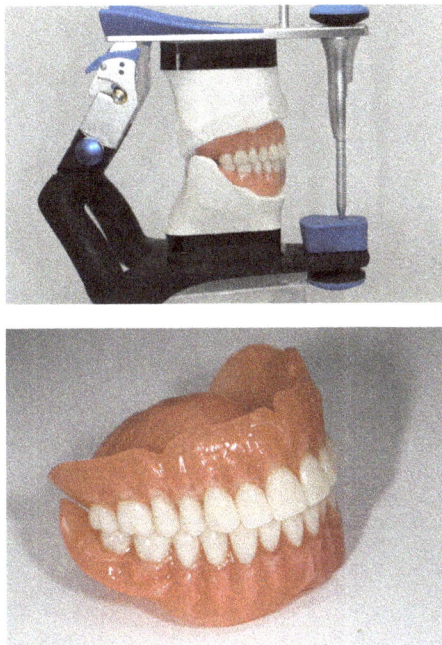

FIGURE 12: Final denture.

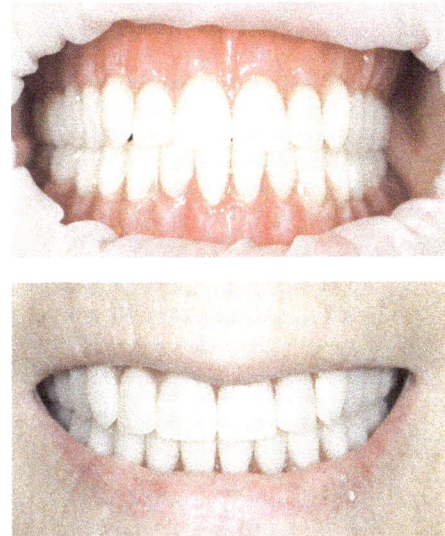

FIGURE 13: Clinical photos of the final denture.

nor was any follow-up necessary, demonstrating the accuracy of the technique (the final denture was a precise replica of the trial, which was approved by the clinician and the patient).

3. Discussion

In the past few years, significant advancements have taken place in the fabrication of complete dentures with the introduction of CAD/CAM technologies. The digital workflow was observed to provide better control of the desired outcomes and also improved the communication between all three parties consisting of the dentist, the patient, and laboratories. It is important to highlight the basic principles for the rehabilitation of the edentulous patient with removable dentures using CAD/CAM technologies and to continue to follow the same principles used to manufacture the analog dentures. With digital dentures, some of the steps that led to failure can be eliminated, like the polymerization shrinkage of the dental base, providing better predictability of the results, high accuracy in denture fit, and easier duplication of dentures [2–5].

The use of CAD/CAM to support the manufacture of removable dentures has been previously reported with different concepts. Some techniques use wax to make the occlusion rims and mill the denture bases with a wax blank for the trial evaluation in the patient mouth. A conventional processing technique is necessary [6]. Another reported system uses a wax occlusion rim for record bases and an anatomic measurement device to complete the OVD record, including centric relation [2]. This technique claimed to decrease the number of clinical appointments but faces the disadvantage of lacking a trial denture, which is considered an important step validating denture goals by patients and dentists before final denture fabrication [1]. The PDC dentures are produced by machining a preformed cylinder of PMMA. This material presents a decrease in the porosity when compared to a conventionally processed denture and a decrease in the retention of *Candida albicans* on the denture base [4]. The conventional denture teeth have their basal surface milled individually and are then bonded chemically to the corresponding sockets.

The PDC workflow presents unique characteristics, because it is a totally wax-free system, which utilizes rapid prototyping to manufacture the occlusion rims, the record of the clinical parameters, and the trial setup for the evaluation of the final design. In this particular case, the first trial, after verifying the occlusion and the eccentric movements, it was decided to make some changes on the tooth position to improve the function and aesthetics. The trial setup was adjusted and a new bite record was made for posterior scanning. The second trial was considered the desirable setup by all the parties involved. The final denture was issued, and at the final appointment no modification was needed on the dentures, demonstrating that successful criteria had been met.

4. Conclusions

A totally wax-free technique for the fabrication of a CAD/CAM denture was described. By using RP, a trial made it possible for all parties to evaluate criteria for successes before the final denture is issued providing control of the outcomes. This clinical report demonstrates that digital denture can be effective and accurate, eliminating or replacing steps that can lead to complications. Since this is a novel approach, further research should provide the limitations of the technique in terms of color stability, stain techniques, and teeth/denture base bond strength. A controlled randomized clinical trial is needed to determine whether CAD/CAM digital dentures are an improvement over conventional methods for removable dentures.

Competing Interests

The authors declare that there are no competing interests regarding the publication of this paper.

References

[1] M. Bilgin, E. Baytaroglu, A. Erdem, and E. Dilber, "A review of computer-aided design/computer-aided manufacture techniques for removable denture fabrication," *European Journal of Dentistry*, vol. 10, no. 2, pp. 286–291, 2016.

[2] L. Infante, B. Yilmaz, E. McGlumphy, and I. Finger, "Fabricating complete dentures with CAD/CAM technology," *Journal of Prosthetic Dentistry*, vol. 111, no. 5, pp. 351–355, 2014.

[3] M. T. Kattadiyil, C. J. Goodacre, and N. Z. Baba, "CAD/CAM complete dentures: a review of two commercial fabrication systems," *Journal of the California Dental Association*, vol. 41, no. 6, pp. 407–416, 2013.

[4] M. T. Kattadiyil, R. Jekki, C. J. Goodacre, and N. Z. Baba, "Comparison of treatment outcomes in digital and conventional complete removable dental prosthesis fabrications in a predoctoral setting," *Journal of Prosthetic Dentistry*, vol. 114, pp. 818–825, 2015.

[5] S. B. M. Patzelt, S. Vonau, S. Stampf, and W. Att, "Assessing the feasibility and accuracy of digitizing edentulous jaws," *Journal of the American Dental Association*, vol. 144, no. 8, pp. 914–920, 2013.

[6] T. Wimmer, K. Gallus, M. Eichberger, and B. Stawarczyk, "Complete denture fabrication supported by CAD/CAM," *Journal of Prosthetic Dentistry*, vol. 115, no. 5, pp. 541–546, 2015.

7

Restoration: Implant with Devastated Platform through Metal Post

Luna Salinas Tatiana and Del Valle Lovato Juan

Central University of Ecuador Dental School, Quito, Ecuador

Correspondence should be addressed to Luna Salinas Tatiana; taty_bel_moon@hotmail.com

Academic Editor: Miguel Peñarrocha

Case Presentation. Implant prostheses are a successful treatment for replacing missing teeth. However, this treatment modality can have biological and mechanical complications causing serious problems for the dentist, as demonstrated in this clinical case. The patient presented with a fractured screw and a severely damaged implant hex connection that corresponded to the second premolar, upper left, stating that she unsuccessfully tried to remove the prosthetic screw, which was most likely to have been loose. After clinical and radiographic review, it was decided to remove small fragments of the fractured prosthetic screw inside the implant head. Removal by conventional methods was unsuccessful but was eventually achieved through use of a bur. Then it was possible to make a cast post (gold-palladium) and develop a fixed prosthesis (silver-palladium), which were attached with luting cement. A cast post (gold-palladium) was made and a fixed prosthesis was developed (silver-palladium), which were attached with luting cement, the same ones that can present mechanical complications such as fractures between the third and fourth thread of the implant, loosening of the abutment, and/or the prosthetic screw in individual crowns, most frequently in partially edentulous patients, mainly in the premolar and molar regions of the maxilla. *Conclusion.* Therefore the present technique used in this case is very simple, noninvasive, and useful to readers.

1. Introduction

Since Branemark introduced the concept of osseointegration, dental implants have been successfully used as a viable treatment for fully and partially edentulous patients [1]. According to Zarb and Schmitt [2] and Wismeyer et al. [3] implant fracture is a rare but significant complication, most of the fractures occurred between the third and fourth thread of the implants. Several authors [4–8] concluded that the loosening of the abutment screw ranged from 2% to 45% and that there was a difference in the incidence of loosening between types of prosthesis; the highest rate was found with single crowns following and overdentures.

The most common complication for a single crown was a prosthetic screw and abutment screw loosening [9], but the prosthetic complications will depend on the number of implants available, size, and arrangement and may cause long-term marginal bone loss, fractures metal fatigue, and/or loss of osseointegration [10, 11].

Hurson [12] states that the nature of loosening is complex because a variety of patterns and occlusal masticatory forces, The clinical studies indicate that between 5% and 45% of loosening or fracture of the components of the implant prosthesis occurs in the first year, Gupta et al. [13].

According to Nergiz et al. [14], screw is the smallest and weakest part between the implant components; therefore it may be lost or broken before other components. Besides the implant systems have such antirotation component as an internal or external hexagon so implants that are not protected against rotation present higher percentage of complications [14].

Jemt [15] states that the screws are typically designed to be the weakest link in the implant-prosthetic system, loosening being an early sign of overload. According to W. Becker and B. E. Becker [16] this loosening in fixed prostheses connected with external hex implants is a phenomenon that occurs most frequently in partially edentulous patients.

Parafunctional habits can be a risk factor related to implant fracture and screw loosening and can create uncontrolled and excessive occlusal loading forces [17]. Indeed some authors state that both the centric and eccentric bruxism can lead to overloading of the implant and metal fatigue as a result of physiological changes of the patient [18, 19].

A higher frequency of screw loosening has been reported for replacement of single crowns in the premolar and molar area than in the anterior region and three times more in the maxilla compared with the mandible [20]. The posterior maxilla had a success rate of 91.4% compared with the maxilla (97%), the posterior mandible (96.3%), and the anterior mandible (97.9%) [21].

Once fracture has been diagnosed, it is possible to proceed to extraction, beginning with the simplest and most conservative method, and trying to respect, as far as possible, the implant head, external hex, and internal thread. Any change in these areas can lead to limitations in future prosthetic use. The methods used to recover the broken fragments or screw are determined according to the location above or below the head of the implant. If a cap screw fracture is above the head of the implant, an explorer, a straight, or a hemostatic probe can succeed, and the tip of the instrument is carefully moved in the opposite direction clockwise on the surface of the segment screw according to Satwalekar et al. [22]. If that procedure is unsuccessful in removing the fragment, Eckert et al. [23] have proposed applying a round bur at high speed to the head of the broken screw and another method is to make a notch in the head fragment, if possible, to attempt to remove the implant fragment by using a screwdriver in reverse. In case of implant fracture, there are two options: (1) complete removal of the implant fractured using explantation drills and (2) the use of the fractured implant in order to place a new prosthesis [24]. Some implant manufacturers offer a kit for this purpose, including a rotary tool to smooth the edges of the fracture and an instrument to create a new internal thread for the implant. Work of Goiato et al. [25] proposes a third option, which is to leave the submerged implant. If the implant is again rehabilitated, noble metal alloys, including gold, palladium, silver, and titanium, should be used. Proper selection and handling of these alloys are essential because the prosthetic restoration and longevity go hand in hand with implants [26, 27].

Finally, although the frequency of fractures of implants is low, treatment planning should include avoiding occlusal overload, in some cases using an occlusal splint to protect the restorations [28].

This report describes the rehabilitation of an implant with screw fracture and severely damaged hex by a cast post.

2. Case Presentation

A 66-year-old female patient who takes bisphosphonates for osteopenia presented at the dental practice in the Postgraduate School of Oral Rehabilitation, Central University of Ecuador, with fracture of the implant prosthetic screw and damaged hex platform (Figure 1).

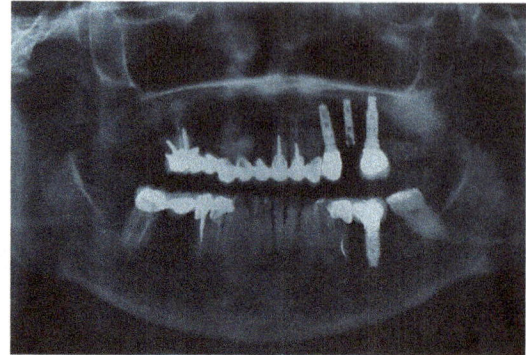

FIGURE 1: Panoramic radiograph. Implant (2.5) with fracture screw and hex devastated platform.

The first step was to attempt extraction of the fragment, beginning with the most conservative and simple method, through dental explorer, without success. Therefore, the fragment was destroyed with a fissure bur, touching the internal threads of the implant, as seen radiographically (Figure 2).

The gum around the implant platform was cut minimally and an acrylic resin impression made of the inside of the implant (DuraLay, Reliance Dental Mfg. Keliance) (Figure 3).

Once the post cast bolt (gold-palladium) was made and its adaptation with wax (Wax Disclosing Kerr) checked radiographically (Figure 4), it was cemented with the following protocol (Figure 5):

(a) The inside of the implant was cleaned, washed, and dried

(b) Hydrofluoric acid gel at 9.6% (EUFAR Laboratories S.A.) was applied to the post for 60 seconds, then washed, and dried

(c) Luting cement (DTK-Klever Bredent, DE) was mixed and placed both on the post and inside the implant

(d) The post was photopolymerized with ultraviolet light (350 to 500 Nm) for 3 minutes

(e) Excess cement was removed

Once the post cemented, cord (Ultradent Ultrapak of two ESPA 00) is placed, printing was performed with heavy and light polyvinyl siloxane (Elite HD + from Zhermack IT) (Figure 6), and metal framework developed (silver-palladium) (Figure 7), by wax (wax Disclosing Kerr) adaptation, and sealing was made.

Finally the prosthetic crown is cemented, after occlusal control, which was allowed to be below 12 micrometers' occlusion (Figure 8) and the patient received information about oral hygiene. After one year of treatment, clinical and radiographic monitoring is performed (Figure 9).

3. Discussion

To Hurson [12] screw loosening is a possible complication of the prosthesis screwed implants, leading to dissatisfaction for the patient and frustration for the dentist, and if left

(a)

(b)

(c)

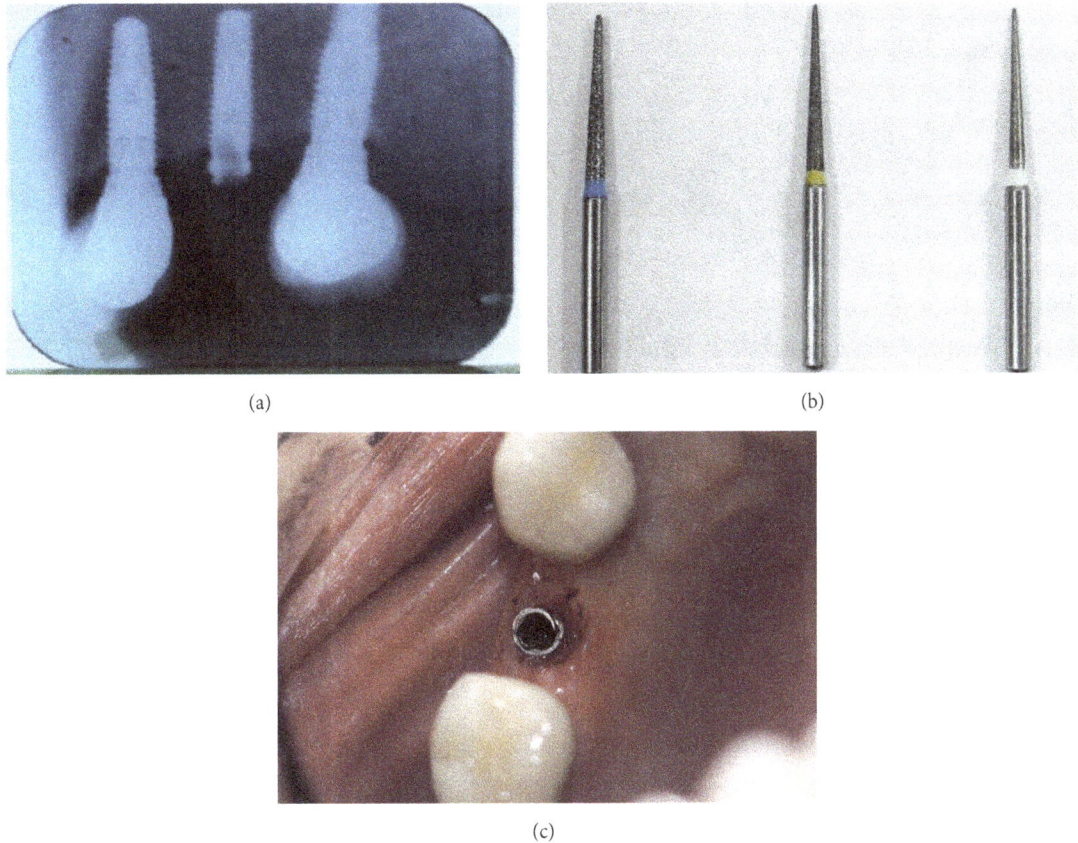

Figure 2: Removal of fracture fragment: (a) radiograph; (b) fissure bur was used to remove the fractured screw; (c) occlusal view.

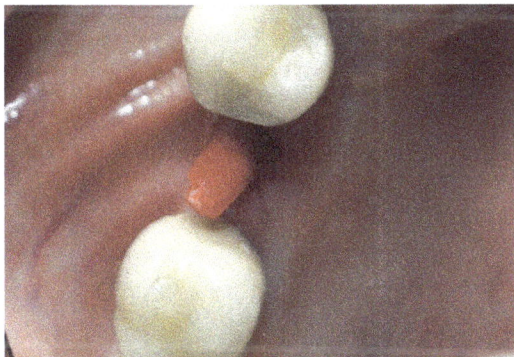

Figure 3: DuraLay post.

untreated it can lead to breakage thereof or one of the implant components becoming more complex and difficulty in solving mechanical complication, as in the present case. Rangert et al. [18] reported that 90% of fractured implants are in the region of the molars and premolars. Similar observations were made by Balshi [24], who found that all implant fractures occurred in the area of the premolars and molars with no distinction between upper and lower jaw. Van Steenberghe et al. [20] state that the first failures occur in the posterior maxilla, with a success rate of 91.4% compared to the previous maxilla with 97%.

In the article by Zarb and Schmitt [2] in which 225 implants were lost, 109 were lost after the prosthetic treatment and generally performed posteriorly. For Jemt [15] they were lost in 1.9% in individual crown on implants. While for Andersson et al. [7] and Haas et al. [8] the most common complication reported with single crowns was a pillar and/or prosthetic screw loosening. A higher frequency of screw loosening according to Ekfeldt et al. [5] and Laney et al. [6] was produced in individual crowns in premolars and molars compared to the previous region. Within the limits of a retrospective study, conducted for W. Becker and B. E. Becker [16] in replacement of molars for implants, it was found that the main complication was loosening gold screws, presented in eight implants (38%) of 21 implants, and one implant was lost and the survival rate was 95.7%.

Jemt [15] stated screws fractured by fatigue occur in the first year of operation, provided that the design of the prosthesis is not appropriate. To Schwarz [10] preload is the only resistance to occlusal forces in implant external hexagon with individual crowns. If occlusal forces exceed this preload, screw loosening and thus its fracture can be produced [11].

In this case, the patient had fracture of the prosthetic screw with damaged external hexagon but had noticed loosening of the screw several times before its fracture; however, it had been decided to maintain the implant within the mouth for further prosthetic rehabilitation as the patient was taking bisphosphonates. The treatment reported here is in contrast

(a)

(b)

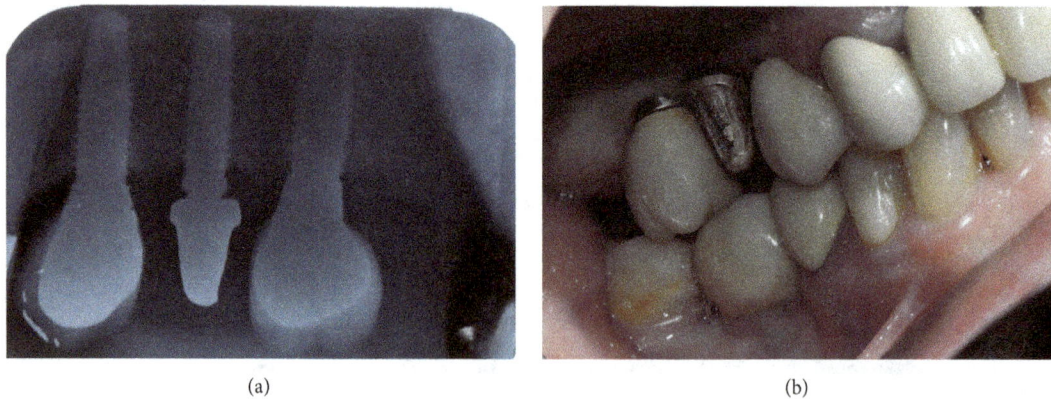

FIGURE 4: Sealing and adaptation were made: (a) radiographic control and (b) disclosing wax verifications.

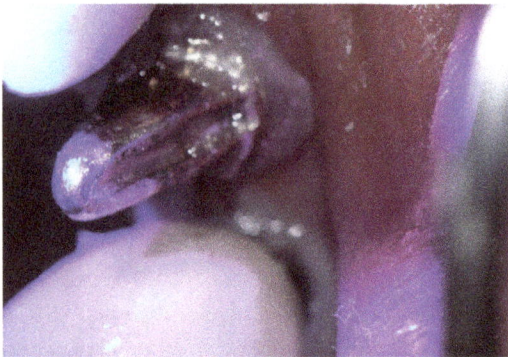

FIGURE 5: Post cement.

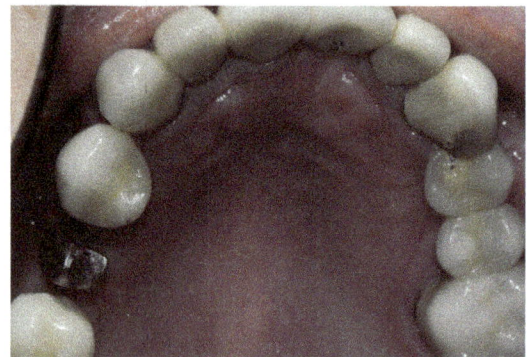

FIGURE 7: Framework sealing and adaptation of metal crown.

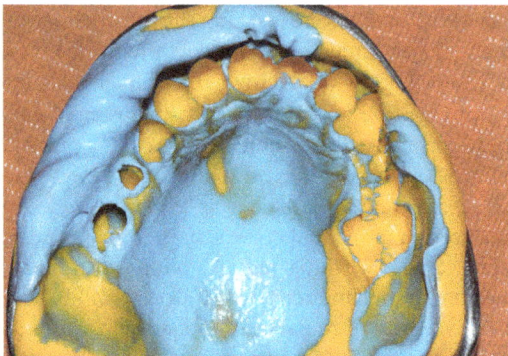

FIGURE 6: Dental impression.

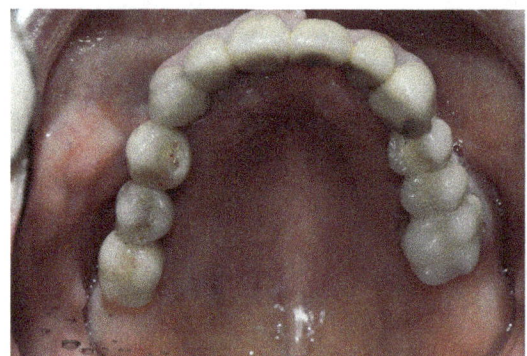

FIGURE 8: Crown cement and occlusal adjustment.

to Gargallo Albiol et al. [19] who conducted an analysis of fracture implants in which 81% was complete removal and subsequent placement of a greater number of implants and larger diameter in the region of premolars and molar. Satwalekar et al. [22] presented a case corresponding screw and fractured the left central incisor, which left it submerged after removing the fractured part implant; then a fixed partial denture was placed. Goiato et al. [25] reported a case of a 58-year-old with implant fractured in a cervical third level in the maxillary first premolar, which was removed trepano in the

same clinical session. Three months later a new implant and prosthesis were put on.

It has been proposed to wear down or attempt to make a notch in the head fragment of the broken screw with a round bur at high speed, depending on the location of the prosthetic screw. In the case reported it was not possible to extract the fragment because it was below the implant head so it was ground down with a bur. The risk of puncturing the implant and bone was controlled radiographically. After achieving the objective, a metal and porcelain post and crown were made.

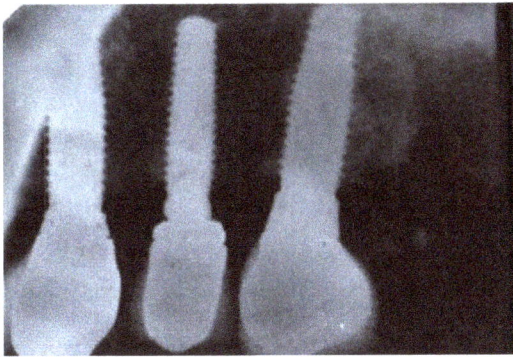

FIGURE 9: Intraoral radiograph at the 1-year follow-up.

Among the advantages of using noble alloys is that they have a lower elastic modulus allowing the occlusal forces to transmit more efficiently to the remaining teeth. Binding of noble metal and porcelain is better than base metal because the oxide layer is thinner. Disadvantage is the high economic cost [26].

Finally, in a monitoring appointment after one year of treatment the patient reported no discomfort. Normality was clinically and radiographically checked.

4. Conclusion

Within the limitations of this case it was possible to conclude that the situations with screws fractured abutment and devastated hexagon can be solved in a time and manner of saving money, with a very useful alternative without the invasive treatment such as removal of the implant and submerging. Therefore the present technique used in this case is very simple, noninvasive, and useful to readers.

Competing Interests

The authors whose names are listed certify that they have no affiliations with or involvement in any organization or entity with any financial interest or nonfinancial interest in the subject matter or materials discussed in this manuscript.

References

[1] P. Bra-nemark, G. A. Zarb, T. Albrektsson, and H. M. Rosen, "Tissue-integrated prostheses. Osseointegration in clinical dentistry," *Plastic and Reconstructive Surgery*, vol. 77, no. 3, pp. 496–497, 1986.

[2] G. A. Zarb and A. Schmitt, "The longitudinal clinical effectiveness of osseointegrated dental implants: the Toronto study. Part I: Surgical results," *The Journal of Prosthetic Dentistry*, vol. 63, no. 4, pp. 451–457, 1990.

[3] D. Wismeyer, M. A. van Waas, and J. I. Vermeeren, "Overdentures supported by ITI implants: a 6.5-year evaluation of patient satisfaction and prosthetic aftercare," *The International journal of oral & maxillofacial implants*, vol. 10, no. 6, pp. 744–749, 1995.

[4] P. A. Fugazzotto, H. J. Gulbransen, S. L. Wheeler, and J. A. Lindsay, "The use of IMZ osseointegrated implants in partially and completely edentulous patients: success and failure rates of 2,023 implant cylinders up to 60+ months in function," *The International Journal of Oral & Maxillofacial Implants*, vol. 8, no. 6, pp. 617–621, 1993.

[5] A. Ekfeldt, G. E. Carlsson, and G. Börjesson, "Clinical evaluation of single-tooth restorations supported by osseointegrated implants: A Retrospective Study," *The International Journal of Oral & Maxillofacial Implants*, vol. 9, no. 2, pp. 179–183, 1994.

[6] W. R. Laney, T. Jemt, D. Harris et al., "Osseointegrated implants for single-tooth replacement: progress report from a multicenter prospective study after 3 years," *The International Journal of Oral & Maxillofacial Implants*, vol. 9, no. 1, pp. 49–54, 1994.

[7] B. Andersson, P. Odman, A. M. Lindvall, and B. Lithner, "Single-tooth restorations supported by osseointegrated implants: Results And Experiences From A Prospective Study After 2 To 3 Years," *The International journal of oral & maxillofacial implants*, vol. 10, no. 6, pp. 702–711, 1995.

[8] R. Haas, N. Mensdorff-Pouilly, G. Mailath, and G. Watzek, "Brånemark single tooth implants: a preliminary report of 76 implants," *The Journal of Prosthetic Dentistry*, vol. 73, no. 3, pp. 274–279, 1995.

[9] C. J. Goodacre, J. Y. Kan, and K. Rungcharassaeng, "Clinical complications of osseointegrated implants," *The Journal of Prosthetic Dentistry*, vol. 81, no. 5, pp. 537–552, 1999.

[10] M. S. Schwarz, "Mechanical complications of dental implants," *Clinical Oral Implants Research*, vol. 11, pp. 156–158, 2000.

[11] T. D. A. P. N. Carneiro, M. S. Prudente, R. S. e Pessoa, G. Mendonça, and F. D. das Neves, "A conservative approach to retrieve a fractured abutment screw—case report," *Journal of Prosthodontic Research*, vol. 60, no. 2, pp. 138–142, 2016.

[12] S. Hurson, "Practical clinical guidelines to prevent screw loosening," *International Journal of Dental Symposia*, vol. 3, no. 1, pp. 22–25, 1995.

[13] S. Gupta, H. Gupta, and A. Tandan, "Technical complications of implant-causes and management: a comprehensive review," *National Journal of Maxillofacial Surgery*, vol. 6, no. 1, pp. 3–8, 2015.

[14] I. Nergiz, P. Schmage, and R. Shahin, "Removal of a fractured implant abutment screw: a clinical report," *Journal of Prosthetic Dentistry*, vol. 91, no. 6, pp. 513–517, 2004.

[15] T. Jemt, "Failures and complications in 391 consecutively inserted fixed prostheses supported by Brånemark implants in edentulous jaws: a study of treatment from the time of prosthesis placement to the first annual checkup," *The International Journal of Oral & Maxillofacial Implants*, vol. 6, no. 3, pp. 270–276, 1991.

[16] W. Becker and B. E. Becker, "Replacement of maxillary and mandibular molars with single endosseous implant restorations: A Retrospective Study," *The Journal of Prosthetic Dentistry*, vol. 74, no. 1, pp. 51–55, 1995.

[17] A. Sánchez-Pérez, M. J. Moya-Villaescusa, A. Jornet-García, and S. Gomez, "Etiology, risk factors and management of implant fractures," *Medicina Oral, Patologia Oral y Cirugia Bucal*, vol. 15, no. 3, pp. e504–e508, 2010.

[18] B. Rangert, P. H. Krogh, B. Langer, and N. Van Roekel, "Bending overload and implant fracture: a retrospective clinical analysis," *The International Journal of Oral & Maxillofacial Implants*, vol. 10, no. 3, pp. 326–334, 1995.

[19] J. Gargallo Albiol, M. Satorres Nieto, J. L. Puyuelo Capablo, M. A. Sánchez Garcés, J. Pi Urgell, and C. Gay-Escoda, "Endosseous dental implant fractures an analysis of 21 cases,"

Medicina Oral, Patologia Oral y Cirugia Bucal, vol. 13, no. 2, pp. 124–128, 2008.

[20] D. Van Steenberghe, R. Jacobs, M. Desnyder, G. Maffei, and M. Quirynen, "The relative impact of local and endogenous patient-related factors on implant failure up to the abutment stage," *Clinical Oral Implants Research*, vol. 13, no. 6, pp. 617–622, 2002.

[21] C. Palma-Carrió, L. Maestre-Ferrín, D. Peñarrocha-Oltra, M. A. Peñarrocha-Diago, and M. Peñarrocha-Diago, "Risk factors associated with early failure of dental implants. A literature review," *Medicina Oral, Patologia Oral y Cirugia Bucal*, vol. 16, no. 4, pp. e514–e517, 2011.

[22] P. Satwalekar, K. Subash Chander, B. Anantha Reddy, N. Sandeep, and T. Satwalekar, "A simple and cost effective method used for removal of a fractured implant abutment screw: a case report," *Journal of International Oral Health*, vol. 5, no. 5, pp. 120–123, 2013.

[23] S. E. Eckert, S. J. Meraw, E. Cal, and R. K. Ow, "Analysis of incidence and associated factors with fractured implants: A Retrospective Study," *International Journal of Oral and Maxillofacial Implants*, vol. 15, no. 5, pp. 662–667, 2000.

[24] T. J. Balshi, "An analysis and management of fractured implants: a clinical report," *International Journal of Oral and Maxillofacial Implants*, vol. 11, no. 5, pp. 660–666, 1996.

[25] M. C. Goiato, M. F. Haddad, H. G. Filho, L. M. R. Villa, D. M. Dos Santos, and A. A. Pesqueira, "Dental implant fractures—aetiology, treatment and case report," *Journal of Clinical and Diagnostic Research*, vol. 8, no. 3, pp. 300–304, 2014.

[26] J. C. Wataha, "Alloys for prosthodontic restorations," *Journal of Prosthetic Dentistry*, vol. 87, no. 4, pp. 351–363, 2002.

[27] R. A. Flinn and P. K. Trojan, *Engineering Materials and Their Applications*, Houghton Mifflin, Boston, Mass, USA, 3rd edition, 1986.

[28] H. J. Conrad, J. K. Schulte, and M. C. Vallee, "Fractures related to occlusal overload with single posterior implants: a clinical report," *Journal of Prosthetic Dentistry*, vol. 99, no. 4, pp. 251–256, 2008.

8

Peri-Implant Bone Loss and Peri-Implantitis

Vanchit John, Daniel Shin, Allison Marlow, and Yusuke Hamada

Department of Periodontics and Allied Dental Program, Indiana University School of Dentistry, Indianapolis, IN 46202, USA

Correspondence should be addressed to Vanchit John; vjohn@iu.edu

Academic Editor: Jamil A. Shibli

Dental implant supported restorations have been added substantially to the clinical treatment options presented to patients. However, complications with these treatment options also arise due to improper patient selection and inadequate treatment planning combined with poor follow-up care. The complications related to the presence of inflammation include perimucositis, peri-implant bone loss, and peri-implantitis. Prevalence rates of these complications have been reported to be as high as 56%. Treatment options that have been reported include nonsurgical therapy, the use of locally delivered and systemically delivered antibiotics, and surgical protocols aimed at regenerating the lost bone and soft tissue around the implants. The aim of this article is to report on three cases and review some of the treatment options used in their management.

1. Introduction

Implant supported restorative treatment has led to increased treatment options for patients who are either partially or completely edentulous. However, it has become evident that while this treatment is successful in many patients, implant supported restorations are not free of postplacement complications. Peri-implantitis is defined as an inflammatory process affecting the supporting hard and soft tissue around an implant in function, leading to loss of supporting bone. Peri-implant mucositis is defined as reversible inflammatory changes of the peri-implant soft tissues without any bone loss [1, 2]. The prevalence of peri-implant mucositis and peri-implantitis has ranged from 19 to 65% and 1 to 47%, respectively [2–4]. The most common etiological factors associated with the development of peri-implantitis are the presence of bacterial plaque and host response [5]. The risk factors associated with peri-implant bone loss include smoking combined with IL-1 genotype polymorphism, a history of periodontitis, poor compliance with treatment and oral hygiene practices, presence of systemic diseases affecting healing, cement left behind following cementation of the crowns, lack of keratinized gingiva, and previous history of implant failure [6].

The treatment of peri-implant disease must include decontamination of previously exposed or infected implant surfaces. However, current evidence has shown that non-surgical therapy for peri-implantitis is minimally effective even with the adjunctive use of locally delivered or systemic antibiotics [5, 6]. Surgical access is usually required. The primary objective of surgical intervention is to allow the surgeon to instrument the implant surface and to perform debridement and decontamination. Decontamination and detoxification of the implant surface can be performed chemically or mechanically. Reported methods include the use of air-power abrasives, lasers, saline wash, ultrasonic use, and the use of chlorhexidine and hydrogen peroxide among others. These are usually combined with flap surgery [4, 7].

Several case report series have shown short- and long-term stability of soft tissue attachment along with radiographic bone fill following surgical procedures that have also included the use of bone regenerative procedures with barrier membranes, bone substitutes, and growth factors, such as enamel matrix derivative or platelet derived growth factors [8, 9]. However, there has been no clear definition in the existing literature on reosseointegration. Simonis et al. [10] conducted a systematic review seeking evidence of reosseointegration after treatment of peri-implantitis on contaminated

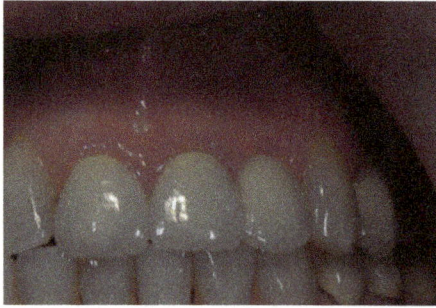

FIGURE 1: Initial presentation of the cantilever bridge in the maxillary anterior region.

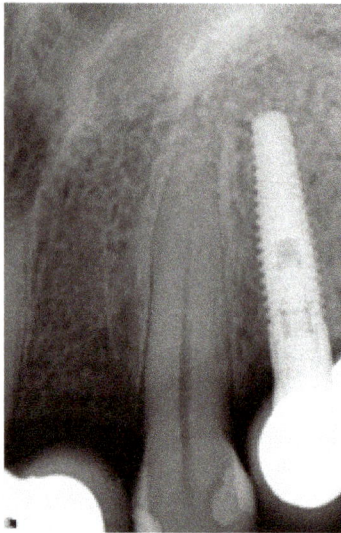

FIGURE 2: Periapical radiograph of the maxillary anterior region.

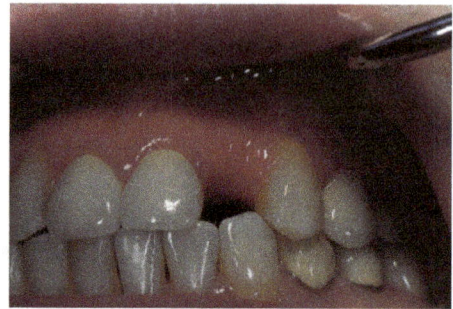

FIGURE 3: Following the sectioning of the cantilever bridge.

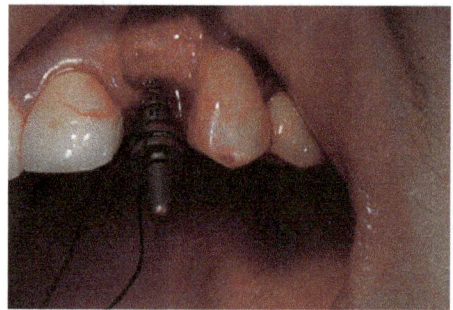

FIGURE 4: Placement of a paralleling pin to check angulation of the implant.

implant surfaces. The authors concluded that reosseointegration is possible on a previously contaminated implant surface. These results were found in experimentally induced peri-implantitis defects following therapy. The amount of reosseointegration varied considerably within and between studies. Implant surface characteristics may influence the degree of reosseointegration. Surface decontamination alone cannot achieve substantial reosseointegration on a previously contaminated implant surface. No method predictably achieved the complete resolution of the peri-implant defect [11]. Esposito indicated in his Cochrane review that there is no reliable evidence suggesting the most effective intervention for treating peri-implantitis [12].

This article discusses two cases of peri-implant bone loss and one case of peri-implantitis. The differentiation in the terms is because in Cases 1 and 2 bone loss around the implant had occurred before the implants were restored. In Case 3, the patient presented with peri-implantitis many years after the implant was placed. The aim of the three case reports is to discuss the treatment of peri-implant bone loss and peri-implantitis to illustrate treatment modalities and to suggest a treatment protocol for surgical regenerative procedures for peri-implant bone loss.

2. Case Reports

Case 1 (Successful Treatment of Peri-Implant Bone Loss). A 48-year-old female, with no significant medical history, presented to the dental office as she was unhappy with her anterior cantilever bridge in the upper anterior region (Figures 1 and 2). Her initial appointment was for a consultation and periodontal exam. Her periodontal findings were normal with only isolated areas of mild gingival inflammation. Following the initial consultation, the patient was referred to a prosthodontist to section the bridge and to fabricate a provisional partial denture and a surgical template for implant placement (Figure 3). The implant was placed using a standard protocol (Figure 4). The implant used was a Straumann Roxolid® implant 3.3 mm in diameter and 10 mm in length. The area was sutured and the patient was given routine postoperative instructions. The patient was prescribed Amoxicillin 500 mg, 21 capsules to take 1 capsule three times a day for 7 days. Pain control included using Ibuprofen 600 mg every 6–8 hours for days 1 and 2 and then as needed after that. Healing appeared to proceed uneventfully (Figures 5 and 6). However, at second-stage surgery, which was done at 3 months following implant placement, vertical bone loss was noted on the mesial and distal aspects of the implant (Figure 7). It was decided to treat the site using the following protocol: the use of titanium curettes to instrument the implant surface and application of ethylenediaminetetraacetic acid (EDTA) twice for 2 minutes. The implant surface was then rinsed with normal saline

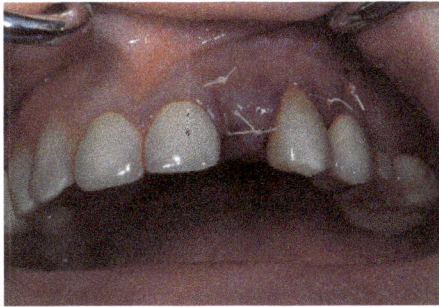

FIGURE 5: Following implant placement and suturing.

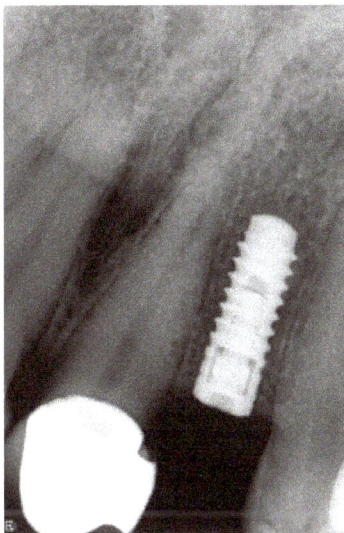

FIGURE 6: Periapical radiograph following implant placement.

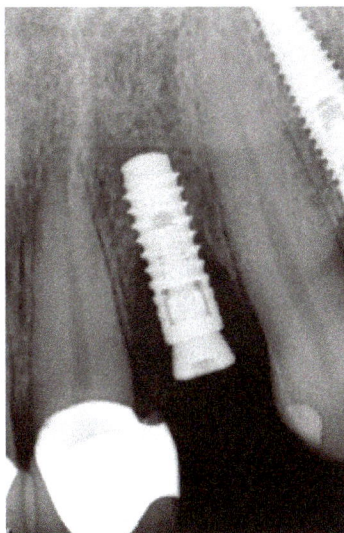

FIGURE 7: Following a healing phase of about 3 months, vertical bone loss around the implant was noted.

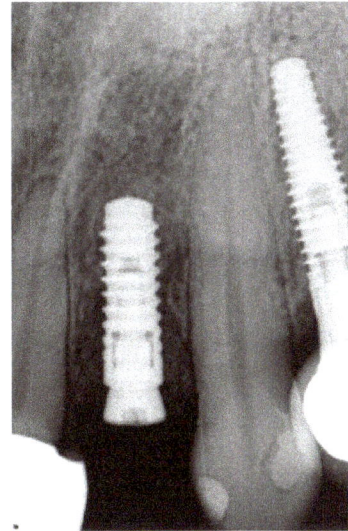

FIGURE 8: Following the treatment of implant site with EDTA, FDBA, and Emdogain®.

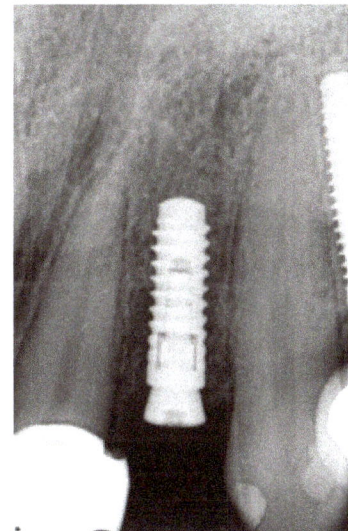

FIGURE 9: PA radiograph 4 months following bone grafting around the implant.

following each application. The site was grafted with freeze-dried bone allograft (FDBA) combined with Emdogain (Figure 8). A similar post-op protocol was followed. Patient called the next day following surgery and indicated that she had fallen at home and hit her lip and that the site of surgery was bleeding. Following another visit, a second dose of antibiotics, Clindamycin 150 mg, 21 caps, 1 capsule three times a day for 7 days, was prescribed. Healing proceeded uneventfully. A periapical radiograph was taken at about 4 months (Figure 9). The patient was referred back to the prosthodontist for the fabrication of a provisional crown (Figures 10 and 11). Following a period of about 4 months, the

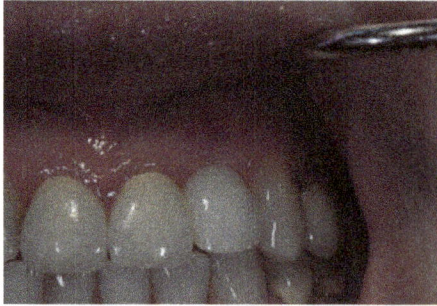

FIGURE 10: Provisional crown on the implant.

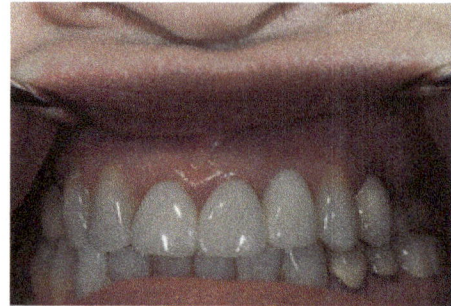

FIGURE 12: Final restoration of the implant in the #10 region.

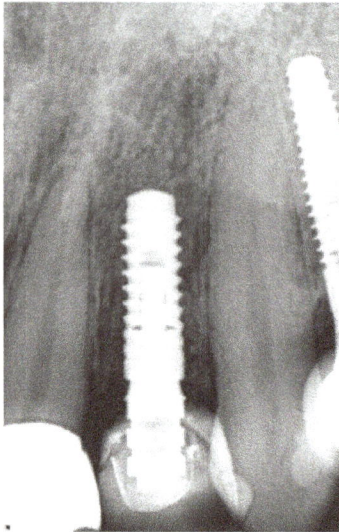

FIGURE 11: PA radiograph of provisional crown.

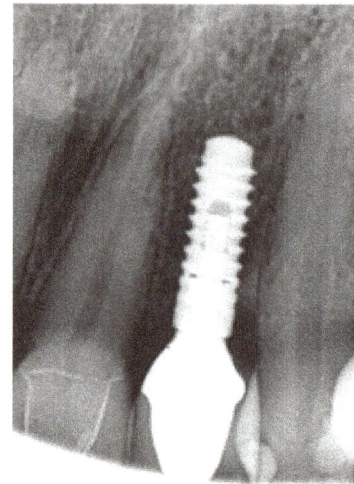

FIGURE 13: One year following implant restoration.

patient had her final restoration fabricated (Figures 12 and 13). She is currently on a 6-month dental prophylaxis schedule.

Case 2 (Successful Treatment of Peri-Implant Bone Loss). A 58-year-old healthy male was referred to the dental clinic to evaluate tooth #18 (Figure 14) which presented with a cracked root and significant interradicular radiolucency. The tooth was deemed to have a "hopeless prognosis." The plan was to extract the tooth and perform "socket grafting" to prepare the site for a future implant supported restoration. The tooth was sectioned and, following extraction, the socket was curetted and then grafted with freeze-dried bone allograft mixed with calcium sulfate. Calcium sulfate was also used as a barrier over the bone graft material (Figure 15). The patient was prescribed Amoxicillin 500 mg, 21 capsules to take 1 capsule three times a day for 7 days. Pain control included using Ibuprofen 600 mg every 6–8 hours for days 1 and 2 and then as needed after that. Following a healing period of four months, a flapless approach was used to place a 4.8 × 8 mm Straumann Roxolid implant in the site (Figure 16). Healing appeared to proceed uneventfully. A similar post-op protocol was followed. However, at second-stage surgery, bone loss was noted around the implant (Figure 17). Just as in Case 1, it was decided to treat the site using the following protocol: the use

of titanium curettes to instrument the implant surface and the application of ethylenediaminetetraacetic acid (EDTA) twice for 2 minutes. The implant surface was then rinsed with normal saline following each application. The site was grafted with freeze-dried bone allograft (FDBA) combined with Emdogain (Figure 18). A similar post-op protocol to what had been done previously was followed. A follow-up radiograph was taken at about 6 months (Figure 19). The patient was then seen by his general dentist and the final crown was fabricated. Healing appeared to be progressing satisfactorily. The crown was fabricated 6 months following surgery to treat peri-implant bone loss. The patient has been followed for one year following the restoration of the implant with satisfactory bone levels being maintained.

Case 3 (Unsuccessful Treatment of Peri-Implantitis). A 50-year-old patient was referred to the dental office to evaluate the peri-implantitis around the implant supported restoration in the #30 region (Figure 20). The implant had been previously placed and restored in a different office in a different state. The patient was not sure how long ago treatment had been completed but reported that it had been at least 5 years since the implant was restored. Patient presented with deep peri-implant probing depths along with presence of

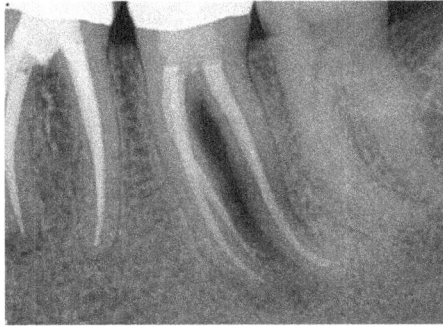

FIGURE 14: Tooth #18 presented with a hopeless prognosis.

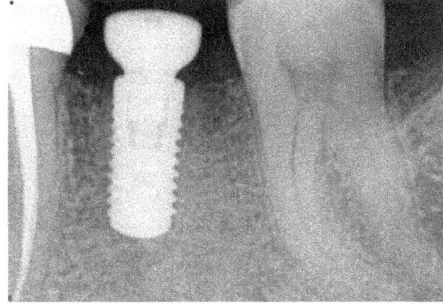

FIGURE 16: Implant was placed at 4 months using a flapless approach.

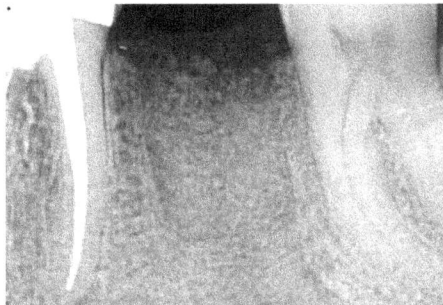

FIGURE 15: Following socket grafting—healing at 3 months.

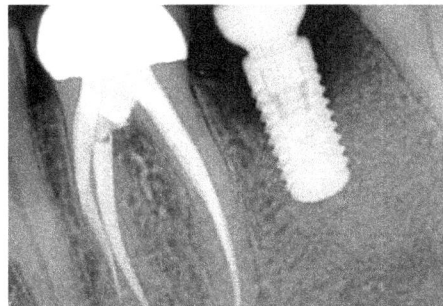

FIGURE 17: Presence of peri-implant bone loss.

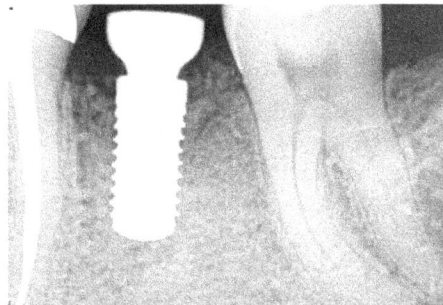

FIGURE 18: Six months following grafting of the site with freeze-dried bone allograft and a resorbable membrane.

exudate that could be expressed when the peri-implant tissues were palpated. The patient did not want to have the implant removed at that time. Initial treatment included a nonsurgical treatment phase that consisted of instrumentation around the implant with an ultrasonic instrument with an implant insert along with a titanium curette followed by subgingival irrigation with chlorhexidine gluconate (0.12%) and the placement of a locally delivered antimicrobial. Minocycline (Arestin®) was placed in the site to help with the healing process. However, the site continued to present with evidence of inflammation. Surgery to access the peri-implant defect was performed 6 months following nonsurgical treatment. The surgical treatment consisted of flap elevation, instrumentation with hand, and ultrasonic instruments, followed by the placement of freeze-dried bone allograft along with platelet-rich plasma. Following early healing, the level of inflammation had reduced. However about 1 year following treatment (Figure 21), there was evidence of increased inflammation along with the presence of some exudate in the site. Nonsurgical treatment was continued and the patient was compliant with keeping his appointments and maintaining his oral hygiene. At each appointment, the patient was counselled to have the implant removed. The patient was reluctant to have the implant removed. However, he finally consented to have the implant removed and the site prepared for a possible future implant supported restoration (Figures 22 and 23). Patient is scheduled to have the procedure done in 2017.

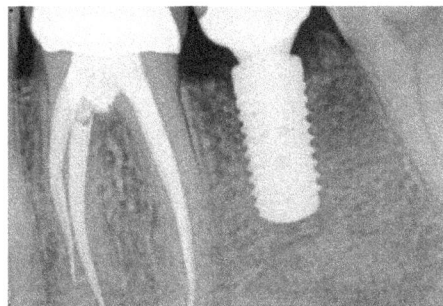

FIGURE 19: The implant was restored following a healing period of 6 months. The patient has been followed for 1 year now.

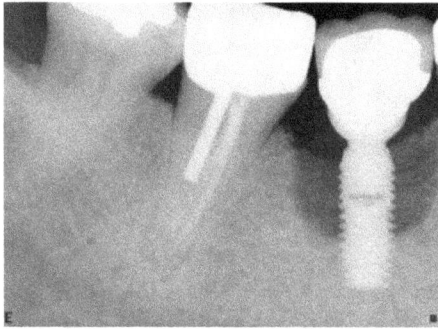

FIGURE 20: Peri-implant bone loss around the implant in the #30 site.

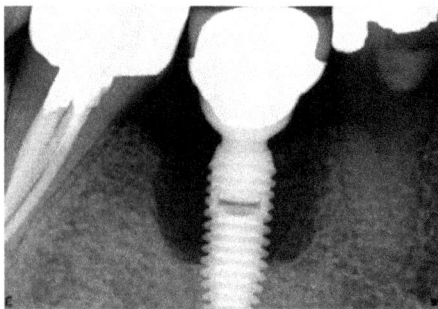

FIGURE 21: One year following treatment. Minimal to no improvement following surgical treatment.

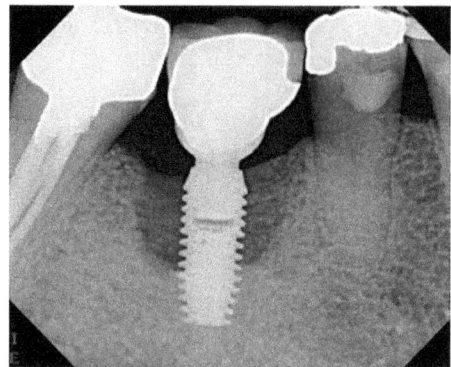

FIGURE 22: Four years following treatment. The site continued to present with inflammation and deep peri-implant probing depths.

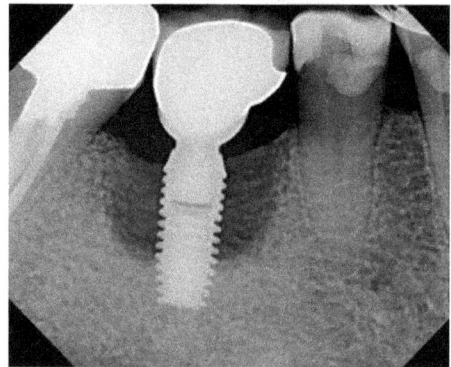

FIGURE 23: Six years following treatment. The patient has finally consented to having the implant removed and the site regrafted and evaluated following healing for possible future implant placement.

3. Discussion

The treatment of peri-implantitis and peri-implant bone loss presents a significant clinical problem facing many clinicians and their patients. The search for predictable treatment protocols is ongoing. Based on the two case reports presented and on the authors experience to date, the use of surface instrumentation of the exposed implants with an ultrasonic instrument using a special insert, combined with the application of EDTA for 2 minutes twice along with the use of Emdogain and freeze-dried bone allograft, has shown positive results.

The major challenge to effectively treating peri-implantitis fundamentally resides in our difficulty of conceptually tying together three equally important determinants that define the success or failure of an implant, that is, "implant survival rate," "implant success rate," and "implant complication rate." Unfortunately, contemporary clinical implant reports tend to heavily stress on the "survival rate" and/or the "success rate" of an implant but very rarely draw attention to the "complication rate" that comes with defining the failure of an implant. This has both good and bad unintended consequences. On the positive side, since both "survival rate" and "success rate" have been shown to be exceptionally high, clinicians are inclined to revolve their entire treatment philosophy around the view that an endosseous implant is the gold standard when it comes to replacing an individual tooth. Yet, on the flip side of the coin, the overreliance of making a treatment decision on the basis of "survival rate" and/or "success rate" *alone* can negatively reinforce the misconceived

assumption that dental implants are infallible. In other words, a dental implant will *never* fail. This notion is far from the truth! And, it becomes even more concerning when one considers that, with the growing number of implants being placed by dentists, there is also a concomitant rise in the number of implant-related complications. Thus, while both "survival rate" and "success rate" are important considerations, the overreliance of building our entire treatment philosophy on these two overarching factors means that we are putting too much weight on the success and/or survivability of the implant, but little on factoring the complications which could have clinically significant consequences on the long-term success and failure of the implant. The importance of the "complication rate" was highlighted in a 10–16-year clinical study which reported the incidence of implant biological complications, namely, peri-implantitis, to be approximately 17% [10]. A similar finding was reported in a recent meta-analysis which revealed a weighted mean prevalence of 22% for peri-implantitis [3]. To put these numbers in perspective, the American Academy of Implant Dentistry (AAID) has reported that approximately 5.5 million implants were placed in the United States in 2006 alone. Thus, using the numbers provided above, it can be inferred that over one million dental implants that were placed ten years ago are at risk of peri-implantitis at present day. This is quite a sobering statistic and, if accurate, is a harbinger of what is to come.

These three case reports are powerful and vivid reminders of the overwhelming destructive consequences of peri-implantitis. At the same time, these case reports illustrate that peri-implantitis—despite being difficult to treat—is still a treatable condition which demands early treatment and early intervention. For instance, Cases 1 and 2 clearly demonstrate that early detection and immediate treatment was critical in arresting peri-implant breakdown and in achieving an optimal regenerative outcome. On the other hand, Case 3 is a prime example of what could possibly happen if surgical intervention is delayed. Over time, the peri-implant infection festers and the prognosis of the implant worsens to the point that any future surgery is for naught. Hence, the common theme from all three cases is that treatment intervention will only have its maximum therapeutic benefits if it is detected early and promptly addressed with appropriate means. Only then can we see an outcome that reverses the effects of peri-implantitis, improves the survivability of the implant, and reduces the risk of complications that could potentially threaten the health of the implant.

Peri-implantitis is a complex multifactorial disease that shares many clinical characteristics and risk factors associated with periodontitis [13, 14]. As such, conventional treatment of peri-implantitis follows along the same lines of surgical treatment of periodontitis. In its most basic form, therapeutic intervention can be subdivided into two phases: (1) the anti-infective phase and (2) the regenerative phase. Similar to treating periodontitis, the primary objective of the anti-infective phase is mechanical decontamination of the implant surface while the primary objective of the regenerative phase is to establish an environment that is conducive to reosseointegration.

From a theoretical standpoint, the rationale for both the anti-infective phase and the regenerative phase has a strong basis. Yet, what remains open to discussion is determining which anti-infective strategy predictably achieves the best therapeutic outcome. Currently, there is no consensus as to which anti-infective strategy is the gold standard. Several conventional anti-infective modalities have been proposed. Mechanical scaling with plastic curettes or titanium curettes and ultrasonic scaling with an implant insert tip are examples of commonly used anti-infective strategies employed to treat peri-implantitis. As shown in the three case reports, the regenerative phase of treatment was preceded by some sort of mechanical debridement and/or ultrasonic debridement of the implant surface. The benefit of employing this type of anti-infective strategy is that it is gentler to the implant surface (less risk of damage to the surface). The limitation, however, is that even with thorough debridement there is no guarantee that the operator can entirely remove the plaque biofilm that has contaminated the implant surface. Furthermore, anti-infective therapy, when done thoroughly and meticulously, can be time-consuming and lead to both patient and operator fatigue. Another recently proposed anti-infective strategy is the use of titanium brushes (Straumann TiBrush™). The titanium brush has a standard dental coupling that fits onto a surgical hand piece while the other side has thin titanium bristles. When activated, the titanium bristles brush the implant surface in a clockwise and counterclockwise manner, thereby sweeping the plaque biofilm away from the implant. The titanium brush appears to be a more efficient means of removing the plaque biofilm when used in conjunction with manual implant scalers. In fact, in a recent preclinical study investigating the *in vivo* effects of the titanium brush on ligature-induced experimental peri-implantitis, it was found that the titanium brush resulted in a statistically significant reduction in inflammation and statistically significant improvement in bony defect fill [15]. While this may be a promising anti-infective strategy, additional studies are required to further support the use of titanium brushes. Other types of anti-infective strategies have been proposed, such as using an air-powder abrasive system with sodium bicarbonate and newer treatment modalities, such as laser therapy and photodynamic therapy. These anti-infective strategies may hold the key to providing results that are superior to conventional therapy. However, like conventional anti-infective strategies, they require further analyses to clarify their impact on halting the devastating consequences of peri-implantitis.

Similar to anti-infective therapy, there is a lack of a gold standard regenerative approach. Current peri-implant regenerative strategies follow along the same path as guided tissue regeneration [7, 10]. Yet, what makes peri-implant regenerative therapy a challenge is the multiple factors that can influence the success or failure of the outcome, namely, surface topography, severity of the peri-implantitis inflammatory lesion, and the therapeutic effectiveness of the type of anti-infective therapy implemented. Ongoing research is being conducted to determine which regenerative protocol offers the best chance in terms of facilitating reosseointegration. But even then, the predictability of a regenerative outcome is predicated on the effectiveness of anti-infective therapy. In all three case reports, the clinician performed exhaustive and thorough surgical debridement of the implant surface. Yet, in spite of the thoroughness of implant debridement, only 2 of the three cases resulted in a successful regenerative outcome. The most plausible explanation would be that anti-infective therapy in Case 3 was inadequate in eliminating the pathogenic plaque biofilm from the roughened implant surfaces. This would suggest that successful treatment of peri-implantitis depends more on the quality of surgical debridement, rather than the selection of a certain type of regenerative material and/or the regenerative technique.

4. Conclusions and Practical Implication

Cases 1 and 2 were examples of patients who presented with evidence of early peri-implant bone loss following implant placement. These patients responded well to the treatment procedures that were aimed at restoring the lost bone tissue. Case 3 was an example of a patient who presented with long-standing inflammation and bone loss. The difference between successful treatment and failure may revolve around the degree of chronicity associated with the bone loss. Early detection and treatment of mucositis, peri-implant bone loss, and peri-implantitis appear to be key factors that determine the prognosis of implant supported restorations. The authors conclude that careful patient selection and experienced clinicians involved with the surgical and restorative phases of treatment combined with regular clinical and radiographic examination around implant supported restorations are the key to long-term clinical and functional success for implant supported restorations.

Competing Interests

The authors declare that there is no conflict of interests regarding the publication of this paper.

References

[1] A.-M. Roos-Jansåker, S. Renvert, and J. Egelberg, "Treatment of peri-implant infections: a literature review," *Journal of Clinical Periodontology*, vol. 30, no. 6, pp. 467–485, 2003.

[2] "Peri-implant mucositis and peri-implantitis: a current understanding of their diagnoses and clinical implications," *Journal of Periodontology*, vol. 84, no. 4, pp. 436–443, 2013.

[3] J. Derks and C. Tomasi, "Peri–implant health and disease. A systematic review of current epidemiology," *Journal of Clinical Periodontology*, vol. 42, supplement 16, pp. S158–S171, 2015.

[4] J. Lindhe and J. Meyle, "Peri-implant diseases: consensus report of the sixth european workshop on periodontology," *Journal of Clinical Periodontology*, vol. 35, no. 8, pp. 282–285, 2008.

[5] S. Renvert, A.-M. Roos-Jansåker, and N. Claffey, "Non-surgical treatment of peri-implant mucositis and peri-implantitis: a literature review," *Journal of Clinical Periodontology*, vol. 35, no. s8, pp. 305–315, 2008.

[6] G. E. Romanos and D. Weitz, "Therapy of peri-implant diseases. Where is the evidence?" *Journal of Evidence-Based Dental Practice*, vol. 12, no. 3, pp. 204–208, 2012.

[7] F. Suarez, A. Monje, P. Galindo-Moreno, and H.-L. Wang, "Implant surface detoxification: a comprehensive review," *Implant Dentistry*, vol. 22, no. 5, pp. 465–473, 2013.

[8] S. J. Froum, S. H. Froum, and P. S. Rosen, "Successful management of peri-implantitis with a regenerative approach: a consecutive series of 51 treated implants with 3- to 7.5-year follow-up," *The International Journal of Periodontics and Restorative Dentistry*, vol. 32, no. 1, pp. 11–20, 2012.

[9] A.-M. Roos-Jansåker, C. Lindahl, G. R. Persson, and S. Renvert, "Long-term stability of surgical bone regenerative procedures of peri-implantitis lesions in a prospective case-control study over 3 years," *Journal of Clinical Periodontology*, vol. 38, no. 6, pp. 590–597, 2011.

[10] P. Simonis, T. Dufour, and H. Tenenbaum, "Long-term implant survival and success: a 10–16-year follow-up of non-submerged dental implants," *Clinical Oral Implants Research*, vol. 21, no. 7, pp. 772–777, 2010.

[11] S. Renvert, I. Polyzois, and R. Maguire, "Re-osseointegration on previously contaminated surfaces: a systematic review," *Clinical Oral Implants Research*, vol. 20, no. 4, pp. 216–227, 2009.

[12] M. Esposito, M. G. Grusovin, and H. V. Worthington, "Treatment of peri-implantitis: what interventions are effective? A Cochrane systematic review," *European Journal of Oral Implantology*, vol. 5, pp. S21–S41, 2012.

[13] L. J. A. Heitz-Mayfield and N. P. Lang, "Comparative biology of chronic and aggressive periodontitis vs. peri-implantitis," *Periodontology 2000*, vol. 53, no. 1, pp. 167–181, 2010.

[14] T. Berglundh, N. U. Zitzmann, and M. Donati, "Are peri-implantitis lesions different from periodontitis lesions?" *Journal of Clinical Periodontology*, vol. 38, no. 11, pp. 188–202, 2011.

[15] C. Carral, F. Muñoz, M. Permuy, A. Liñares, M. Dard, and J. Blanco, "Mechanical and chemical implant decontamination in surgical peri-implantitis treatment: preclinical 'in vivo' study," *Journal of Clinical Periodontology*, vol. 43, no. 8, pp. 694–701, 2016.

9

Nonneoplastic Tongue Swellings of Lymphatic and Lymphocytic Origin

Manar A. Abdul Aziz[1] and Nermin M. Yussif[2]

[1]Oral Pathology Department, Faculty of Oral & Dental Medicine, Cairo University, Cairo, Egypt
[2]National Institute of Laser Enhanced Sciences (NILES), Cairo University, Cairo, Egypt

Correspondence should be addressed to Nermin M. Yussif; dr_nermin_yusuf@yahoo.com

Academic Editor: Giuseppe Alessandro Scardina

Tongue is formed of a mass of muscles and salivary gland embedded in anterior highly vascular and posterior lymphoid stroma and covered by specialized surface epithelium. Growths from all of these heterogonous components may occur resulting in a wide variation in clinical features and behavior, ranging from self-limiting to aggressive lesions. Therefore, surgical excision is the treatment of choice. The aim of the current study is to report three different lesions that came to the Oral Surgery Department in the Faculty of Oral and Dental Medicine, Cairo University. Following clinical and histopathological examination, the diagnosis of reactive lymphoproliferative lesion, cystic lymphoepithelial lesion, and developmental lymphatic vessel malformation was reached.

1. Introduction

Tongue is a unique vital structure that favors great importance to the oral health. It usually appears at the fourth week of fetus intrauterine life. The anterior two-thirds of the tongue is formed by the fusion of both primary pharyngeal arches and tuberculum impar. While the posterior one-third arises from the 2nd, 3rd, and 4th pharyngeal arches [1].

Tongue is a highly vascular and muscular organ that is involved in a mucous sac [1]. This sac is smooth in relation to the ventral surface of the tongue and rough containing variant types of lingual papillae in relation to the dorsal surface. The ventral surface is more vascular than the dorsal one with thin webbed projections (plica fimbriata) arising within the lingual frenum while the dorsal surface is divided by groove into papillary anterior two-thirds and lymphoid posterior one-third. Lymphoid tissue is found in the posterior one-third of the tongue. It is a part of Waldeyer ring [2].

Its nomenclature as a muscular hydrostat arises from its ability to move and to give skeletal support for this motion. These hydrostatic properties are related to the specialized muscle arrays and muscle fibers. Therefore, tongue controls critical function such as speech, taste sensation,

swallowing, and cleansing of the oral cavity. Tongue provides clue and reflection about the systemic condition. If lingual deformation or pathology occurs, these functions become impaired [1]. This developing pathology differs from congenital abnormalities and idiopathic lesions into infections and carcinogenic disorders. Tongue lesions may be short-term or long-term lesions which are classified according to their location, nature, composition, depth, and behavior. They are commonly classified into developmental, reactive, benign, or malignant lesions. The color and consistency differ from one lesion to another (Table 1). Recognition and diagnosis of these lesions require adequate knowledge about the basic anatomy of the tongue, comprehensive examination, and proper history. As a rule, most of the tongue lesions resolve fast as regards the high blood supply unless they have to be biopsied to exclude the malignancies [3, 4].

Lymphangiomas are congenital malformations that are derived from the lymphatic vessels. They are mainly related to the head and neck. There are various theories that explain their origin. They are mainly formed due to defect occurring during embryogenesis. They can be capillary, cavernous, or cystic [6]. Intraoral lymphangiomas are rare and arise mainly in the buccal mucosa, lips, palate, and lateral and

TABLE 1: Different types of tongue swellings adapted from Neville et al. [5].

Tongue swelling	Common site	Nature
Squamous cell papilloma	Tip	Benign neoplasm
Verruca vulgaris	Tip	Reactive
Granular cell tumor	Dorsal surface	Benign neoplasm
Sialithiasis	Ventral surface	Reactive
Salivary gland neoplasms	Anterior two-thirds	Benign and malignant lesion
Irritational fibroma	Lateral side	Reactive
Squamous cell carcinoma	Lateral and ventral surfaces	Malignant neoplasm
Lymphoepithelial cyst	Posterolateral and ventral surfaces	Reactive
Lymphoid hyperplasia	Posterolateral side	Reactive
Lymphoma	Posterior third	Malignant neoplasm
Haemangioma	Anterior two-thirds	Developmental
Lymphangioma	Dorsal surface	Developmental

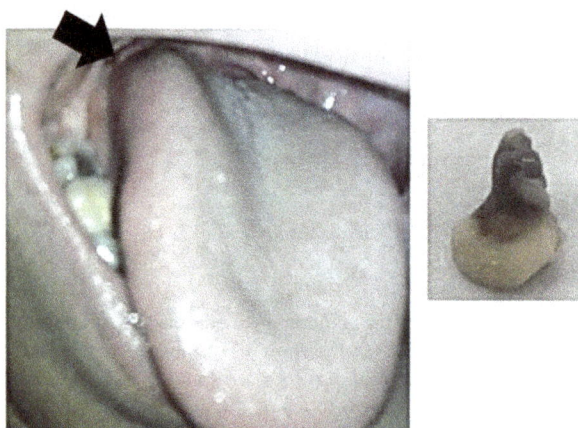

FIGURE 1: Clinical aspect of lymphoepithelial cyst in relation to the right lateral tongue border and macroscopic picture of the submitted biopsy.

posterior surface of the tongue. The main problem caused by such lesions is macroglossia that causes limitation of tongue movement, bleeding on trauma, and sleeping apnea. They may be superficial or deep. Superficial lesions usually appear as a pebbly surface which may affect the surface texture and color. On the other hand, the deep lesions do not exhibit change in the tongue surface or color but cause diffuse enlargement. Depending on their location, size, depth, and accessibility, they can be removed using conventional blade technique, cryotherapy, or laser. Sclerotherapy can also be used with inaccessible lesions [7].

Lymphoepithelial cyst is rare idiopathic intraoral condition. It usually arises in relation to the lateral and ventral surface of the tongue [8, 9]. Although palate is not a common location of this type of cysts, it may arise in relation to palatine tonsils and hard and soft palate. There is no age or sex predilection. It is painless lesion unless traumatized. Its treatment is restricted to the surgical excision [10–12].

Lymphoid hyperplasia is one of the rare lymphoproliferative lesions. Although it has common clinical and histopathological features with oral carcinoma, it is benign in nature. It usually appears as painless malignant-like ulcer [13, 14].

2. Case 1

A fifty-eight-year-old female patient came to the Department of Oral and Maxillofacial Surgery, Faculty of Dental Medicine, Cairo University, complaining of a swelling in the right side of the tongue. The presence of this swelling caused also difficulty in speech and deglutition.

Upon clinical examination, a well-circumscribed pinkish white nodule approximately 1×1 cm in size and round in shape was noted on the right lateral border of posterior third of the tongue (Figure 1). The surface was smooth. Upon palpation, it was soft and nontender.

As a differential diagnosis, fibroma, lymphoid hyperplasia, lymphoepithelial cyst, choristoma, lymphoma, and salivary gland neoplasm were included.

The excisional biopsy was performed at the Oral Surgery Department and the surgical specimen was submitted for microscopic examination in the Department of Oral and Maxillofacial Pathology, Faculty of Dental Medicine, Cairo University. In macroscopic examination, the specimen was received as one mass that appeared rounded in shape of about 1.0×1.2 cm in size with a narrow stump of about 1.0×0.6 cm.

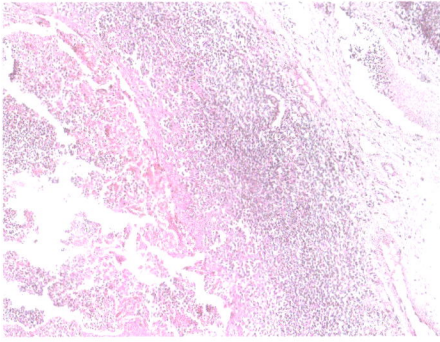

FIGURE 2: Photomicrograph of lymphoepithelial cyst showing cystic cavity lined by keratinized epithelium and filled with desquamated keratin intermixed with lymphocytes (H&E ×100).

The specimen was whitish in color and soft in consistency (Figure 1).

Histopathological examination revealed a cystic cavity lined by orthokeratinized stratified squamous epithelium with uneven thickness. Within the lumen, keratin sloughs interspersed with lymphocytes were observed. The connective tissue wall contained well-demarcated aggregates of lymphocytes. Few germinal centers were detected within the lymphoid tissue. The lesion was covered by keratinized stratified squamous epithelium (Figure 2). Immunohistochemical reaction to CD3 and CD20 showed normal appearance of germinal center excluding the malignant nature of the lesion. The final diagnosis was designated as an oral lymphoepithelial cyst.

3. Case 2

A sixty-year-old female patient came to the Department of Oral and Maxillofacial Surgery, Faculty of Dental Medicine, Cairo University, complaining of bilateral swellings in the tongue. The patient noticed the enlargement of the left side mass.

On clinical examination, well-circumscribed red nodules approximately 1 × 1 cm and 1.5 × 1.25 cm in size were noted on the right and left lateral borders of posterior third of the tongue, respectively (Figure 3). The surface was smooth. Upon palpation, they were soft and nontender. Reactive or hamartomatous lesions were expected.

The excisional biopsy from the left side was removed in Oral Surgery Department and submitted for microscopic examination in the Department of Oral and Maxillofacial Pathology, Faculty of Dental Medicine, Cairo University. In macroscopic examination, the specimen was received as two small pieces of 0.5 × 1 and 0.8 × 1 cm in size, reddish in color, and soft in consistency.

Histopathological examination revealed a hyperplastic lymphatic tissue containing aggregations of lymphocytes that form germinal centers in some areas. The lesion was covered by hyperplastic keratinized stratified squamous epithelium (Figure 3). The final diagnosis was designated as a lymphoid hyperplasia.

4. Case 3

A ten-year-old female patient came to the Department of Oral and Medicine, Faculty of Dental Medicine, Cairo University, complaining of a swelling and multiple red areas on the dorsal surface of the tongue.

On clinical examination, well-circumscribed bluish nodule approximately 1.2 × 1.2 cm in size was noted on the right dorsal surface of the tongue (Figure 4). The surface was smooth. Upon palpation, it was soft and nontender. In addition, four depapillated red areas were detected in dorsal and lateral surfaces of tongue. The lingual mass was excised and submitted for pathological examination. In macroscopic examination, the received specimen was as 1 × 1 cm in size, bluish in color, and soft in consistency.

Histopathological examination revealed numerous variably sized lymphatic vessels, some of which contain coagulated lymph. The lesion was covered by keratinized stratified squamous epithelium (Figure 4). The final diagnosis was designated as a lymphangioma.

Five days later, the healing of the area of surgery was reexamined and the disappearance of red areas was noticed (Figure 4).

5. Discussion

Swellings in the posterior part of the tongue present a diagnostic and therapeutic dilemma due to their different histogenesis, nature, and subsequently behavior. Slowly growing, painless nonulcerative growths are usually benign while presence of pain, bleeding, ulcer, and induration are characteristic for malignancy. However, some overlapping clinical features are encountered. Therefore, biopsy is usually required to differentiate benign lesions from premalignant and malignant lesions [3, 7, 15].

Oral lymphoepithelial cysts (OLC) are rare lesions arising commonly in the floor of the mouth followed by lateral border and ventral surface of the tongue. Few cases were also reported in soft and hard palate, retromolar area, palatoglossal arch, and palatine tonsil [12, 16, 17].

Despite early description of this type of cysts, the pathogenesis is still debatable. Sethi and Patankar have suggested that oral lymphoepithelial cyst is a pseudocyst caused by obstruction in the crypt of tonsil orifice [16], while Bhaskar identified the ectopic glandular epithelium present within lymphoid tissue of oral mucosa, when undergoing cystic changes, as an origin of lymphoepithelial cyst [8].

The LC can occur in any age with the majority of cases being usually diagnosed in the second and third decade with a slight male predilection [11, 12].

As noticed in our case, clinically, OLC appears as a solitary small soft swelling usually with the color similar to that of adjacent mucosa. However, in some cases, it may appear as yellow papule due to the presence of keratin in its lumen, which leads to a creamy or cheesy appearance.

Histopathologically, the OLC reveals a cystic cavity lined by a stratified squamous epithelium with desquamated keratin in the lumen. The connective tissue wall is usually formed of diffuse lymphoid tissue with frequently observed germinal centers. Our case showed all of these features [12].

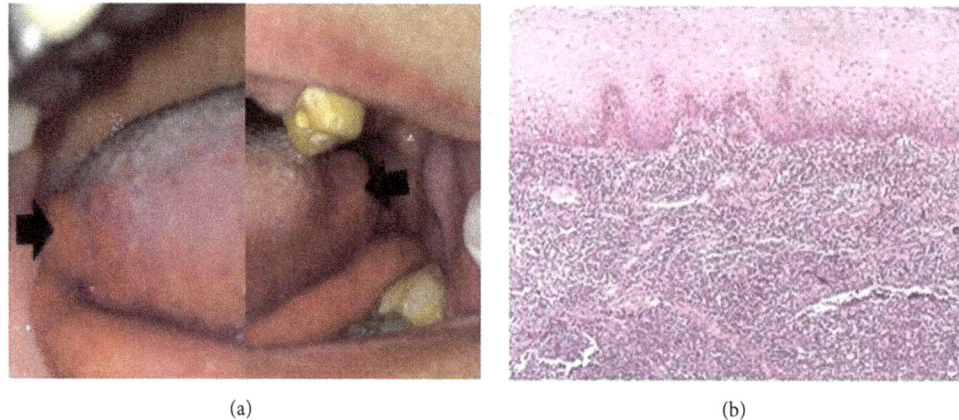

(a)   (b)

FIGURE 3: (a) Clinical aspect of bilateral lymphoid hyperplasia in relation to the posterior part of lateral border of the tongue. (b) Photomicrograph of lymphoid hyperplasia showing lymphocytic proliferation in subepithelial and deep connective tissue (H&E ×100).

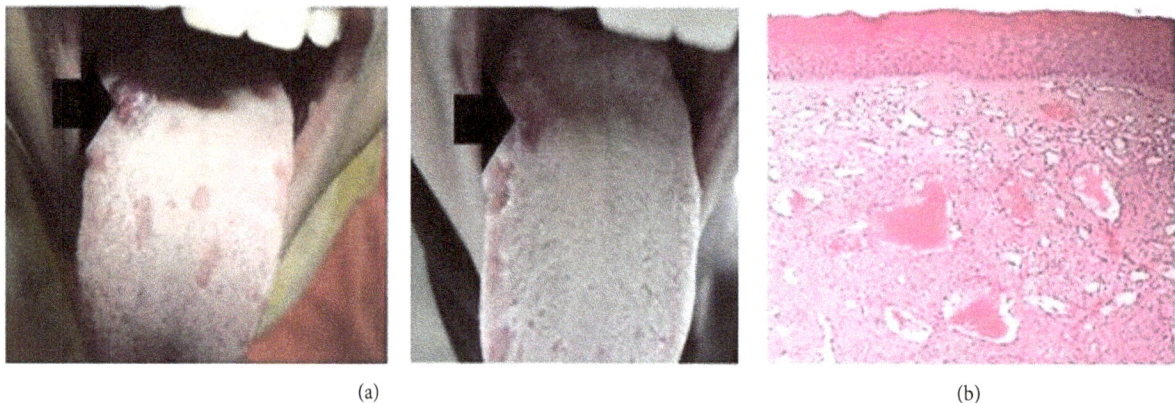

(a)   (b)

FIGURE 4: (a) Pre- and postoperative clinical pictures of lymphangioma in relation to the right posterior area of the dorsal surface of the tongue. (b) Photomicrograph of lymphangioma showing numerous subepithelial lymphatic vessels, some of which contain coagulated lymph (H&E ×100).

Surgical excision is usually done to be examined and exclude the malignant probabilities. Rare recurrence rate was reported with no malignant transformation potentiality [11, 16].

Lymphoid hyperplasia (LH) is an uncommon benign entity related to a rapid proliferation of lymphocytes contained within or outside of lymph nodes. The majority of existing head and neck reports are of hyperplasia in the oral cavity, namely, of the mucosa overlying the hard palate. The exact etiology is not clearly understood, but the reactive nature is strongly suggested [14].

It was called pseudolymphoma due to the great similarity between their clinical and histological pictures [13].

LH affects commonly older female. It may arise as a unilateral, painless, slow-growing, nonulcerated mass. But multifocal lesions were also reported. Histologically, LH is formed of dense lymphoid hyperplasia within the papillary and deep submucosa. Occasionally, germinal centers may also be seen. Absence of cellular monotony and signs of malignancy supports the exclusion of lymphoma [13, 14].

In our case, an old nonsmoker female patient was complaining of slowly growing bilateral swellings in posterior part of lateral borders of the tongue.

Histologically, the examined specimen showed dense lymphoid hyperplasia with few germinal centers covered by hyperplastic stratified squamous epithelium. No signs of malignancy were detected. Both clinical and histological pictures were consistent with previously reported data.

Lymphangiomas are benign, hamartomatous proliferations of lymphatic vessels. They most likely represent developmental malformations that arise from sequestrations of lymphatic tissue that do not communicate normally with the rest of the lymphatic system [18, 19].

They appear in the first few years of life, grow slowly, and sometime resolve spontaneously. They were classified according to the size of lymphatic vessels into lymphangioma simplex (capillary lymphangioma), which consists of small lymphatic capillaries, cavernous lymphangioma, which contains dilated lymphatic vessels, and cystic lymphangioma (cystic hygroma), which exhibits large, macroscopic cystic spaces [19].

However, all of these variants of vessels may be found within the same lesion. Like our case, oral lymphangioma occurs frequently on anterior two-thirds of the tongue with superficial location and pebbly surface. However, deeply located lesions were also reported that cause diffuse swelling, termed macroglossia [18, 19].

Histopathological features of our case revealed small capillary sized lymphatic vessels containing proteinaceous fluid and occasional lymphocytes. These vessels were superficially located just beneath the epithelial surface. The most probable type is capillary lymphangioma.

The other clinical finding noticed in the same patient was the presence of red areas that resolved spontaneously. It met the features of geographic tongue.

Geographic tongue is also known as benign migratory glossitis or erythema migrans. It is benign self-limiting condition of unknown etiology that is characterized by depapillated red areas and requires no treatment except reassurance. Mild sensitivity to hot or spicy foods was reported [3].

6. Conclusion

Histological examination is only safer way to determine the exact nature of the tongue swellings for the selection of appropriate treatment.

Competing Interests

The authors declare that there is no conflict of interests regarding the publication of this paper.

References

[1] R. J. Gilbert, V. J. Napadow, T. A. Gaige, and V. J. Wedeen, "Anatomical basis of lingual hydrostatic deformation," *The Journal of Experimental Biology*, vol. 210, no. 23, pp. 4069–4082, 2007.

[2] M. Can, S. Atalgin, S. Ates, and L. Takci, "Scanning electron microscopic study on the structure of the lingual papillae of the Karacabey Merino sheep," *Eurasian Journal of Veterinary Sciences*, vol. 32, no. 3, 2016.

[3] B. V. Reamy, R. Derby, and C. W. Bunt, "Common tongue conditions in primary care," *American Family Physician*, vol. 81, no. 5, pp. 627–634, 2010.

[4] A. Sunil, J. Kurien, A. Mukunda, A. Basheer, and Deepthi, "Common superficial tongue lesions," *Indian Journal of Clinical Practice*, vol. 23, no. 9, pp. 534–542, 2013.

[5] B. Neville, D. Damm, C. Allen, and J. Bouquot, *Oral and Maxillofacial Pathology*, Elsevier, New York, NY, USA, 3rd edition, 2015.

[6] B. Radhika and A. Lankupalli, "Lesions of lip and tongue," *Journal of Dental and Medical Sciences*, vol. 13, no. 2, pp. 1–5, 2014.

[7] S. Bansal, S. Dhingra, R. Kanojia, and A. Gupta, "Lymphangioma neck presenting as a secondary lesion of the tongue," *Online Journal of Health and Allied Sciences*, vol. 11, no. 1, article 18, 2012.

[8] S. N. Bhaskar, "Lymphoepithelial cysts of the oral cavity: report of twenty-four cases," *Oral Surgery, Oral Medicine, Oral Pathology*, vol. 21, no. 1, pp. 120–128, 1966.

[9] K. M. A. Pereira, C. F. W. Nonaka, P. P. D. A. Santos, A. M. C. De Medeiros, and H. C. Galvão, "Unusual coexistence of oral lymphoepithelial cyst and benign migratory glossitis," *Brazilian Journal of Otorhinolaryngology*, vol. 75, no. 2, p. 318, 2009.

[10] C. M. Flaitz, "Oral lymphoepithelial cyst in a young child," *Pediatric Dentistry*, vol. 22, no. 5, pp. 422–423, 2000.

[11] X. Yang, A. Ow, C.-P. Zhang et al., "Clinical analysis of 120 cases of intraoral lymphoepithelial cyst," *Oral Surgery, Oral Medicine, Oral Pathology and Oral Radiology*, vol. 113, no. 4, pp. 448–452, 2012.

[12] L. M. De Sousa, A. F. M. Albuquerque, P. G. B. Silva et al., "Unusual occurrence of tongue sensorial disorder after conservative surgical treatment of Lymphoepithelial cyst," *Case Reports in Dentistry*, vol. 2015, Article ID 352463, 6 pages, 2015.

[13] S. Carnelio and G. Rodrigues, "Benign lymphoid hyperplasia of the tongue masquerading as carcinoma: case report and literature review," *The Journal of Contemporary Dental Practice*, vol. 6, no. 3, pp. 111–119, 2005.

[14] N. B. Sands and M. Tewfik, "Benign lymphoid hyperplasia of the tongue base causing upper airway obstruction," *Case Reports in Otolaryngology*, vol. 2011, Article ID 625185, 2 pages, 2011.

[15] S. Verghese, V. Rupa, and S. Kurian, "Schwannoma of the base of tongue," *Indian Journal of Otolaryngology and Head and Neck Surgery*, vol. 48, no. 3, pp. 228–229, 1996.

[16] N. Sethi and S. Patankar, "Oral lymphoepithelial cyst: a case report," *International Journal of oral and Maxillofacial Pathology*, vol. 2, no. 4, pp. 80–82, 2011.

[17] A. Saneem, V. Sadesh, K. Velaven, G. R. Sathyanarayanan, J. Roshni, and E. Elavarasi, "Lymphoepithelial cyst of the submandibular gland," *Journal of Pharmacy & Bioallied Sciences*, vol. 6, no. 1, pp. S185–S187, 2014.

[18] S. Kheur, S. Routray, Y. Ingale, and R. Desai, "Lymphangioma of tongue: a rare entity," *Indian IJDA*, vol. 3, no. 3, 2011.

[19] M. Goswami, S. Singh, A. Singh, and S. Gokkulakrishnan, "Lymphangioma of the tongue," *National Journal of Maxillofacial Surgery*, vol. 2, no. 1, pp. 86–88, 2011.

10

Palatal Swelling: A Diagnostic Enigma

Ramalingam Suganya,[1] Narasimhan Malathi,[1] Harikrishnan Thamizhchelvan,[1] Subramaniam Ramkumar,[2] and G. V. V. Giri[2]

[1]*Department of Oral Pathology and Microbiology, Faculty of Dental Sciences, Sri Ramachandra University, Tamil Nadu, India*
[2]*Department of Oral and Maxillofacial Surgery, Faculty of Dental Sciences, Sri Ramachandra University, Tamil Nadu, India*

Correspondence should be addressed to Ramalingam Suganya; drsuganyapavendhan@yahoo.com

Academic Editor: Luis M. J. Gutierrez

Giant cell tumor (GCT) of bone is a giant-cell-rich bony lesion associated with abundant multinucleated osteoclast-type giant cells. It is a primary neoplasm of bone with characteristic clinical, radiological, and pathological features. It is an expansive and lytic lesion without periosteal reaction and prominent peripheral sclerosis. Giant cells are also seen in other diseases like giant cell granuloma of the jaws, traumatic bone cyst, aneurysmal bone cyst, and jaw tumor of hyperparathyroidism. We present a unique case of GCT of palate in a 30-year-old female.

1. Introduction

Giant cell tumor of bone or Osteoclastoma is a benign giant cell tumor characterized by mononuclear cells proliferation intermixed with multinucleated osteoclast-like giant cells. However, because of their unpredictable nature, these lesions are no longer termed as "Benign." The mononuclear cells, although considered to be nonneoplastic and reactive in nature, they are seen in distant lung metastases [1].

2. Case Report

A 30-year-old female patient reported to the Department of Oral Pathology, with a swelling over the left side of the palate. Past history revealed that the patient had initially noticed the swelling 6 weeks ago. She had consulted a private dentist when the swelling was approximately 1.5 × 1.5 cm in size and had no associated symptoms (Figures 1 and 2). She was advised a biopsy, report of which revealed a histopathological diagnosis of Hemangioendothelioma. She then reported to our hospital for management of the same. On taking an elaborate history, difficulty eating and brushing was revealed. On extra oral examination, a firm swelling extending 1 cm from ala of the nose on the left side anteriorly up to 3 cm from the tragus of the left ear posteriorly was noted. On intraoral examination, a massive, solitary proliferative growth measuring 2.5 cm × 3 cm with irregular margins, extending from the left maxillary canine region up to the posterior part of the hard palate, was evident. The lesion was crossing the midline at the midpalatal region. Mucosa over the swelling was erythematous in appearance and the labial, buccal, and palatal sulci were obliterated due to buccopalatal expansion. It appeared that, at this stage, the swelling had increased in size from its initial description. Computed tomography (CT) findings revealed a heterogenous, well-defined, intensely enhancing lesion measuring 3 × 4.1 × 4.3 cm (cc × ap × trans) seen involving the left side of buccal mucosa and hard palate (Figures 3(a) and 3(b)). Laterally, an erosion of alveolar process of maxilla on left side and involvement of levator anguli oris muscle were seen, with no evidence of neovascularity. The H&E section (provided by the previous hospital of consultation) did not reveal a concrete picture of Hemangioendothelioma. An IHC analysis for CD 34 of the incisional biopsy also revealed a negativity for the tumor cells ruling out the provisional diagnosis of Hemangioendothelioma (Figures 4, 5, and 6). Based on the clinical manifestations and investigatory findings, the patient was referred to the Department of Oral and Maxillofacial Surgery for further surgical management. Partial alveolectomy of left maxillary region was planned.

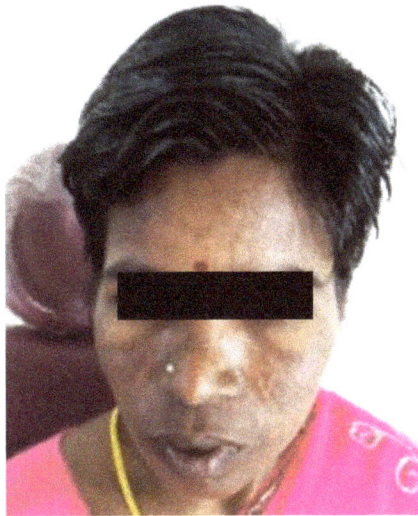

FIGURE 1: Swelling in the left maxillary region.

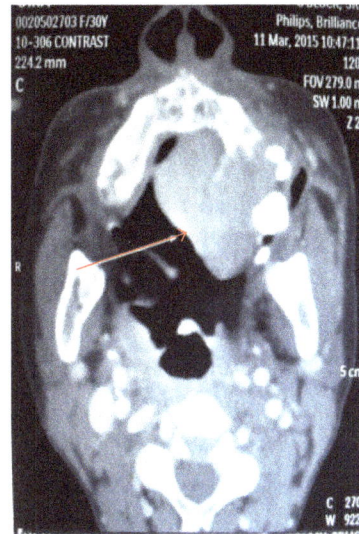

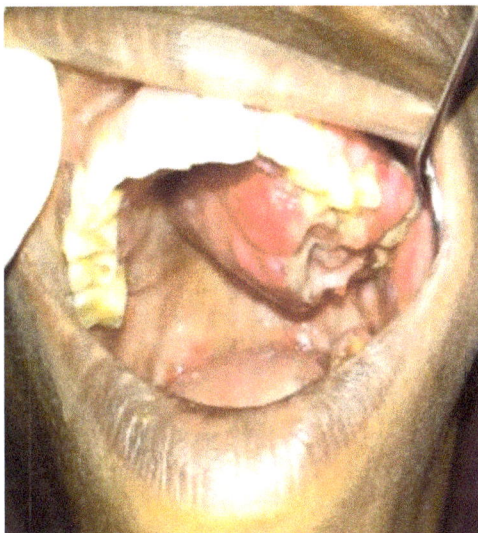

FIGURE 2: Proliferative growth of size 6 cm × 5 cm with irregular margins, extending from the 24 region up to the posterior part of the hard palate crossing the midline.

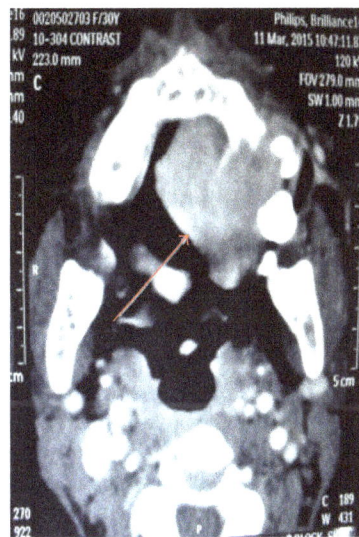

(a)

(b)

FIGURE 3: Heterogenous, well-defined, intensely enhancing lesion measuring 3 × 4.1 × 4.3 cm (cc × ap × trans) seen involving left side of buccal mucosa and the hard palate with displacement of lingual septum to right.

Patient was placed in supine position and GA was administered. Right nasotracheal intubation was done. Considering the angiomatous nature of the lesion in maxilla, prior to Maxillectomy, the ECA was exposed and held for immediate ligation in case of untoward hemorrhage. The surgery was done as two stages: (1) neck and (2) maxilla.

Skin incision was placed on Resting Skin Tension Line on the left side of the neck, followed by layer-by-layer dissection. Weber-Ferguson incision was placed on the left side and layer-by-layer dissection done to locate the left maxillary buttress region. Osteotomy was done at Lefort I level from left pyriform aperture to maxillary tuberosity region. After complete excision of the lesion with adequate clearance, an obturator was placed over a Bismuth Iodide Paraffin Paste

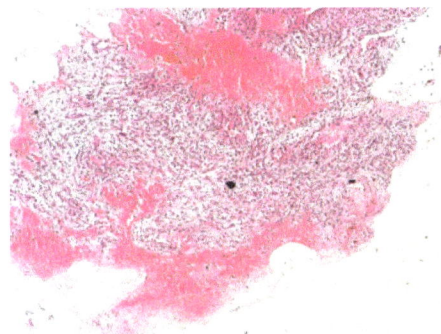

FIGURE 4: H&E 10x view showing vascular stroma with proliferation of spindle cells intermixed with extravasated RBCs.

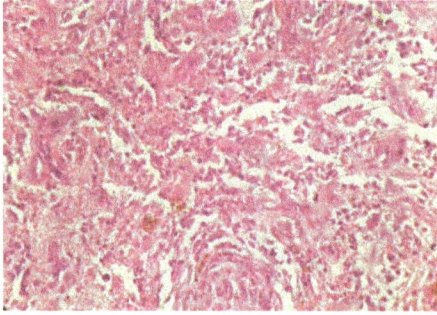

FIGURE 5: H&E 40x view showing anastomosing vascular channels lined by atypical endothelial cells.

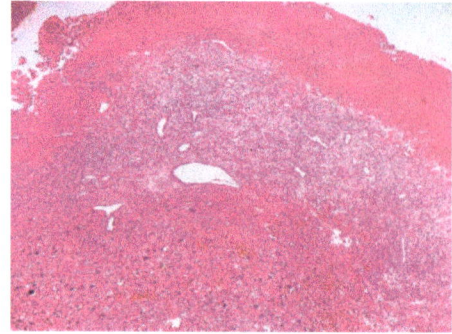

FIGURE 6: Immunohistochemical staining: showing positivity for endothelial cells to CD34 and negativity for tumor cells.

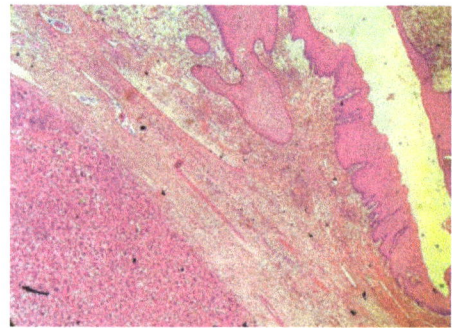

FIGURE 7: H&E 10x view vascular stroma with multinucleated giant cells.

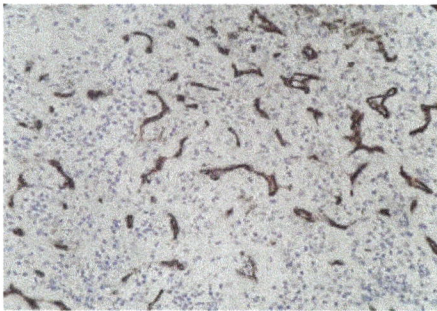

FIGURE 8: H&E 10x view overlying epithelium, connective tissue capsule, neoplastic areas showing proliferation of stromal cells, and multinucleated giant cells.

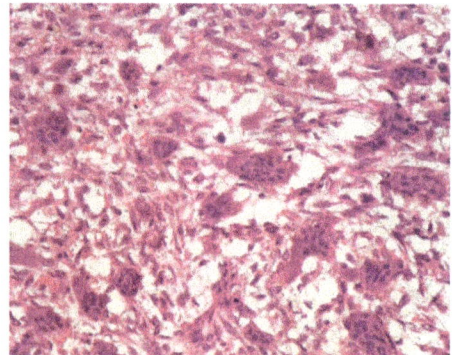

FIGURE 9: H&E 40x view showing multinucleated giant cells with agglomerate of nuclei in the center with a clear cytoplasmic halo.

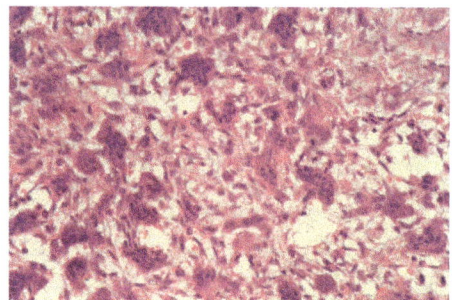

FIGURE 10: H&E 40x view showing cellular pleomorphism and mitotic activity.

pack. The resected tumor was sent for histopathological examination.

Histopathological examination of the soft tissues revealed an encapsulated mass comprising stratified squamous epithelium and underlying richly cellular connective tissue stroma, containing plenty of multinucleated giant cells and dilated blood capillaries. H&E 40x view showed multinucleated giant cells with agglomeration of around 20–40 hyperchromatic nuclei in the center surrounded by clear cytoplasm and pleomorphic proliferating stromal cells. Some of the sections showed the increased vascularity with extravasation of red blood cells. Cellular pleomorphism and mitotic figures with an average of 4 per high power view were also seen which indicates local aggressiveness of this lesion (Figures 7, 8, 9, and 10). The level of serum alkaline phosphate was highly increased (320 U/L) (normal level: 45–129 U/L). A final diagnosis of giant cell tumor was given based on these characteristic findings: the characteristic appearance of proliferating stromal cells, presence of multinucleated giant cells, occurrence of cellular atypia and mitotic activity, CT, and laboratory findings. There was no evidence of recurrence in eleven months of follow-up.

3. Discussion

Giant cell tumor is rare and benign tumor of bone. It occurs in approximately one person per million per year [1]. Histologically, the giant cells are larger with more nuclei and evenly distributed. They may occasionally undergo malignant

TABLE 1: Literature review of previously reported cases of oral cavity with treatment aspects.

S. number	Authors	Year	Gender/age	Site	Follow-up	Recurrence	Treatment
1	Koszel et al. [2]	2011	17 M	Maxillary alveolar process	2 years	No recurrence	Surgical removal
2	Pradhan et al. [3]	2003	19/F	Jaw bones, orbit	Every 6 months	No recurrence	Subciliary, transperiosteal anterior orbitotomy
3	Giri et al. [4]	2015	12/F	Mandible	3 years	No recurrence	Surgical resection
4	Anand et al. [5]	2001	20/M	Hard palate	Eight months	No recurrence	Surgical excision
5	Mishra and Shukia [6]	1999	6/M	Upper alveolus, cheek	3 years	No recurrence	Surgical removal
6	Saha et al. [7]	2012	45/M	Maxilla	—	No recurrence	Partial anterolateral maxillectomy

transformation [8]. It involves head and neck region, proximal tibia, distal femur, proximal humerus, and distal radius. Peak incidence is seen between 20 and 45 years of age [9]. Our case was reported in a 30-year-old female which involves palatal region of maxilla.

Based on clinical features and radiological and histological features, staging classification was initially proposed by Campanacci [10], which is nearly equivalent with the staging system of Enneking et al. [11]. The Enneking classification of GCT of bones is described as Stages I, II, and III and Malignant. Occurrence of obvious hemorrhage and various types of major cells like mononuclear cells of macrophage/monocyte lineage, multinucleated giant cells, and stromal cells are characteristically seen in giant cell tumor of bone [9].

Giant cell tumor of bone causes localised severe intractable epistaxis, proptosis, visual defects, hearing loss, tinnitus, reduced joint mobility, and swelling [12]. In our patient, lesion arising from palatal region of maxilla showed pain, swelling of involved region with oozing of blood, and difficulty in swallowing.

The classic radiological findings of giant cell tumor often reveal a well-circumscribed lytic lesion enclosed by minimal or no sclerosis. Tumors may break through the cortex and invade the adjacent soft tissues. A CT scan of lesion shows soft tissue mass, bony destruction, perforation of cortex, extension toward adjacent anatomic structures, resorption of teeth, and perforation of bundle bone [13]. A CT scan taken in our patient also revealed similar findings.

The appearance of gross findings of GCT of bone is variable. It is generally soft, purple-red to brown, and meaty and may be uniform or variegated in aspect, with small, spongy yellow foci or extensive areas of cystic changes [1]. In our case, grossed specimen demonstrated with blackish brown, soft to firm in consistency.

Metastasis in GCTs ranges from 1 to 6%. Lung is the main site where metastasis usually occurs [9]. Mean interval among the commencement of tumor and recognition of lung metastases is about 4-5 years [14].

The level of serum alkaline phosphate in our case was 320 U/L (normal level: 45–129 U/L). Histochemical and quantitative chemical methods show high levels of alkaline phosphate in relation to osteogenic matrix of giant cell tumor [15].

Giant cells can also be found in certain other giant cell lesions such as central giant cell granuloma, brown tumors of hyperparathyroidism, and aneurysmal bone cysts [12].

Central giant cell granuloma is a proliferative lesion, which is usually seen in young females. Clinically, it appears that destructive lesion, definite loculations and histopathological presence of proliferating spindle-shaped fibroblasts, collagen fibers, deposits of hemosiderin, patchy distribution of multinucleated giant cells, and signs of bleeding into mass are present usually on maxilla followed by mandible, whereas in our case there was no definite loculations noted [16].

Brown tumors of hyperparathyroidism show bone cysts, bone resorption, and generalized osteopenia. The most common sites are ribs, clavicle, pelvic girdle, and mandible. Deposits of hemosiderin and vascularity and presence of hemorrhage are responsible for arriving at a diagnostic terminology as "brown tumor." Histologically, these tumors are characterized by several osteoclast-like multinucleated giant cells interspersed with infiltration of hemorrhage and deposits of hemosiderin [17].

Aneurysmal bone cysts are usually seen in vertebral column and mandible. They consist of blood filled spaces separated by fibrous septa, multinucleated giant cells, and osteoid and presence of hemosiderin and bone formation. Conventional type of ABC shows soft tissue invasion, expansive and rapid growing destructive lesion causing cortical perforation, whereas in our case absence of blood filled spaces and hemosiderin pigments were seen [18].

Treatment of GCT usually consists of intralesional curettage with autograft reconstruction [19] and wide surgical resection and placement of cement, polymethyl methacrylate [9] (Table 1).

Alcohol, hydrogen peroxide, zinc chloride, and phenol are usually applied to the lesional site. Application of hydrogen peroxide raises the infiltration of phenol into adjacent tissues. Low recurrences rate has been related to chemical adjuvants. Embolisation can be achieved by polyvinyl alcohol particles, coils, and gelfoam. Serial embolisation in large cortical effects has reduction in morbidity rate, preserve function, and relieve pain [9].

4. Conclusion

Various bone tumors reveal multinucleated giant cells which often should be differentiated from GCT. Early diagnosis of GCT can be done with evaluation of all the radiographic, biochemical, and histopathological limits. To attain a proper diagnosis, careful histopathological assessment is mandatory. Our case describes the difficulty in diagnosing giant cell tumors from various other lesions with which they contribute to similar behaviour, histopathology, and prognosis.

Competing Interests

The authors declare that there is no conflict of interests regarding the publication of this paper.

References

[1] A. L. Folpe and C. Y. Inwards, *Bone and Soft Tissue Pathology: A Volume in the Foundations in Diagnostic Pathology Series*, Elsevier Health Sciences, 2009.

[2] U. O. Koszel, M. Rahnama, A. Szyszkowska, and M. Lobacz, "Giant cell tumor of the Maxilla—case report and long term follow up results," *Annales Universitatis Mariae Curie Sklodowska Lubin Polonia*, vol. 24, no. 4, 2011.

[3] E. Pradhan, J. K. Shrestha, and P. C. Karmacharya, "An unusual presentation of giant cell tumour (osteoclastoma)," *Kathmandu University Medical Journal*, vol. 1, no. 3, pp. 190–192, 2003.

[4] G. V. V. Giri, G. Sukumaran, C. Ravindran, and M. Narasimman, "Giant cell tumor of the mandible," *Journal of Oral and Maxillofacial Pathology*, vol. 19, no. 1, p. 108, 2015.

[5] T. S. Anand, D. Kumar, S. Kumar, and K. Agarwal, "Giant cell tumor of hard palate," *Indian Journal of Otolaryngology and Head and Neck Surgery*, vol. 53, no. 4, pp. 299–300, 2001.

[6] A. Mishra and G. K. Shukia, "True giant cell tumour of maxilla," *Indian Journal of Otolaryngology and Head & Neck Surgery*, vol. 51, no. 4, pp. 59–62, 1999.

[7] S. Saha, S. Sen, V. Padmini Saha, and S. Pal, "Giant cell tumor of the maxilla," *Philippine Journal of Otolaryngology Head and Neck Surgery*, vol. 27, no. 2, pp. 24–27, 2012.

[8] R. Sarkar, "Pathological and clinical features of primary osseous tumours of the jaw," *Journal of Bone Oncology*, vol. 3, no. 3-4, pp. 90–95, 2014.

[9] A. López-Pousa, J. M. Broto, T. Garrido, and J. Vázquez, "Giant cell tumour of bone: new treatments in development," *Clinical and Translational Oncology*, vol. 17, no. 6, pp. 419–430, 2015.

[10] M. Campanacci, "Giant-cell tumor and chondrosarcomas: grading, treatment and results (studies of 209 and 131 cases)," in *Malignant Bone Tumors*, pp. 257–261, Springer, Berlin, Germany, 1976.

[11] W. F. Enneking, S. S. Spanier, and M. Goodman, "A system for the surgical staging of musculoskeletal sarcoma," *Clinical Orthopaedics and Related Research*, vol. 153, pp. 106–120, 1980.

[12] S. R. Park, S. M. Chung, J.-Y. Lim, and E. C. Choi, "Giant cell tumor of the mandible," *Clinical and Experimental Otorhinolaryngology*, vol. 5, no. 1, pp. 49–52, 2012.

[13] D. W. Kufe, R. E. Pollock, R. R. Weichselbaum et al., Eds., *Holland-Frei Cancer Medicine*, BC Decker, Hamilton, Canada, 6th edition, 2003.

[14] C.-C. Chen, C.-T. Liau, C.-H. Chang, Y.-H. Hsu, and H.-N. Shih, "Giant cell tumors of the bone with pulmonary metastasis," *Orthopedics*, vol. 39, no. 1, pp. e68–e73, 2016.

[15] O. Bodansky, *Biochemistry of Human Cancer*, Elsevier, 2012.

[16] U. H. Uzbek and I. Mushtaq, "Giant cell granuloma of the maxilla," *Journal of Ayub Medical College, Abbottabad*, vol. 19, no. 3, pp. 93–95, 2007.

[17] A. D. Shetty, J. Namitha, and L. James, "Brown tumor of mandible in association with primary hyperparathyroidism: a case report," *Journal of International Oral Health: JIOH*, vol. 7, no. 2, pp. 50–52, 2015.

[18] G. Bharadwaj, N. Singh, A. Gupta, and A. Sajjan, "Giant aneurysmal bone cyst of the mandible: a case report and review of literature," *National Journal of Maxillofacial Surgery*, vol. 4, no. 1, p. 107, 2013.

[19] A. Puri and M. Agarwal, "Treatment of giant cell tumor of bone: current concepts," *Indian Journal of Orthopaedics*, vol. 41, no. 2, pp. 101–108, 2007.

11

Presurgical Cone Beam Computed Tomography Bone Quality Evaluation for Predictable Immediate Implant Placement and Restoration in Esthetic Zone

Corina Marilena Cristache

Faculty of Midwifery and Medical Assisting, "Carol Davila" University of Medicine and Pharmacy,
8 Blvd Eroilor Sanitari, 050474 Bucharest, Romania

Correspondence should be addressed to Corina Marilena Cristache; corinacristache@gmail.com

Academic Editor: Yuk-Kwan Chen

Despite numerous advantages over multislice computed tomography (MSCT), including a lower radiation dose to the patient, shorter acquisition times, affordable cost, and sometimes greater detail with isotropic voxels used in reconstruction, allowing precise measurements, cone beam computed tomography (CBCT) is still controversial regarding bone quality evaluation. This paper presents a brief review of the literature on accuracy and reliability of bone quality assessment with CBCT and a case report with step-by-step predictable treatment planning in esthetic zone, based on CBCT scans which enabled the clinician to evaluate, depending on bone volume and quality, whether immediate restoration with CAD-CAM manufactured temporary crown and flapless surgery may be a treatment option.

1. Introduction

Nowadays, cone beam computed tomography (CBCT) systems replaced multislice computed tomography (MSCT) for dental treatment and planning due to many advantages offered, including a lower radiation dose to the patient, shorter acquisition times [1, 2], affordable cost, better resolution, and sometimes greater details [3, 4]. CBCT uses isotropic voxels and, as a result, measurements are precise and considered 1:1; therefore study models and 3D printing or milling surgical templates can be fabricated with great accuracy [5]. Despite these preference factors, the reliability, consistency, and accuracy of CT numbers derived from CBCT imaging systems in bone quality evaluation remain controversial [6]. Therefore gray values resulting from the CBCT scan are referred to as voxel values (VVs) and not HU. The imprecision of the intensity values of CBCT systems is commonly attributed to differences in characteristics of the devices (kVp, mA, exposure time), the imaging parameters (voxel size), and the position or field of view (FOV) of the area being evaluated [7, 8].

Several studies [6–9] performed on homogenous phantoms and nonhomogenous materials (similar to human tissues) using different CBCT scanners demonstrated linear correlation between CBCT gray scale and HU.

Other studies [10–13] focused on investigating the relation between bone characteristics obtained from CBCT scan and primary stability of the implants found a direct correlation between VVs, insertion torque value (ITV), and implant stability quotient (ISQ).

Moreover, González-García and Monje [14] were the first authors to report that a strong positive correlation was present between radiological bone density (RBD) assessed by CBCT and bone density assessed by micro-CT (considered "gold-standard" for evaluating bone morphology) at the site of dental implants in the native maxillary bones. They also stated that preoperative estimation of density values by CBCT was a reliable tool to objectively determine bone density.

Based on the previous experience by González-García [14], his group also supported later the use of CBCT as preoperative tool for implant treatment planning because it

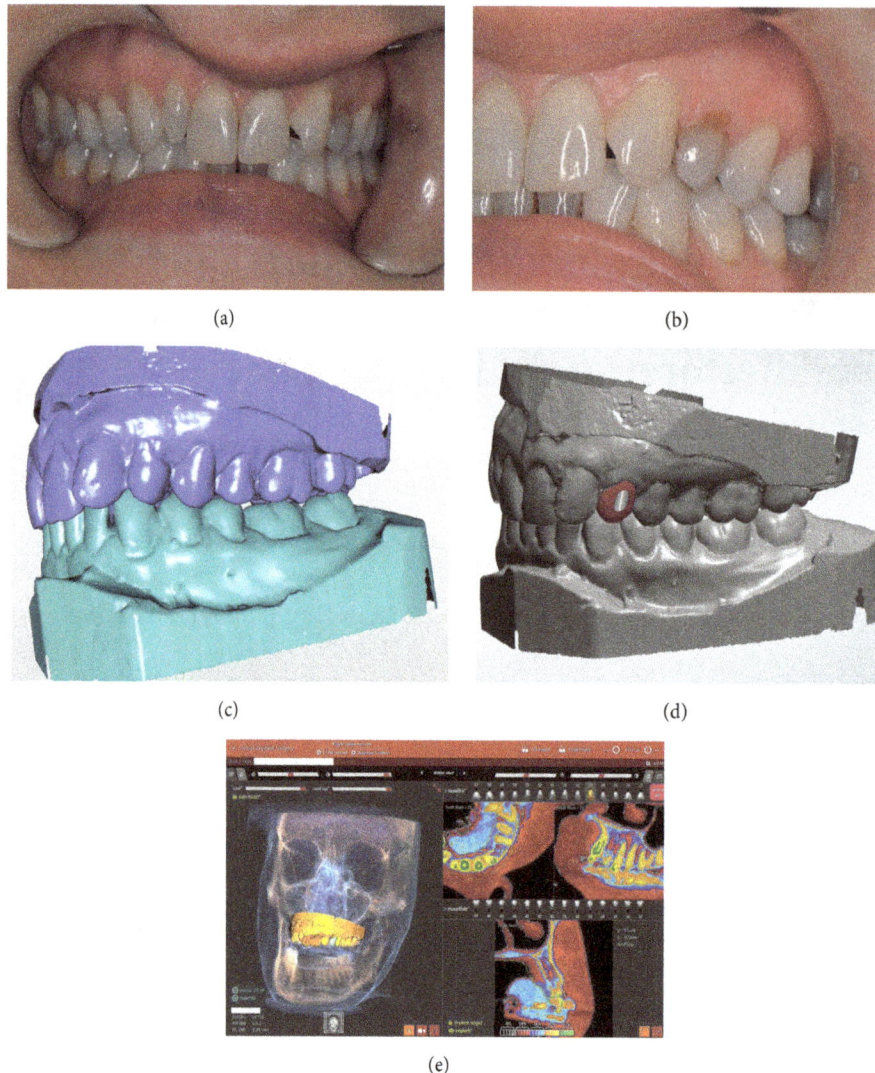

(a)

(b)

(c)

(d)

(e)

FIGURE 1: (a) At the clinical oral examination a retained #63 with complete transposition of #23 is observed. On the right maxillary arch a peg lateral incisor is present. (b) #63 with gingival margin lower than transposed #25. Gingival biotype was determined as being thick. (c) Scanned models in intercuspal position. Distovestibular rotation of transposed #23 is observed. (d) Digital wax-up of the maxillary canine implant crown according to the planned position. (e) Print-screen of the treatment plan. Bone characteristics can be observed and buccal plate can be measured in R2GATE software.

was shown to be reliable to assess atrophic posterior maxilla density and microarchitecture [15].

But the final decision on the safety of immediate loading should be evaluated at the time of surgery upon measuring primary implant stability by ITV and/or ISQ.

The aim of the clinical report presented is to describe a sequence of minimally invasive treatment procedures for predictable immediate placement and restoration of a dental implant replacing a temporary maxillary canine. Decision of immediate implant placement in fresh extraction socket and restoration was based upon an CBCT evaluation of bone characteristics (volume and quality) prior to implant surgery.

2. Case Presentation

A 31-year-old woman was referred by her general dentist to our dental implant department after being evaluated by the orthodontist. The clinical and radiological examination revealed a retained upper left primary canine tooth, agenesis of #22, permanent cusped (#23) in transposition with mesiovestibular rotation. On the contralateral side a peg lateral incisor (#12) was present. Patient's request was replacing #63 with an implant and reproducing its shape with no prior orthodontic treatment. The mid-facial gingival margin of #63 was slightly lower than transposed #23 and that of the contralateral tooth (Figures 1(a) and 1(b)). The gingival tissue surrounding the crown was measured with a periodontal probe and characterized as thick [16]. Interproximal papilla was present and underlying bone level was at 1.5 mm from the margin, based on probing.

There were no medical contraindications, and patient agreed with dental implant treatment and signed the written consent form.

2.1. Treatment Protocol. Alginate and Tropicalgin (Zhermack, Italy) impression of the surgical site and the opposite arch for stone models was taken using standard trays. Maximum intercuspal position was registered with vinyl polysiloxane bite registration material (Regisil, Dentsply, USA). For diagnostic accuracy a radiopaque stent, R2 tray® (Megagen, Korea), was customized on the maxillary arch with non-radiopaque silicon impression material (Speedex, Coltene, Switzerland). A medium volume CBCT using ProMax 3D (Planmeca, Finland) with the characteristics of rotation of 360 degrees, height and diameter of 160 mm and 160 mm, voxel size of 0.3 mm, and the exposure factors of 110 kV and 2 mA was performed.

A series of axially sliced image data were obtained and exported to a personal computer in DICOM (Digital Imaging and Communications in Medicine) format.

Stone models alone, maximum intercuspal position, and R2 tray were scanned using a D 700 3D scanner (3Shape, Denmark) and imported as STL (Standard tessellation language) files (Figure 1(c)).

On the scan models, a virtual wax-up was designed with the use of 3Shape® CAD (Computer Aided Design) software and saved as STL file (Figure 1(d)).

2.2. Matching CT and Models Scan Data. DICOM files obtained from CBCT and STL files were imported in a treatment plan software R2GATE® version 1.0 (Megagen, Korea) and implant insertion was planned according to the final restoration and bone anatomy.

2.3. Treatment Planning. To facilitate bone quality assessment the "Digital Eye" option of R2GATE treatment planning software was used. This option provides automat conversion of CBCT gray scale in 5 basic colors, corresponding to the 256 shades of gray, from the CBCT scan, visible on computer monitors. In figures treatment plan on R2GATE software 1.0 is illustrated (Figure 1(e)).

The temporary screw-retained crown was designed according to the planned position of the implant and was sent as STL file for evaluation by the patient and the restorative team (Figure 1(e)).

2.4. Manufacturing of the Stereolithographic Surgical Template and Temporary Screw-Retained Crown. Surgical template was printed according to the established position of the implant, which was simulated in alveolar bone by the R2GATE software based on the obtained CBCT data, estimated bone quantity and quality, and digital wax-up of the future prosthetic reconstruction. Screw-retained provisional was manufactured according to the planed implant position and delivered before surgery with the computer aided design

and manufacturing (CAD-CAM) surgical template (Figures 2(a) and 2(b)).

2.5. Surgery and Provisional Crown. Atraumatic extraction of the primary canine using periotomes was performed (Figures 2(c) and 2(d)). Care was taken not to damage the labial bone, the socket was irrigated with saline, and the site was examined to verify an intact buccal plate. A 10 mm with 3,5 mm diameter Megagen AnyRidge® (Korea) was inserted flapless, under local anesthesia, according to the planned 3D position with the use of the stereolithographic template (Figure 2(e)).

Insertion drill sequence was recommended by the manufacturer according to the bone characteristics evaluated with the aid of the CBCT in order to acquire maximum bone to implant contact. Torque insertion value was 65N cm resulting in a good primary stability. The space between the inner surface of the labial osseous wall and the labial surface of the implant was filled with resorbable bovine bone graft material (Cerabone, Botiss, Germany). After implant insertion the prefabricated provisional crown was screwed into the implant and occlusal adjustments were performed (Figure 3(a)).

Eight weeks after implant surgery, after uneventful osseointegration, the provisional crown was unscrewed and an excellent healing of dentogingival complex and papilla preservation were observed (Figure 3(b)). Digital impression was performed (Figure 3(c)) and a CAD-CAM zirconia customized abutment and ceramic crown were manufactured according to patient's request (Figure 3(d)).

Patient was very pleased with the final result (Figures 4(a) and 4(b)).

At the annual recall the implant showed no signs of complications nor infection (Figure 4(c)). Clinical assessment of pink esthetic score (PES) [17] and white esthetic score (WES) [18], utilized to objectively evaluate single tooth implant restoration, rated 14/14 and 9/10, respectively, due to minor discrepancies between the two canines (left and right). On the CBCT evaluation no buccal bone resorption was observed after one year of function (Figure 4(d)).

3. Discussions

Primary implant stability is the key factor for immediate restoration and it is obvious that attention should be paid to the local bone quantity and quality during the presurgical planning phase [19].

For bone volume, it is well known that CBCT provides submillimeter isotropic voxels allowing accurate measurements, with minimal magnification and distortion (error less than 0.1 mm) [4], allowing safe dental implant insertion [20, 21].

Bone quality on CBCT, prior to implant placement, even though not being quantifiable in reproducible unit (e.g., HU), can be reliably evaluated by assessing radiographic bone density (RBD) as demonstrated by González-García and his group in both nonatrophic [14] and atrophic maxilla [15]. The authors compared architectural metric parameters, bone volume (BV) and total volume (TV) on micro-CT bone

(a)

(b)

(c)

(d)

(e)

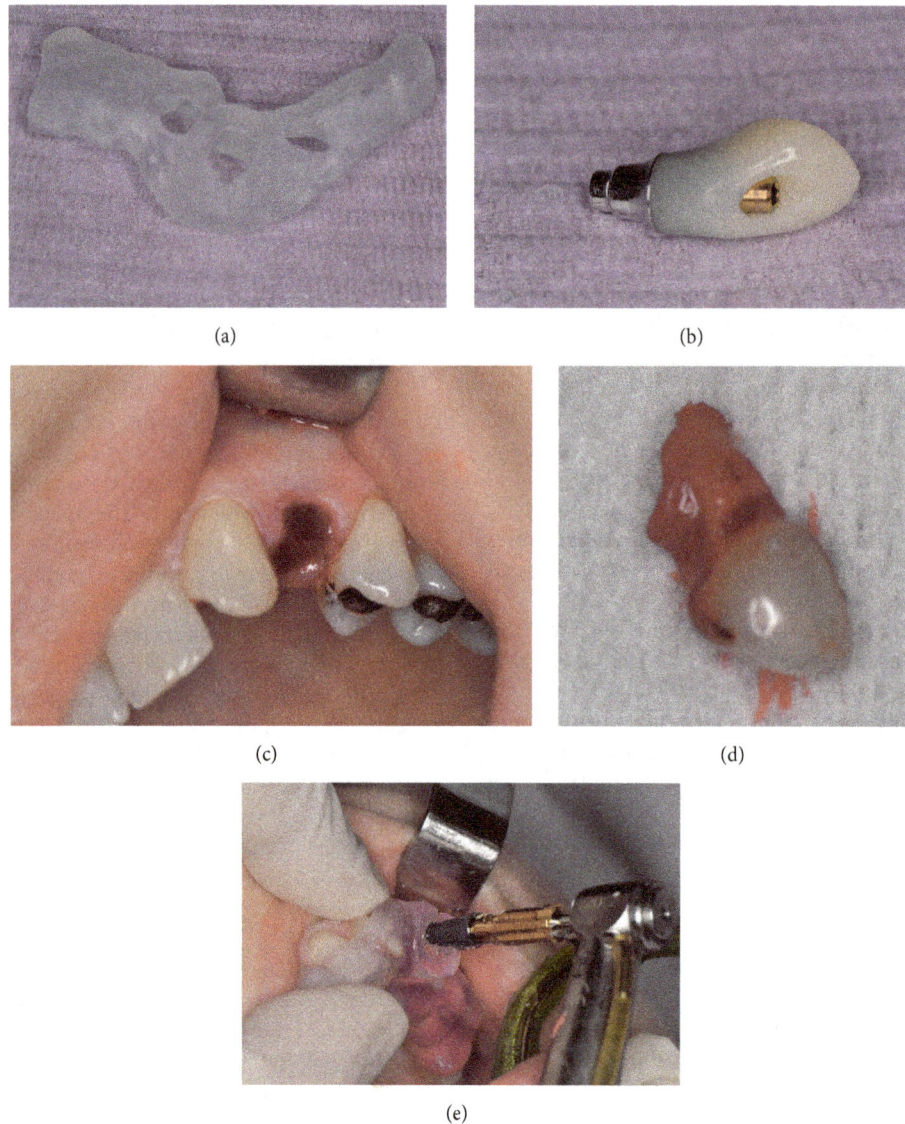

FIGURE 2: (a) 3D printed surgical template. (b) Temporary screw-retained crown manufactured before surgery according to the planned implant position. (c) Atraumatic extraction of #63. (d) #63 after extraction with almost no root resorption. (e) Flapless dental implant insertion utilizing the stereolithographic surgical template.

biopsies at implant sites to radiologic bone density (RBD) measured on CBCT, and found a high positive correlation between RBD and BV/TV ($r = 0.858$) [14]. Moreover, they established, in pristine maxillary bone, some regression equations allowing clinicians to preoperatively estimate the microstructure of the maxillary bone based on a mean bone density value assessed by CBCT [22].

According to González-García and Monje [14], preoperative estimation of density values by CBCT is a reliable tool to objectively determine bone density. Therefore a temporary crown can be manufactured prior to implant insertion to facilitate immediate implant restoration especially for the high requirements in esthetic zone [23].

The implant treatment planning software utilized (R2GATE) allowed the clinician to better evaluate bone quality by using "Digital Eye" option. Due to the fact that the

eye and the monitor display are not able to handle 4096 (2^{12}) shades of gray obtained from a CBCT scan (computer monitor is able to display only 255 shades of gray and human eye can clearly distinguish between 8 and 16 [24]), the R2GATE software automatically converts gray shades, measuring X-ray absorption, in a range of 5 basic colors. Human eye sensitivity is limited for gray shades but is able to distinguish 128 fully saturate hues and with the addition of white light to hue enables discernment of a number of 350.000 shades, 20.000 times more than shades of gray [24, 25].

Intensity transformations are the most commonly used image processing techniques, enabling image data adjustments for better visualization. Therefore a scale has to be mapped to display intensity values that extends from 0 to 255 and the conversion is usually done with a linear function. For

(a)

(b)

(c)

(d)

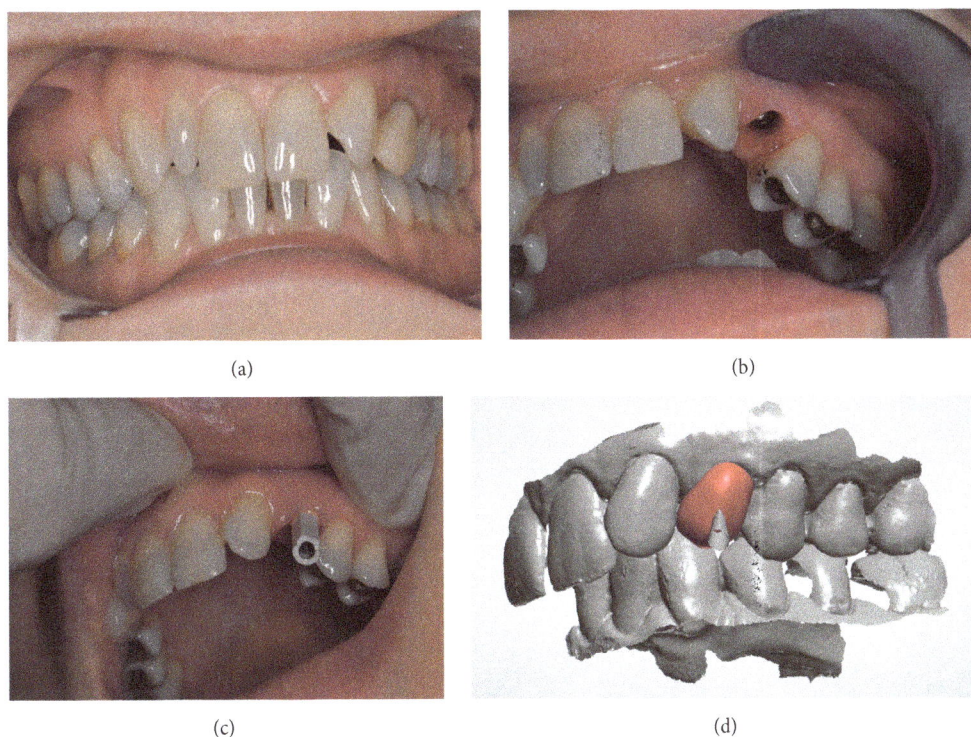

FIGURE 3: (a) Patient after surgery with the temporary crown screwed into the implant. (b) Eight weeks after implant surgery, temporary crown was removed and dentogingival complex was successfully preserved. (c) Digital impression with scannable coping screwed into the implant. (d) Digital wax-up of the final crown.

example, a function to convert the voxel values lying between a lower limit A and an upper limit B to a scale of 255 gray values has a window with $W = B - A$ and a window level (or center) $L = (A + B)/2$. As the window with W decreases, the contrast in the displayed image increases. As the window level (L) moves up (down), the image becomes darker (lighter). This operation is called windowing (leveling) and adjusts brightness and contrast for a better visualization, without changing the original data of the CBCT [26]. Windowing allows a better evaluation of voxel values (VVs) from the CBCT, facilitating predictable treatment planning. R2GATE software, used for treatment planning in the presented case report, allows changing the values of colors displayed on the screen (contrast control) using windowing in order to better visualize the volume of interest, outbalancing the limitations of human eyes and computer monitors.

Moreover, the color-coded bone density assessment enables the clinician to establish an individualized drilling protocol in order to improve dental implant primer stability.

The use of a guided surgical approach through a computerized simulation enables the implant placement to be provided with around 98% accuracy [27, 28]. Guided surgery is advantageous for conventional implant placement, immediate implant placement, and potential immediate provisionalisation.

The advantage of single stage immediate implant placement is more predictable preservation of the peri-implant gingival tissue [29] with less patient discomfort and less treatment time [30].

The criteria and techniques for proper immediate implant placement have previously been established and reported with successful long-term outcomes [31, 32]. Some aspects for treatment's success are mandatory: at least 2 mm of buccal plate to avoid soft and hard tissue recession [33], positioning the implant with sufficient primary stability in the extraction socket [32], without flap elevation, thick gingival biotype if possible [34, 35], ideally 3D positioning of the implant, grafting the gap between the buccal wall and the implant [36], and using a provisional crown immediately after implant insertion for maintaining soft tissue contours [31].

In order to compensate for the expected horizontal bone resorption of the buccal plate, the use of bone substitutes, with a low resorption rate, to fill the gap has been shown to reduce this resorption significantly and therefore their use should be advocated when the esthetic demands are high [37].

Immediate implant placement and restoration not only reduced the number of necessary surgeries but also decreased treatment time and costs and is recommended to be utilized each time local and systemic condition permits [38].

4. Conclusions

This case report presented step by step a straightforward, predictable, treatment planning, based on CBCT scans, which enables the clinician to evaluate whether immediate restoration and flapless surgery may be a treatment option and allows CAD-CAM manufacturing of a temporary crown

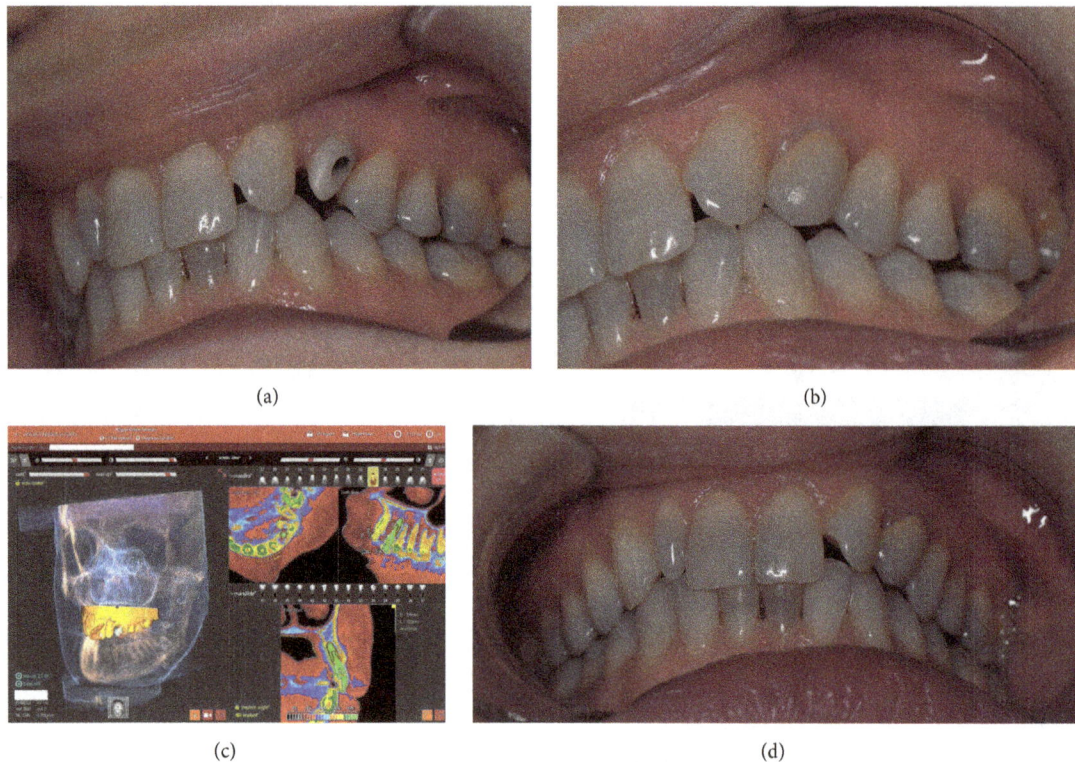

(a)

(b)

(c)

(d)

FIGURE 4: (a) Zirconia customized abutment screwed on the implant. (b) Final full ceramic crown cemented. (c) CBCT at one-year follow-up. No bone resorption was noticed. (d) Final crown at 1-year follow-up. Distal and mesial papilla are present. PES and WES scored 14/14 and 9/10, respectively. WES score is 9 due to nonperfect resemblance of the restored canine. The patient's option was reproducing a canine crown resembling a premolar and not #13.

with adequate subgingival contour in order to preserve soft tissue architecture.

The decision of immediate implant placement and manufacturing provisional crown can rely on CBCT bone quality assessment during the presurgical implant-planning phase [19].

The use of CBCT gray scale automate conversion in 5 colors and the windowing process allows the clinician for a better evaluation of bone characteristics for a precise implant planning and crown fabrication. But final decision on immediate restoration can be taken only at the time of surgery, after objective evaluation of primary implant stability.

Competing Interests

The author declares that she has no competing interests.

References

[1] X. Liang, R. Jacobs, B. Hassan et al., "A comparative evaluation of cone beam computed tomography (CBCT) and multi-slice CT (MSCT) Part I. On subjective image quality," *European Journal of Radiology*, vol. 75, no. 2, pp. 265–269, 2010.

[2] X. Liang, I. Lambrichts, Y. Sun et al., "A comparative evaluation of Cone beam computed tomography (CBCT) and multi-slice CT (MSCT). Part II: on 3D model accuracy," *European Journal of Radiology*, vol. 75, no. 2, pp. 270–274, 2010.

[3] M. Loubele, M. E. Guerrero, R. Jacobs, P. Suetens, and D. Van Steenberghe, "A comparison of jaw dimensional and quality assessments of bone characteristics with cone-beam CT, spiral tomography, and multi-slice spiral CT," *International Journal of Oral and Maxillofacial Implants*, vol. 22, no. 3, pp. 446–454, 2007.

[4] K. Hashimoto, S. Kawashima, M. Araki, K. Iwai, K. Sawada, and Y. Akiyama, "Comparison of image performance between cone-beam computed tomography for dental use and four-row multidetector helical CT," *Journal of Oral Science*, vol. 48, no. 1, pp. 27–34, 2006.

[5] C. E. Misch, *Dental Implant Prosthetics*, Elsevier Health Sciences, 2014.

[6] P. Bujtár, J. Simonovics, G. Zombori et al., "Internal or in-scan validation: a method to assess CBCT and MSCT gray scales using a human cadaver," *Oral Surgery, Oral Medicine, Oral Pathology and Oral Radiology*, vol. 117, no. 6, pp. 768–779, 2014.

[7] T. Razi, M. Niknami, and F. Alavi Ghazani, "Relationship between hounsfield unit in CT scan and gray scale in CBCT," *Journal of Dental Research, Dental Clinics, Dental Prospects*, vol. 8, no. 2, pp. 107–110, 2014.

[8] D. Seriwatanachai, S. Kiattavorncharoen, N. Suriyan, K. Boonsiriseth, and N. Wongsirichat, "Reference and techniques used in alveolar bone classification," *Journal of Interdisciplinary Medicine and Dental Science*, vol. 3, no. 2, article 172, 2015.

[9] M. Cassetta, L. V. Stefanelli, A. Pacifici, L. Pacifici, and E. Barbato, "How accurate is CBCT in measuring bone density?

A comparative CBCT-CT in vitro study," *Clinical Implant Dentistry and Related Research*, vol. 16, no. 4, pp. 471–478, 2014.

[10] M. Á. Fuster-Torres, M. Peñarrocha-Diago, D. Peñarrocha-Oltra, and M. Peñarrocha-Diago, "Relationships between bone density values from cone beam computed tomography, maximum insertion torque, and resonance frequency analysis at implant placement: a pilot study," *The International Journal of Oral & Maxillofacial Implants*, vol. 26, no. 5, pp. 1051–1056, 2011.

[11] K. Isoda, Y. Ayukawa, Y. Tsukiyama, M. Sogo, Y. Matsushita, and K. Koyano, "Relationship between the bone density estimated by cone-beam computed tomography and the primary stability of dental implants," *Clinical Oral Implants Research*, vol. 23, no. 7, pp. 832–836, 2012.

[12] S. Lee, B. Gantes, M. Riggs, and M. Crigger, "Bone density assessments of dental implant sites: 3. Bone quality evaluation during osteotomy and implant placement," *International Journal of Oral and Maxillofacial Implants*, vol. 22, no. 2, pp. 208–212, 2007.

[13] F. Salimov, U. Tatli, M. Kürkçü, M. Akoglan, H. Öztunç, and C. Kurtoglu, "Evaluation of relationship between preoperative bone density values derived from cone beam computed tomography and implant stability parameters: a clinical study," *Clinical Oral Implants Research*, vol. 25, no. 9, pp. 1016–1021, 2014.

[14] R. González-García and F. Monje, "The reliability of cone-beam computed tomography to assess bone density at dental implant recipient sites: a histomorphometric analysis by micro-CT," *Clinical Oral Implants Research*, vol. 24, no. 8, pp. 871–879, 2013.

[15] A. Monje, F. Monje, R. González-García, P. Galindo-Moreno, F. Rodriguez-Salvanes, and H.-L. Wang, "Comparison between microcomputed tomography and cone-beam computed tomography radiologic bone to assess atrophic posterior maxilla density and microarchitecture," *Clinical Oral Implants Research*, vol. 25, no. 6, pp. 723–728, 2014.

[16] J. Y. K. Kan, T. Morimoto, K. Rungcharassaeng, P. Roe, and D. H. Smith, "Gingival biotype assessment in the esthetic zone: visual versus direct measurement," *The International Journal of Periodontics & Restorative Dentistry*, vol. 30, no. 3, pp. 237–243, 2010.

[17] R. Fürhauser, D. Florescu, T. Benesch, R. Haas, G. Mailath, and G. Watzek, "Evaluation of soft tissue around single-tooth implant crowns: the pink esthetic score," *Clinical Oral Implants Research*, vol. 16, no. 6, pp. 639–644, 2005.

[18] U. C. Belser, L. Grütter, F. Vailati, M. M. Bornstein, H.-P. Weber, and D. Buser, "Outcome evaluation of early placed maxillary anterior single-tooth implants using objective esthetic criteria: a cross-sectional, retrospective study in 45 patients with a 2- to 4-year follow-up using pink and white esthetic scores," *Journal of Periodontology*, vol. 80, no. 1, pp. 140–151, 2009.

[19] R. Pauwels, R. Jacobs, S. R. Singer, and M. Mupparapu, "CBCT-based bone quality assessment: are hounsfield units applicable?" *Dentomaxillofacial Radiology*, vol. 44, no. 1, Article ID 20140238, 2015.

[20] R. A. Mischkowski, R. Pulsfort, L. Ritter et al., "Geometric accuracy of a newly developed cone-beam device for maxillofacial imaging," *Oral Surgery, Oral Medicine, Oral Pathology, Oral Radiology and Endodontology*, vol. 104, no. 4, pp. 551–559, 2007.

[21] W. C. Scarfe, Z. Li, W. Aboelmaaty, S. A. Scott, and A. G. Farman, "Maxillofacial cone beam computed tomography: essence, elements and steps to interpretation," *Australian Dental Journal*, vol. 57, supplement 1, pp. 46–60, 2012.

[22] A. Monje, R. González-García, F. Monje et al., "Microarchitectural pattern of pristine maxillary bone," *The International journal of oral & maxillofacial implants*, vol. 30, no. 1, pp. 125–132, 2015.

[23] D. P. Tarnow, J. M. Pérez, S. S. Ghamid et al., "A new technique to identify the location of the mucogingival junction on computer tomographic scans before implant placement," *Implant Dentistry*, vol. 24, no. 3, pp. 338–342, 2015.

[24] F. Dambrosio, D. Amy, and A. Colombo, "B−mode color sonographic images in obstetrics and gynecology: preliminary report," *Ultrasound in Obstetrics and Gynecology*, vol. 6, no. 3, pp. 208–215, 1995.

[25] K. A. Comess, K. W. Beach, T. Hatsukami, D. E. Strandness Jr., and W. Daniel, "Pseudocolor displays in B-mode imaging applied to echocardiography and vascular imaging: an update," *Journal of the American Society of Echocardiography*, vol. 5, no. 1, pp. 13–32, 1992.

[26] C. C. Shaw, *Cone Beam Computed Tomography*, Taylor & Francis, 2014.

[27] M. M. Soares, N. D. A. Harari, E. S. E. Cardoso, M. C. O. Manso, M. B. A. Conz, and G. M. A. Vidigal, "An in vitro model to evaluate the accuracy of guided surgery systems," *The International Journal of Oral & Maxillofacial Implants*, vol. 27, no. 4, pp. 824–831, 2012.

[28] J. Brief, D. Edinger, S. Hassfeld, and G. Eggers, "Accuracy of image-guided implantology," *Clinical Oral Implants Research*, vol. 16, no. 4, pp. 495–501, 2005.

[29] T. De Rouck, K. Collys, I. Wyn, and J. Cosyn, "Instant provisionalization of immediate single-tooth implants is essential to optimize esthetic treatment outcome," *Clinical Oral Implants Research*, vol. 20, no. 6, pp. 566–570, 2009.

[30] D. M. Ravindran, U. Sudhakar, T. Ramakrishnan, and N. Ambalavanan, "The efficacy of flapless implant surgery on soft-tissue profile comparing immediate loading implants to delayed loading implants: a comparative clinical study," *Journal of Indian Society of Periodontology*, vol. 14, no. 4, pp. 245–251, 2010.

[31] D. P. Tarnow, S. J. Chu, M. A. Salama et al., "Flapless postextraction socket implant placement in the esthetic zone: part 1. The effect of bone grafting and/or provisional restoration on facial-palatal ridge dimensional change-a retrospective cohort study," *The International Journal of Periodontics & Restorative Dentistry*, vol. 34, no. 3, pp. 323–331, 2014.

[32] D. Schwartz-Arad and G. Chaushu, "The ways and wherefores of immediate placement of implants into fresh extraction sites: a literature review," *Journal of Periodontology*, vol. 68, no. 10, pp. 915–923, 1997.

[33] U. Grunder, "Crestal ridge width changes when placing implants at the time of tooth extraction with and without soft tissue augmentation after a healing period of 6 months: report of 24 consecutive cases," *The International Journal of Periodontics & Restorative Dentistry*, vol. 31, no. 1, pp. 9–17, 2011.

[34] J. C. Kois and J. Y. Kan, "Predictable peri-implant gingival aesthetics: surgical and prosthodontic rationales," *Practical Procedures & Aesthetic Dentistry*, vol. 13, no. 9, pp. 691–722, 2001.

[35] J. C. Kois, "Predictable single-tooth peri-implant esthetics: five diagnostic keys," *Compendium of Continuing Education in Dentistry*, vol. 25, no. 11, pp. 895–896, 2004.

[36] M. G. Araújo, E. Linder, and J. Lindhe, "Bio-Oss® Collagen in the buccal gap at immediate implants: a 6-month study in the dog," *Clinical Oral Implants Research*, vol. 22, no. 1, pp. 1–8, 2011.

[37] F. Vignoletti and M. Sanz, "Immediate implants at fresh extraction sockets: from myth to reality," *Periodontology 2000*, vol. 66, no. 1, pp. 132–152, 2014.

[38] B. Atalay, B. Öncü, Y. Emes, Ö. Bultan, B. Aybar, and S. Yalçn, "Immediate implant placement without bone grafting: a retrospective study of 110 cases with 5 years of follow-up," *Implant Dentistry*, vol. 22, no. 4, pp. 360–365, 2013.

12

Traumatic Foreign Body into the Face

Maysa Nogueira de Barros Melo,[1] **Lidyane Nunes Pantoja,**[2]
Sara Juliana de Abreu de Vasconcellos,[2] **Viviane Almeida Sarmento,**[1]
and Christiano Sampaio Queiroz[1]

[1]*Federal University of Bahia, Salvador, BA, Brazil*
[2]*Department of Diagnostics and Therapeutics, Dentistry School, The Federal University of Bahia, Araújo Pinho Avenue, No. 62, 40110-150 Canela, Salvador, BA, Brazil*

Correspondence should be addressed to Maysa Nogueira de Barros Melo; maysa.nogueira.melo@gmail.com

Academic Editor: Leandro N. de Souza

This paper describes a case of mouth opening limitation, secondary to a facial trauma by cutting-piercing instrument, whose fragments had not been diagnosed in the immediate posttrauma care. Description of an unusual surgical maneuver and a literature review are presented.

1. Introduction

Punctate and incised/piercing wounds are described as injuries that occur because of perforating and cutting/piercing instruments such as knives and splinters, which violate cutaneous or mucosal barriers [1]. Foreign bodies or their fragments—resulting from fracture of these instruments—although often found in the oral cavity and maxillofacial region [2], are rarely reported in the literature [3].

These lesions may represent a challenging situation for the oral maxillofacial surgeon due to many factors, such as object size, difficult access, and the proximity of the foreign body to vital structures [4].

Occasionally, foreign bodies may remain impacted for some time, causing persistent and distressing symptoms [5]. Some of them may remain in situ for clinical reasons [6] and removing them could bring more harm than benefits. Most of them, however, are removed before the onset of complications, remarkably infection [7].

It is essential to find exactly where the foreign body is located before its removal [4]. It is therefore important to perform imaging examination, as plain radiographs, computed tomography (CT scans), magnetic resonance imaging (MRI),

and ultrasound, depending on the location and composition of the foreign body [8, 9]. These should be recent at the time of surgery, because of the migration risk to adjacent areas [10, 11].

Treatment of punctate and cutting-incised wounds on the face includes suturing, bone fracture reductions and fixation, and, in severe cases, facial reconstruction [12].

This paper describes a case of limited mouth opening, secondary to facial trauma by cutting-incised object (glass), whose fragments had not been diagnosed in the immediate posttrauma care, remaining in the region of the infratemporal fossa. A brief literature review is also presented.

2. Literature Review

Foreign bodies are often found in facial wound but rarely reported in the literature [3]. Some authors believe that the head is the body region most frequently affected by trauma, and facial involvement is very common due to the face exposure [13].

According to Sastry et al. (1995) [14], the lodgment of foreign body in an area like infratemporal fossa is quite rare and only few cases have been reported in the literature so far.

TABLE 1: Indications to remove facial foreign bodies.

Remove	Do not remove
Organic [16]	Inorganic [16]
Freely palpable [16]	Posterior orbit (organic or inorganic) [16]
Anterior orbit (organic or inorganic) [16]	Proximity to vital structures [15]
Reactivity, heavy contamination, or toxicity [17]	Absence of imaging exams [17]
Intra-articular location, persistent pain [17]	Risk of iatrogenic injury [4]
Infection, psychological distress [17]	Absence of symptoms [17]
Impairment of mechanical function [17]	Unknown precise location [17]

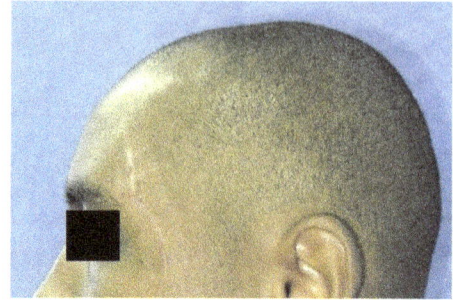

FIGURE 1: Clinical preoperative aspect (scar on the temporal region).

TABLE 2: Facial foreign bodies common sites.

Authors	Region
Perumall et al. 2014 [16]	Intraorbital/mandible/frontal bone
Wulkan et al. 2005 [15]	Infratemporal fossa
Vikram et al. 2012 [17]	Zygomatic
Sajad et al. 2011 [4]	Infratemporal fossa
Moretti et al. 2012 [18]	Periorbital

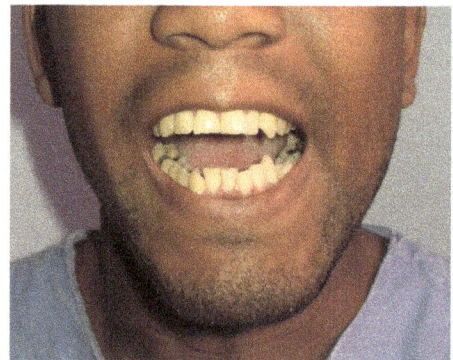

FIGURE 2: Opening mouth limitation.

Wulkan et al. (2005) [15] also report complications associated with the foreign body removing due to its critical structures: excessive hemorrhage, infection, pain, swelling, and trismus.

There are some indications to foreign body removing, listed in Table 1, and foreign body most common sites according to the literature are found in Table 2.

3. Case Report

Male patient, brunette skin, 28 years old, attended the outpatient clinic of the Department of Oral & Maxillofacial Surgery of Santo Antônio Hospital (affiliated to Federal University of Bahia), complaining about progressive mouth opening limitation after assault by a cutting-piercing instrument, 35 days before.

Clinical examination revealed a hypochromic linear scar on the left temporal region, corresponding to the aggression site (Figure 1). Suture was performed in immediate posttrauma care, without imaging exams and the patient did not remember the type of object that stroked him. Unilateral paralysis of the scalp muscle was noticed, configuring frontal branch injury of the seventh cranial nerve pair. No signs of facial fractures were observed. The mouth opening—the main complaint—was restricted, with interincisal distance of approximately 24 mm (Figure 2). When asked about tetanus prophylaxis, the patient said he had been vaccinated in less than a 10-year period.

The computed tomography (CT) scan showed two rectangular hyperdense images: one medially to the zygomatic arch and the other one medially to the mandibular ramus (Figure 3). We removed the foreign bodies under general anesthesia via preauricular access with temporal extension. We chose this access over an approach by the entry scar, because the object fragments were distant from the entrance site.

During the intraoperative exploration, there was difficulty in locating the object fragments. A zygomatic arch ostectomy was made then, after which a colorless fragment of hard consistency and smooth surface—possibly glass—was palpable and carefully removed (Figure 4). Further exploration allowed us to locate and remove the second fragment.

We performed osteosynthesis of the zygomatic arch with two stainless steel wires. Irrigation and aspiration of the operative site with posterior suture of the tissue planes finalized the surgical procedure.

The first postsurgical review followed a week later. Mouth opening had a slight improvement (28 mm of interincisal distance) and CT showed infratemporal fossa without foreign body fragments (Figure 5). Physiotherapy was initiated two weeks after the surgery. Forty-five days after the operation, we observed a mouth opening of 31 mm (Figure 6).

4. Discussion

Punctate and cutting-incised wounds can be considered one of the most devastating attacks because of the emotional consequences and the possibility of deformity [19]. This case exemplifies the deforming character of these lesions, illustrated by the presence of extensive hypertrophic scar in the left temporal region.

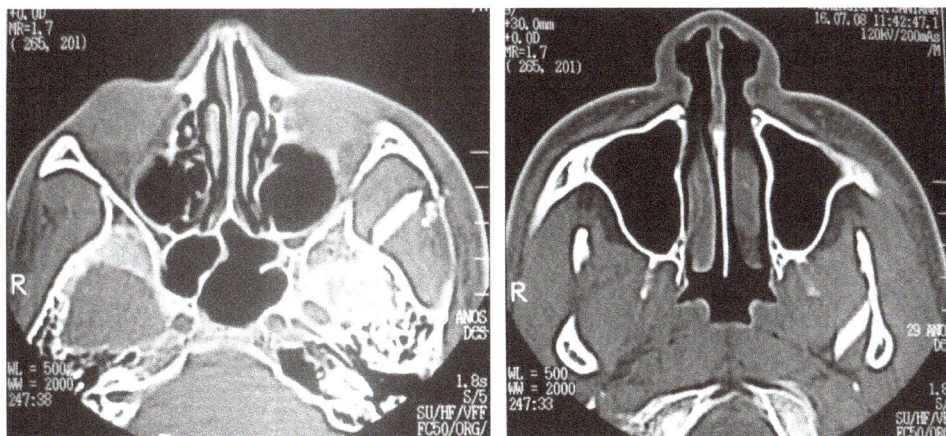

FIGURE 3: Computed tomography scan (hyperdense images medially to left zygomatic arch near to mandibular ramus).

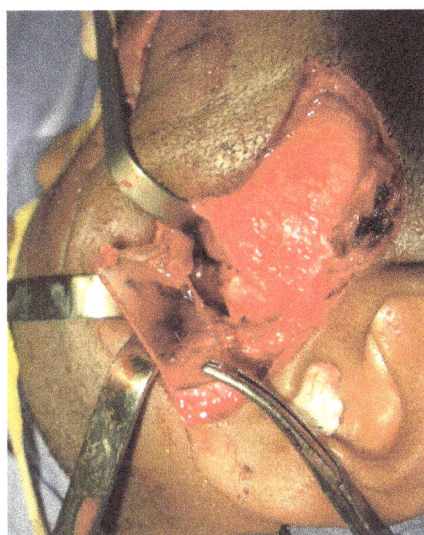

FIGURE 4: First foreign body removal.

That patient belongs to gender and age group (20–39 years) most affected by facial trauma, and the etiology of the trauma that attacked him (interpersonal violence) fits as the most frequent [20].

The prompt removal of foreign bodies from the intimacy of body parts may not occur due to a misdiagnosis or absence of symptoms [7]. That is what happened in the reported case: the glass fragments in the infratemporal fossa were not found in immediate posttrauma care and the patient sought treatment only when he realized the limitation of mouth opening. The delay in treating these cases can lead to definitive limitations or even death [20]. Unlike in more commonly observed cases [9], no infection was found.

As recommended by Shinohara et al. [20], the following steps were made: access, foreign body removal, exploration of the wound, irrigation, and suturing, in addition to certifying about tetanus prophylaxis [21] and use of antimicrobials [16].

Metallic objects and glass splinters as foreign bodies as in this case are more frequent and well tolerated by the body, while organic materials cause more inflammation and

can lead to serious complications [18, 22]. Metal objects are most commonly readily diagnosed by physical examination or conventional imaging studies. Glass fragments, however, may have diagnosis delayed until the appearance of clinical complications such as skin lesions, cellulite [23], or granuloma [24]. Mouth opening limitation was the complication observed in this case. Not performing imaging tests on the patient's initial care was a major factor to the misdiagnosis. Knowing the object that caused the injury is very important to choose the type of imaging test to be requested. Glass fragments would hardly be properly diagnosed by plain radiographs [17].

The limitation of mouth opening after trauma with cutting-piercing instruments is a sign that may suggest infection by *Clostridium tetani* [25, 26]. Thus, the maxillofacial surgeon should consider this possibility if local factors justifying this sign cannot be found. In the reported case, glass fragments were this cause, probably due to fibrosis of the injured musculature, inflammatory reaction to foreign bodies, or even foreign bodies acting as physical barriers to mandible movement.

The treatment of cutting-piercing wound victims with retention of foreign bodies in the maxillofacial region should be often conducted by a multidisciplinary team including maxillofacial surgeons, radiologists, otolaryngologists, ophthalmologists, and vascular surgeons, due to the possibility of profuse bleeding during or after removal of the foreign body [20]. In this case, the surgery was uneventful, but it did require caution in handling the foreign body, since the sharp borders of the glass could cause vessel damage during removal. The chosen approach was closer to the foreign body and avoided esthetical losses on the scar area. The same approach was described by Sajad et al. in 2011 [4] to solve a similar clinical situation. According to Wulkan et al. 2005 [15], little is known about the best strategy for removing foreign bodies in infratemporal regions.

5. Conclusion

Foreign bodies misdiagnosed causes complicated medical problems and sometimes the surgical operations are

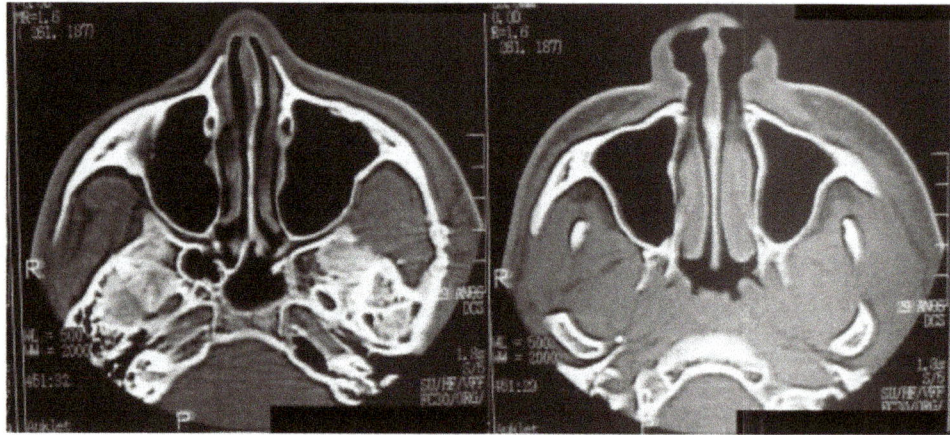

FIGURE 5: Postoperative computed tomography images.

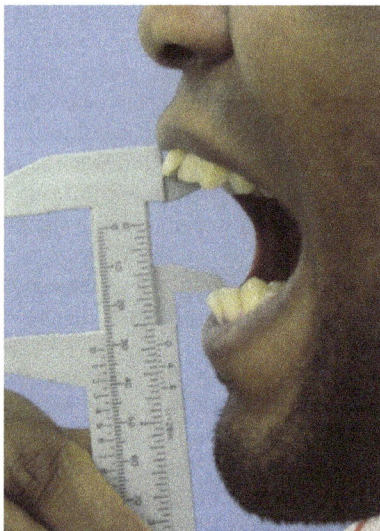

FIGURE 6: Mouth opening at 45th postoperative day.

necessary. When they are in infratemporal fossa—a closed anatomic space that includes neurovascular vital structures—it is important to provide a safe and effective solution, as showed in the reported case.

On trismus complaint cases, they should be included in the differential diagnosis, especially in patients with recent past history of trauma.

Additional Points

Institution/Department to Which the Work Should Be Attributed. Department of Diagnostics and Therapeutics, Dentistry School of the Federal University of Bahia, address: Av. Araújo Pinho, No. 62, Canela, 40110-150 Salvador, Bahia, Brazil.

Competing Interests

The authors guarantee the absence of conflict of interests in this paper.

References

[1] B. A. Ueeck, "Penetrating injuries to the face: delayed versus primary treatment—considerations for delayed treatment," *Journal of Oral and Maxillofacial Surgery*, vol. 65, no. 6, pp. 1209–1214, 2007.

[2] G. Eggers, C. Haag, and S. Hassfeld, "Image-guided removal of foreign bodies," *British Journal of Oral and Maxillofacial Surgery*, vol. 43, no. 5, pp. 404–409, 2005.

[3] W. C. Cavalcante, H. A. Coelho, A. I. T. Neto, L. C. S. Santos, and M. C. Carvalho, "Corpo estranho na intimidade dos ossos da face: relato de caso," *Revista de Cirurgia e Traumatologia Buco-Maxilo-Facial*, vol. 10, no. 1, pp. 97–102, 2010.

[4] M. Sajad, M. A. Kirmani, and A. R. Patigaroo, "Neglected foreign body infratemporal fossa, a typical presentation: a case report," *Indian Journal of Otolaryngology and Head and Neck Surgery*, vol. 63, no. 1, pp. 96–98, 2011.

[5] B. Teng, J. Yang, Q. Feng, Y. Wang, and X. Xin, "Removal of infratemporal fossa foreign body under C-arm," *Journal of Craniofacial Surgery*, vol. 25, no. 4, pp. 1313–1314, 2014.

[6] P.-J. Holmes, J. R. Miller, R. Gutta, and P. J. Louis, "Intraoperative imaging techniques: a guide to retrieval of foreign bodies," *Oral Surgery, Oral Medicine, Oral Pathology, Oral Radiology and Endodontology*, vol. 100, no. 5, pp. 614–618, 2005.

[7] P. D. Robinson, V. Rajayogeswaran, and R. Orr, "Unlikely foreign bodies in unusual facial sites," *British Journal of Oral and Maxillofacial Surgery*, vol. 35, no. 1, pp. 36–39, 1997.

[8] P. R. Gaitonde and A. S. Davies, "Foreign body in the floor of the orbit," *British Journal of Oral and Maxillofacial Surgery*, vol. 38, no. 4, pp. 404–405, 2000.

[9] M. Cameron and B. Phillips, "Snookered! Facial infection secondary to occult foreign body," *International Journal of Oral and Maxillofacial Surgery*, vol. 35, no. 4, pp. 373–375, 2006.

[10] K. S. Oikarinen, T. M. Nieminen, H. Mäkäräinen, and J. Pyhtinen, "Visibility of foreign bodies in soft tissue in plain radiographs, computed tomography, magnetic resonance imaging, and ultrasound: an *in vitro* study," *International Journal of Oral and Maxillofacial Surgery*, vol. 22, no. 2, pp. 119–124, 1993.

[11] M. Krimmel, C. P. Cornelius, S. Stojadinovic, J. Hoffmann, and S. Reinert, "Wooden foreign bodies in facial injury: a radiological pitfall," *International Journal of Oral and Maxillofacial Surgery*, vol. 30, no. 5, pp. 445–447, 2001.

[12] S. M. Chung, H. S. Kim, and E. H. Park, "Migrating pharyngeal foreign bodies: a series of four cases of saw-toothed fish bones," *European Archives of Oto-Rhino-Laryngology*, vol. 265, no. 9, pp. 1125–1129, 2008.

[13] M. A. Cohen and G. Boyes-Varley, "Penetrating injuries to the maxillofacial region," *Journal of Oral and Maxillofacial Surgery*, vol. 44, no. 3, pp. 197–202, 1986.

[14] S. M. Sastry, C. M. Sastry, B. K. Paul, L. Bain, and H. R. Champion, "Leading causes of facial trauma in the major trauma outcome study," *Plastic and Reconstructive Surgery*, vol. 95, no. 1, pp. 196–197, 1995.

[15] M. Wulkan, J. G. Parreira Jr., and D. A. Botter, "Epidemiology of facial trauma," *Revista da Associacao Medica Brasileira*, vol. 51, no. 5, pp. 290–295, 2005.

[16] V. V. Perumall, P. Sellamuthu, R. Harun, and M. S. Zenian, "Posterior intraorbital metallic foreign body: a case discussion," *Medical Journal of Malaysia*, vol. 69, no. 2, pp. 89–91, 2014.

[17] A. Vikram, A. Mowar, and S. Kumar, "Wooden foreign body embedded in the zygomatic region for 2 years," *Journal of Maxillofacial and Oral Surgery*, vol. 11, no. 1, pp. 96–100, 2012.

[18] A. Moretti, M. Laus, D. Crescenzi, and A. Croce, "Peri-orbital foreign body: a case report," *Journal of Medical Case Reports*, vol. 6, article 91, 2012.

[19] K. Takaoka, S. Hashitani, Y. Toyohara, K. Noguchi, and M. Urade, "Migration of a foreign body (staple) from the oral floor to the submandibular space: case report," *British Journal of Oral and Maxillofacial Surgery*, vol. 48, no. 2, pp. 145–146, 2010.

[20] E. H. Shinohara, L. Heringer, and J.P. J. De Carvalho, "Impacted knife injuries in the maxillofacial region: report of 2 cases," *Journal of Oral and Maxillofacial Surgery*, vol. 59, no. 10, pp. 1221–1223, 2001.

[21] M. Alves, E. Canoui, L. Deforges et al., "An unexpected trismus," *The Lancet*, vol. 380, no. 9840, p. 536, 2012.

[22] F. H. Casanova, P. A. Mello Filho, D. M. Nakanami, and P. G. Manso, "Corpo estranho orgânico intra-orbitário: avaliação tomográfica e conduta," *Arquivos Brasileiros de Oftalmologia*, vol. 64, no. 4, pp. 297–301, 2001.

[23] J. D. Bullock, R. E. Warwar, G. B. Bartley, R. R. Waller, and J. W. Henderson, "Unusual orbital foreign bodies," *Ophthalmic Plastic and Reconstructive Surgery*, vol. 15, no. 1, pp. 44–51, 1999.

[24] V. Á. S. Silveira, E. D. Do Carmo, C. E. Dias Colombo, A. S. R. Caval-cante, and Y. R. Carvalho, "Intraosseous foreign-body granuloma in the mandible subsequent to a 20-year-old work-related accident," *Medicina Oral, Patologia Oral y Cirugia Bucal*, vol. 13, no. 10, pp. E657–E660, 2008.

[25] A. W. Paterson, W. Ryan, and V. V. Rao-Mudigonda, "Trismus: or is it tetanus? A report of a case," *Oral Surgery, Oral Medicine, Oral Pathology, Oral Radiology and Endodontology*, vol. 101, no. 4, pp. 437–441, 2006.

[26] A. Van Driessche, B. Janssens, Y. Coppens, C. Bachmann, and J. Donck, "Tetanus: a diagnostic challenge in the western world," *Acta Clinica Belgica*, vol. 68, no. 6, pp. 416–420, 2013.

13

The Diagnosis and Treatment of Multiple Factitious Oral Ulcers in a 6-Year-Old Boy

Priscilla Santana Pinto Gonçalves,[1] Daniela Alejandra Cusicanqui Mendez,[1] Paulo Sérgio da Silva Santos,[2] José Humberto Damante,[2] Daniela Rios,[1] and Thiago Cruvinel[1]

[1]*Department of Pediatric Dentistry, Orthodontics and Public Health, Bauru School of Dentistry, University of São Paulo, Bauru, SP, Brazil*

[2]*Department of Surgery, Stomatology, Pathology and Radiology, Bauru School of Dentistry, University of São Paulo, Bauru, SP, Brazil*

Correspondence should be addressed to Thiago Cruvinel; thiagocruvinel@fob.usp.br

Academic Editor: Samir Nammour

Factitious ulcers are characterized by self-inflicted lesions with multifactorial origin. These lesions are frequently found in head, neck, and hands. This report shows a 6-year-old boy diagnosed with factitious oral ulcers that occurred after the self-biting of buccal vestibule and nail-scratching of gingival tissue. Clinically, a significant swelling was observed, hard on palpation, located at the right lower third of the face, next to the posterior area of the mandible. In the intraoral examination, ulcers at different healing stages were noted on the swelling area. During the anamnesis, the father reported a change in his familial structure that triggers psychological stress, providing the clues to the presumptive diagnosis of factitious oral ulcers. We prescribed the topical use of Gingilone® three times a day to control the local pain and inflammation. At 7-day follow-up, we noticed the reduction of extraoral swelling and the initial healing of the ulcers. The presumptive diagnosis was confirmed at 30-day follow-up, with the lasting remission of oral lesions. The treatments of factitious oral ulcers should be individually tailored for each patient, focused on a multidisciplinary approach, including psychotherapy and periodic clinical control. To the best of our knowledge, gaps of evidence lead to the lack of standardized clinical protocols on this issue.

1. Introduction

The factitious ulcers are characterized by self-inflicted lesions related to multifactorial origin, such as accidents and/or chronic habits [1]. Such lesions are frequently located on head, neck, and hands [2]; the dentists can easily detect factitious oral ulcers in their daily clinical routine [1, 3].

People more susceptible to develop factitious ulcer include individuals with syndromes, insensitivity to congenital pain, intellectual disability, autism, or schizophrenia, besides children from unstructured families, homeless people, drug addicts, and sexual abuse victims [2, 4, 5]. The individuals with emotional or psychological disturbances may develop masochistic attitudes towards self-harm [1, 3, 4], with the purpose of seeking their family attention [4].

The factitious ulcers in nonsyndromic individuals are either intentional (functional) or unintentional (organic) [2]. The intentional self-harm occurs in individuals with psychological/emotional disturbances who seek help or attention [2]. The unintentional self-harm appears during stressful situations related to chronic deleterious habits, such as bruxism, thumb, or lip sucking, and the *morsicatio buccarum* [6]. These habits begin from an initial accidental injury that continues to damage, not allowing the natural healing of lesion [6, 7].

The prevalence of factitious ulcers among nonsyndromic individuals seems to be higher among children, teenagers, and young people (17 to 38%) compared to adults (4%) [2]. Also, females are more prone to have self-harm episodes [8]. The ulcers are located in any anatomic structure of oral

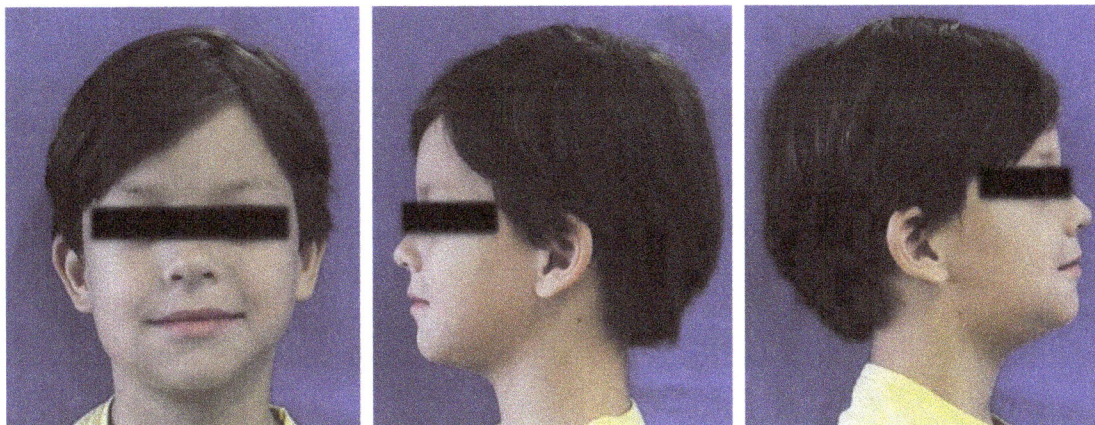

FIGURE 1: The initial clinical aspect of the child. Note the presence of swelling on the right lower third of the face.

cavity [6]. Nevertheless, the lower lip and the tongue are most affected by biting [2]. The treatments vary according to the lesion severity and the frequency of the self-harm act, being based on psychological, pharmacological, and physical restrain and, in severe cases, dental extraction of the teeth near the injury [9].

This report shows a singular clinical case of factitious oral ulcers in a 6-year-old boy without systemic disease.

2. Case Presentation

A 6-year-old boy accompanied by his father came to the Clinics of Pediatric Dentistry and Stomatology of the Bauru School of Dentistry, University of São Paulo (FOB-USP). The father previously signed the free consent form, authorizing the treatment and the publication of this case. During the anamnesis, the father reported that they first sought a doctor suspecting of parotiditis that was not confirmed. The doctor referred the child to the dentist. Then, the father reported his concern with an abnormal tumescence that appeared in the right side of the boy's face two days ago. This lesion was associated with pain on palpation. Other relevant clinical findings were the allergy to insect bites and tonsillectomy performed eight months ago. The boy was not under medical treatment or medication use.

The extraoral clinical examination revealed that the patient had a significant swelling, hard on palpation, in the right lower third of the face, next to the posterior area of the mandible's body (Figure 1). In the intraoral examination, we noted a dental caries lesion on the left second primary molar (#75). Notwithstanding, either other alterations in hard and soft tissues or premature occlusal contacts were not found at the right side of the mandibular arch (Figures 2 and 3). The oral mucosa located on the swelling area had ulcers at different healing stages (Figure 4). The boy affirmed that he did not remember when the lesions had started, reporting pain only on palpation. The analysis of an orthopantomography confirmed no bone or tooth alterations that could justify the swelling.

During the session, the boy was very quiet and cooperative, demonstrating his shy behavior. In the anamnesis, the

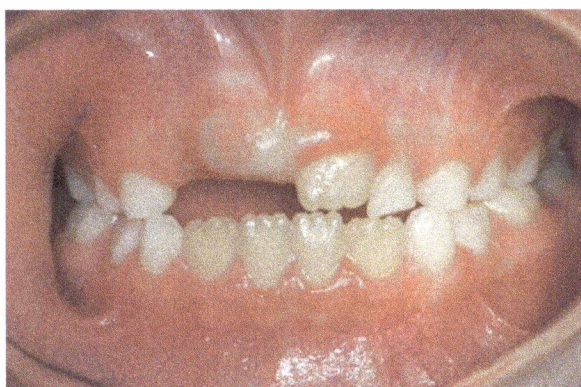

FIGURE 2: Frontal clinical view of the maxillary and mandibular arches.

father reported two significant facts: (1) a recent change in his familial structure, when his daughter left home after her marriage; (2) the very close relationship between his children. At that moment, we suggested the hypothesis of self-harm for attention, which led to the presumptive diagnosis of factitious oral ulcers. The lesions were probably produced by self-biting of buccal vestibule and nail-scratching of gingival tissue. These hypotheses were supported by additional reports, describing the boy's habit of introducing his fingers into the mouth, in the same side where the ulcers were observed.

We established the treatment for pain and inflammation control, by the topical application of Gingilone ointment (hydrocortisone acetate 5.0 mg/g, neomycin sulfate 5.0 mg/g, troxerutin 20.0 mg/g, ascorbic acid 0.50 mg/g, and benzocaine 2.0 mg/g, Cosmed Indústria de Cosméticos e Medicamentos S.A., Tamboré, Barueri, São Paulo, Brazil) on the ulcers, in the regime of three times a day for one week. After that, the patient was advised to return periodically until a conclusive diagnosis.

At 7-day follow-up appointment, we observed the swelling regression during the extraoral examination. The intraoral examination revealed the initial healing of the ulcers. At 30-day follow-up appointment, we observed the total

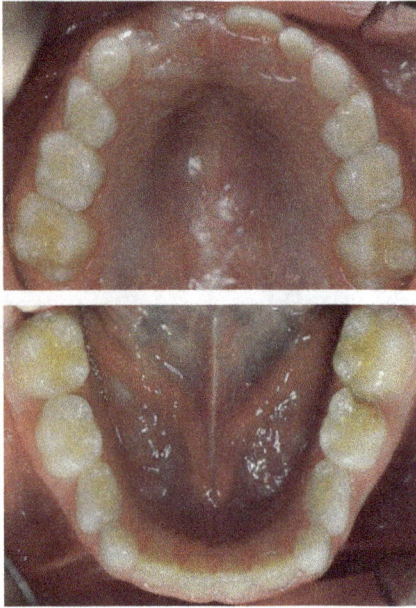

FIGURE 3: Maxillary and mandibular occlusal views. Note the presence of a dental caries lesion developed on the hypomineralized distal-occlusal surface of tooth #75. There is no evidence of clinical alterations in the right mandibular teeth and mucosa.

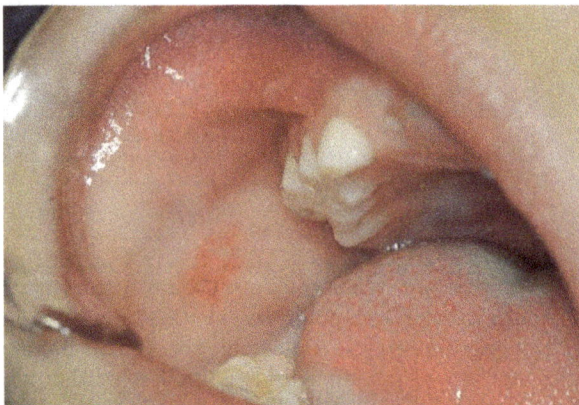

FIGURE 4: The initial clinical aspect of the ulcerated mucosa. Note the presence of factitious oral ulcers and localized swelling. The lesions were produced by self-biting of buccal vestibule and nail-scratching of gingival tissue.

remission of the swelling and ulcers on the right side of the mandible (Figures 5 and 6). Thus, the diagnosis of factitious oral ulcers was clinically confirmed by the case resolution.

At this moment, the patient is being periodically monitored to observe the possible recurrence of lesions. We recommended that the parents seek specialized psychological treatment to help the boy with the new family routine.

3. Discussion

Self-harm is the aggressive manifestation of the individual with psychological and emotional disturbances [3]. It results in physical damage and pain performed by the individual him/herself [1]. The nonsyndromic factitious ulcers are either intentional or unintentional [2]. The latter is generally related to deleterious habits as lip/thumb sucking, bruxism, nail/other object biting [6].

This present clinical case of factitious oral ulcers was linked directly to the boy's emotional stress caused by a change in his family dynamics. The comprehensive anamnesis provided useful information reported by the father and was of major importance to determine the lesion etiology [4]. Stewart and Kernohan [10] classified the oral factitious ulcer in three types: (A) those not related to a preexisting lesion; (B) secondary lesions caused by chronic habits; (C) lesions of difficult diagnosis due to unknown etiology. This case report showed a type (C) lesion, because of lack of chronic habits or previous lesions, which was confirmed by the emotional and psychological cause. Kwon et al. [11] reported that the differential diagnosis in children is very challenging because they do not provide clear information on their emotional state.

The literature reports the presence of factitious ulcers on oral mucosa and face [7]. Most of the cases is reported in women who injured the oral and perioral structures with the nails, periodically returning to the dentist without knowing to explain how the lesions appear [4, 6, 7]. To the best of our knowledge, the literature lacks reports on the presence of swelling close to the site of the factitious ulcers. Probably, these clinical signs occurred due to an inflammatory response to self-harm. The presence of local infection was discarded because we did not observe important signs as hyperthermia, flushing, and/or face heat.

The clinical treatment of individuals with factitious ulcers is problematic because of the behavior of patients, normally very quiet and shy, reluctant in accepting the self-harm as the cause of the lesion itself [7, 11]. In these cases, the discontinuity of the harmful habits is the target of the treatment planning, which should consider the severity, intensity, and the frequency of the self-harm actions [11, 12]. The multidisciplinary treatment involving dentists, psychologists, and psychiatrist is essential in most severe cases [4, 6, 7, 9, 11].

In clinical failures, the use of mouthguards could be an alternative to restrict the deleterious habits, by the introduction of a customized mouthguard with lingual and labial barriers [13]. This appliance can avoid that the individual interpose the lip, cheek, and tongue between the tooth arches [11, 13], preventing the continuity of self-harm [13]. It is worth noting that the mouthguards do not treat the problem origin. Even the extraction of some or all teeth may be considered as an invasive alternative treatment to avoid persistent self-harm problems in cases without remission [13]. However, this treatment approach is not well accepted by parents.

In this present case, intraoral devices were not necessary to prevent self-harm. We achieved a satisfactory result by a clinical control of lesions with minimal intervention. The instruction of parents and the use of an anti-inflammatory ointment were enough to promote the healing of ulcers and the prevention of their recurrence. Besides, we emphasized the mandatory importance of oral hygiene to prevent secondary infections.

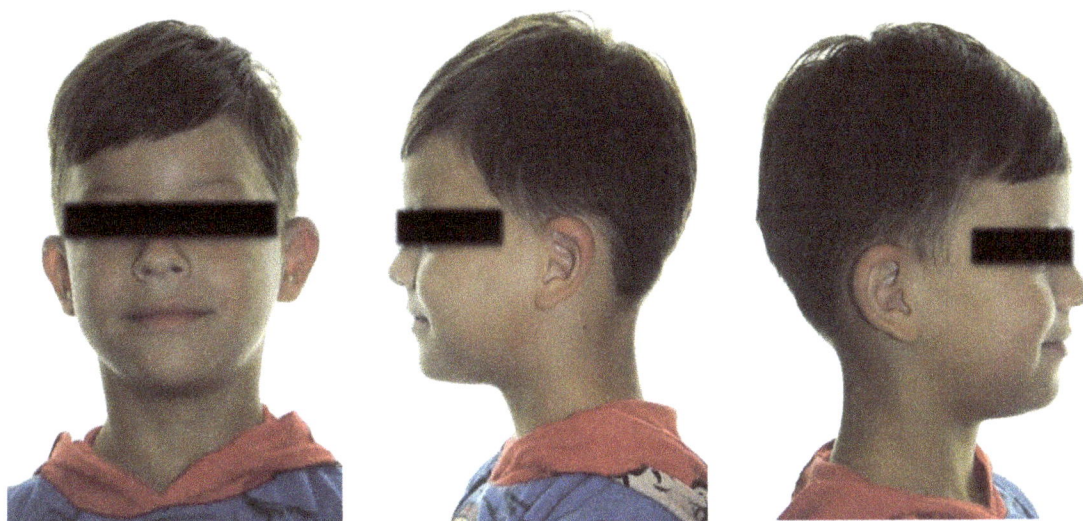

FIGURE 5: The clinical aspect of the boy at 30-day follow-up appointment.

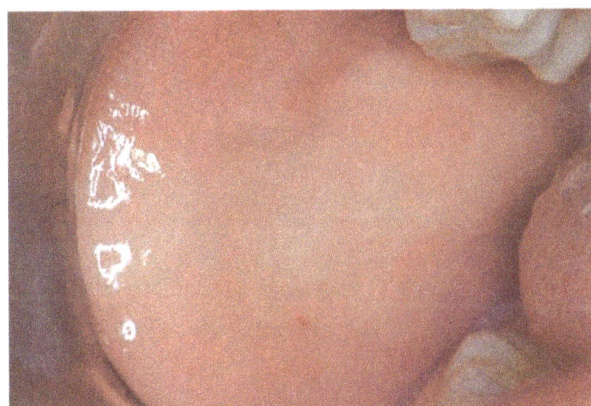

FIGURE 6: The clinical aspect of health mucosa at 30-day follow-up appointment.

A comprehensive anamnesis associated with clinical examinations is important to the correct diagnosis and proper treatment of factitious oral ulcers. The early diagnosis of lesions and the recognition of their risk factors enable a more conservative clinical approach and the maintenance of the anatomical and physiological health of oral and perioral structures. Due to the lack of available literature on this topic, the establishment of a standardized treatment protocol is difficult. To achieve successful outcomes, the treatments of factitious oral ulcers should be individually tailored for each patient, with focus on a multidisciplinary approach, including psychotherapy and periodic clinical control of possible recurrences.

Competing Interests

The authors declare that there is no conflict of interests regarding the publication of this paper.

References

[1] R. R. Kashyap and R. S. Kashyap, "Self-inflicted injury as a potential trigger for carcinoma of lip—a case report," *Gerodontology*, vol. 30, no. 3, pp. 236–238, 2013.

[2] J. Limeres, J. F. Feijoo, F. Baluja, J. M. Seoane, M. Diniz, and P. Diz, "Oral self-injury. An update," *Dental Traumatology*, vol. 29, no. 1, pp. 8–14, 2013.

[3] E. D. Klonsky, "Non-suicidal self-injury in United States adults: prevalence, sociodemographics, topography and functions," *Psychological Medicine*, vol. 41, no. 9, pp. 1981–1986, 2011.

[4] A. T. Zonuz, N. Treister, F. Mehdipour, R. M. Farahani, R. S. Tubbs, and M. M. Shoja, "Factitial pemphigus-like lesions," *Medicina Oral, Patología Oral Y Cirugía Bucal*, vol. 12, no. 3, pp. E205–E208, 2007.

[5] L. F. Guimarães, M. E. Janini, Á. S. B. Vieira, L. C. Maia, and L. G. Primo, "Self-inflicted oral trauma in a baby with Moebius syndrome," *Journal of Dentistry for Children*, vol. 74, no. 3, pp. 224–227, 2007.

[6] A. Dilsiz and T. Aydin, "Self-Inflicted gingival injury due to habitual fingernail scratching: a case report with a 1-year follow up," *European Journal of Dentistry*, vol. 3, no. 2, pp. 150–154, 2009.

[7] K. Kotansky, M. Goldberg, H. C. Tenenbaum, and D. Mock, "Factitious injury of the oral mucosa: a case series," *Journal of Periodontology*, vol. 66, no. 3, pp. 241–245, 1995.

[8] T. S. Barbosa, P. M. Castelo, M. S. Leme, and M. B. D. Gavião, "Associations between oral health-related quality of life and emotional statuses in children and preadolescents," *Oral Diseases*, vol. 18, no. 7, pp. 639–647, 2012.

[9] G. Ragazzini, A. Delucchi, E. Calcagno, R. Servetto, and G. Denotti, "A modified intraoral resin mouthguard to prevent self-mutilations in Lesch-Nyhan patients," *International Journal of Dentistry*, vol. 2014, Article ID 396830, 6 pages, 2014.

[10] D. J. Stewart and D. C. Kernohan, "Self-inflicted gingival injuries. Gingivitis artefacta, factitial gingivitis," *The Dental practitioner and dental record*, vol. 22, no. 11, pp. 418–426, 1972.

[11] I. J. Kwon, S. M. Kim, H. K. Park, H. Myoung, J. H. Lee, and S. K. Lee, "Successful treatment of self-inflicted tongue trauma

patient using a special oral appliance," *International Journal of Pediatric Otorhinolaryngology*, vol. 79, no. 11, pp. 1938–1941, 2015.

[12] M. C. Munerato, S. P. Moure, V. Machado, and F. G. Gomes, "Self-mutilation of tongue and lip in a patient with simple schizophrenia," *Clinical Medicine and Research*, vol. 9, no. 1, pp. 42–45, 2011.

[13] A. Arhakis, N. Topouzelis, E. Kotsiomiti, and N. Kotsanos, "Effective treatment of self-injurious oral trauma in Lesch-Nyhan syndrome: a case report," *Dental Traumatology*, vol. 26, no. 6, pp. 496–500, 2010.

14

Disseminated Histoplasmosis with Oral Manifestation in an Immunocompetent Patient

Debopriya Chatterjee,[1] Aishwarya Chatterjee,[2] Manoj Agarwal,[3] Meetu Mathur,[4] Setu Mathur,[1] R. Mallikarjun,[5] and Subrata Banerjee[6]

[1]Department of Periodontics, Government Dental College, Jaipur, India
[2]SMS Dental Department, SMS Medical College, Jaipur, India
[3]Department of Endodontics, Government Dental College, Jaipur, India
[4]Department of Endodontics, Rajasthan Dental College, Jaipur, India
[5]Department of Prosthodontics, AB Shetty Dental College, Karnataka, India
[6]Department of Medicine, SMS Medical College, Jaipur, India

Correspondence should be addressed to Debopriya Chatterjee; banerjee.debo@gmail.com

Academic Editor: Adriano Loyola

A case of disseminated histoplasmosis (DH) in a 60-year-old female patient is reported from Jaipur, Rajasthan, India. The patient presented with multiple papules on the skin surrounding the lips, face, torso, trunk, and back. She also complained of growth in the palate. Histoplasmosis was confirmed by biopsy and histopathology of skin and palatal lesions. This case report highlights the presenting features and occurrence of histoplasmosis in nonendemic region in India.

1. Introduction

Histoplasmosis is a dimorphic fungus, which grows in the yeast form in infected tissues. It was first identified by Samuel Darling in 1905, hence known as Darling's disease. Infection is mainly caused by inhalation of droppings from infected birds or bats. *Histoplasma capsulatum* mainly infects the lungs and passes asymptomatically to involve the skin and reticuloendothelial system [1].

Clinically, histoplasmosis has been classified as (i) primary acute pulmonary, (ii) chronic pulmonary, (iii) disseminated form, and (DH) occurring in infants, elderly, or immunocompromised patients [2]. In human immunodeficiency virus (HIV) positive patients, 95% of histoplasmosis appears as disseminated infection. Occurrence of disseminated form of histoplasmosis is very rare in HIV seronegative patients [3].

The manifestations of disseminated form of histoplasmosis are fever, weakness, weight loss, hepatosplenomegaly, and mucocutaneous lesions. The oral lesions may occur in any part of the oral cavity and the lesions vary from nodules to painful shallow or deep ulcers [4]. The incidence of oral manifestation is 25–45% in the disseminated form of the disease [3].

Skin lesions range from papules and plaques with or without crusts, pustules and nodules to mucosal ulcers and erosions, molluscum contagiosum-like lesions, acneiform eruptions, erythematous papules, and keratotic plaques [5].

Although worldwide in distribution, in India, histoplasmosis seems to be prevalent in the Gangetic delta. Panja and Sen reported the first case of disseminated histoplasmosis from Calcutta in 1954 and since then individual cases have been reported from various states, mostly from West Bengal. Among the forms of histoplasmosis reported from India, disseminated histoplasmosis is the rarest [1].

2. Case Report

A 60-year-old female was referred from a private practitioner to Dental Department of SMS Medical College Jaipur, with swelling of lower limbs and abdomen for past 3 months. She

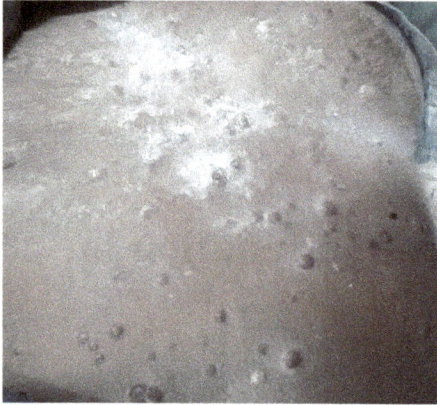

FIGURE 1

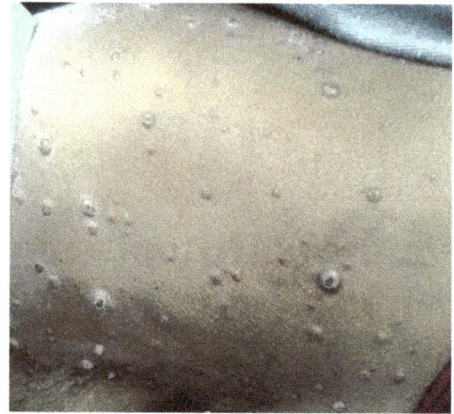

FIGURE 3

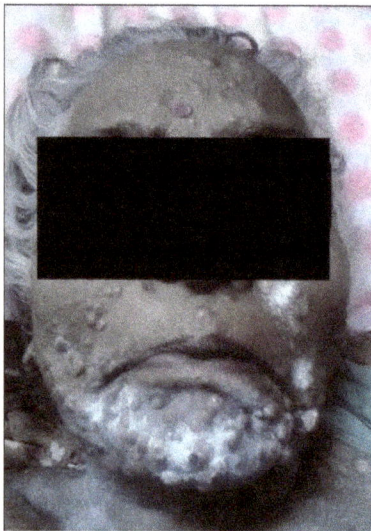

FIGURE 2

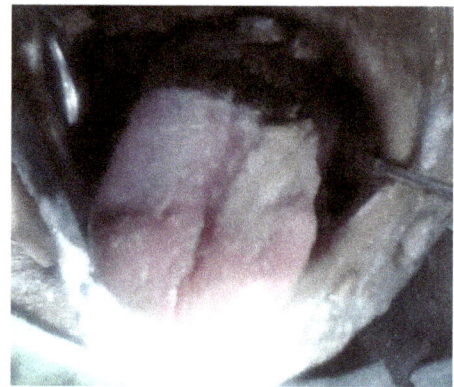

FIGURE 4

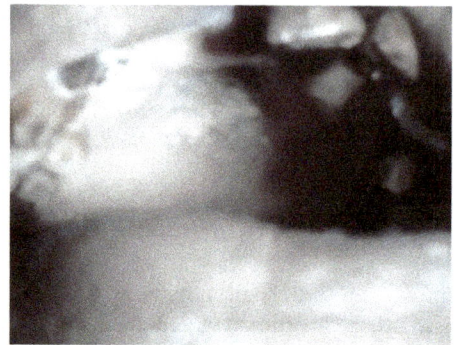

FIGURE 5

also complained of difficulty in breathing during exertion. Patient did not have any significant familial history. At presentation, the patient had skin warts which were generalized and tender [Figures 1, 2, and 3]. Clinical examination revealed distended abdomen with splenomegaly and hepatomegaly.

Oral examination revealed ulcerated and necrotic lesions located on the labial mucosa, dorsal surface of tongue, and hard and soft palate [Figures 4 and 5]. The lesions were covered by a pseudomembrane and were painful to palpation. Bilateral submandibular lymphadenopathy was noted. Extraoral examination revealed multiple nodular lesions on the chin, face, and the lips, which were tender to palpation. Multiple nodules were seen on the ventral surface of the forearm and dorsal aspect of thigh. There was a rise in local temperature of the nodules in comparison to the surrounding skin. A firm consistency was felt while palpating these lesions.

Routine investigations revealed random blood sugar was 130 mg/dl (normal range 79–140 mg/dl). Serum creatinine was 1 mg/dl. Serum urea was 30 mg/dl (normal range 15–39 mg/dl). Serum albumin was 3.2 g/dl (normal range 3.5–5.0 g/dl). Serum triglycerides levels were 189 mg/dl (normal range 36–175 mg/dl). Serum VLDL was 38 mg/dl (normal

range < 35 mg/dl), haemoglobin was 7.9 gm/dl (normal range 14.0–18.0 gm/dl), and platelet count was 1 lakh/ml (normal range 1.4–4.4 lakh/ml). Levels of urea, creatinine, bilirubins, alkaline phosphatase, and cortisol were normal. Urine examination revealed protein was positive; RBC and pus cell count was 2–4.

The X-ray of the paranasal sinuses, chest, and abdominal ultrasonography did not demonstrate alterations.

Lab investigation revealed no malarial parasites in peripheral blood smear. Febrile agglutination tests for typhoid, brucellosis, and infectious mononucleosis were negative. Antibodies to HIV were negative.

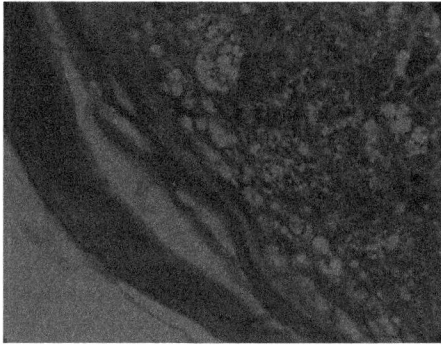

FIGURE 6

An incisional biopsy of the palatal lesion showed the presence of epithelioid cell granulomas in the connective tissue with numerous histiocytes, many of which formed multinucleated giant cells. The cytoplasm of the histiocytes showed the presence of small round to oval basophilic bodies surrounded by a clear halo, which is the characteristic feature of *Histoplasma capsulatum*. *H. capsulatum*-like yeasts were demonstrated by Periodic Acid Schiff stain. Biopsy of the skin revealed the same histopathologic features [Figure 6].

Antifungal therapy was started with intravenous liposomal amphotericin B at 0.7 mg/kg/day administered for 15 days. Patient's respiratory symptoms showed marked improvement. Oral and cutaneous lesions showed signs of remission. The patient was followed up for 6 months after cessation of therapy, but there was no recurrence. The treatment was tolerated well, with no side effects.

3. Discussion

H. capsulatum is an intracellular organism. The target organ is reticuloendothelial system and involving the spleen liver, kidney, and CNS. *H. capsulatum* exists as a saprophyte in nature and found in soil, particularly when contaminated with chicken feathers or droppings. By airborne route the spores are infectious to humans [4].

Histoplasmosis is seldom reported from India, due to its varied clinical presentation and lack of awareness amongst dermatologists. Panja and Sen first reported histoplasmosis from India in 1959. *Histoplasma capsulatum* is endemic in certain North Indian states like West Bengal, where a study showed a prevalence of skin positivity of 9.4% to histoplasmin antigen. There are a few sporadic case reports from South India as well [6].

The clinical features simulate other systemic febrile illnesses and most of the times the initial diagnosis is either tuberculosis or malignancy. When it is involving the oral cavity, the most commonly involved sites are tongue, palate, buccal mucosa, gingiva, and pharynx and the differential diagnoses should include squamous cell carcinoma, hematologic malignancy, tuberculosis, other deep fungal infections, oral lesions of Crohn's disease, necrotizing sialometaplasia of the palate, and chronic traumatic ulcers. The palatal ulcers present in our case report resembled squamous cell carcinoma and also the patient had respiratory symptoms similar to tuberculosis [7].

Biopsy of a mucosal or cutaneous lesion might be the most rapid method of arriving at a specific diagnosis of disseminated histoplasmosis [8]. The spores of *H. capsulatum* are visualized in sections stained with hematoxylin and eosin and special stains like Periodic Acid Schiff (PAS).

Antifungal medications are used to treat severe cases of acute histoplasmosis and all cases of chronic and disseminated disease. Amphotericin B is still the drug of choice for disseminated histoplasmosis. For patients who cannot tolerate amphotericin B, itraconazole is an effective and alternative therapy and it may be given as a prophylaxis for patients with advanced HIV infection [9]. Histoplasmosis has been reported in immunocompetent and immunocompromised individuals with the disseminated forms being more common in the latter group [1].

To the best of our knowledge, only one case [10] of disseminated histoplasmosis with oral manifestation has been reported in immunocompetent individual from India.

4. Conclusion

Progressive disseminated histoplasmosis is a rare entity among immunocompetent individuals from nonendemic regions. Subjects from endemic regions and around livestock do report occurrences of the disease sporadically. The presenting features of exanthema of the skin and enanthema in the oral cavity are reported for the first time from a nonendemic region in an immunocompetent individual. Histoplasmosis as a differential diagnosis should be kept in mind when diagnosing cases with similar presentations. Early diagnosis and prompt treatment provide alleviation of symptoms and a favourable outcome. However, late presentation at end stages does not respond to medications and may lead to loss of life.

Competing Interests

The authors declare that they have no competing interests.

References

[1] S. Subramanian, O. C. Abraham, P. Rupali, A. Zachariah, M. S. Mathews, and D. Mathai, "Disseminated histoplasmosis," *Journal of Association of Physicians of India*, vol. 53, pp. 185–189, 2005.

[2] S. L. Hernández, S. A. López de Blanc, R. H. Sambuelli et al., "Oral histoplasmosis associated with HIV infection: a comparative study," *Journal of Oral Pathology & Medicine*, vol. 33, no. 8, pp. 445–450, 2004.

[3] S. Vidyanath, P. M. Shameena, S. Sudha, and R. Nair, "Disseminated histoplasmosis with oral and cutaneous manifestations," *Journal of Oral and Maxillofacial Pathology*, vol. 17, no. 1, pp. 139–142, 2013.

[4] O. G. Ferreira, S. V. Cardoso, A. S. Borges, M. S. Ferreira, and A. M. Loyola, "Oral histoplasmosis in Brazil," *Oral Surgery, Oral Medicine, Oral Pathology, Oral Radiology, and Endodontics*, vol. 93, no. 6, pp. 654–659, 2002.

[5] V. S. Cunha, M. S. Zampese, V. R. Aquino, T. F. Cestari, and L. Z. Goldani, "Mucocutaneous manifestations of disseminated histoplasmosis in patients with acquired immunodeficiency syndrome: particular aspects in a Latin-American population," *Clinical and Experimental Dermatology*, vol. 32, no. 3, pp. 250–255, 2007.

[6] S. A. Joshi, A. S. Kagal, R. S. Bharadwaj, S. S. Kulkarni, and M. V. Jadhav, "Disseminated histoplamosis," *Indian Journal of Medical Microbiology*, vol. 24, no. 4, pp. 297–298, 2006.

[7] N. Golda and M. Feldman, "Histoplasmosis clinically imitating cutaneous malignancy," *Journal of Cutaneous Pathology*, vol. 35, no. 1, pp. 26–28, 2008.

[8] D. E. Elder, R. Elenitsas, B. L. Johnson Jr., and G. F. Murphy, "Fungal diseases," in *Lever's Histopathology of the Skin*, pp. 623–624, Lippincott Williams & Wilkins, Philadelphia, Pa, USA, 9th edition, 2005.

[9] L. J. Wheat, "Histoplasmosis: a review for clinicians from non-endemic areas," *Mycoses*, vol. 49, no. 4, pp. 274–282, 2006.

[10] S. Vidyanath, P. M. Shameena, S. Sudha, and R. G. Nair, "Disseminated histoplasmosis with oral and cutaneous manifestations," *Journal of Oral and Maxillofacial Pathology*, vol. 17, no. 1, pp. 139–142, 2013.

15

Perioprosthetic and Implant-Supported Rehabilitation of Complex Cases: Clinical Management and Timing Strategy

**Luca Landi,[1] Stefano Piccinelli,[1] Roberto Raia,[1]
Fabio Marinotti,[2] and Paolo Francesco Manicone[1,3]**

[1]Studio di Odontoiatria Ricostruttiva, Rome, Italy
[2]Dental Laboratory Technician, Studio di Odontoiatria Ricostruttiva, Rome, Italy
[3]Institute of Clinical Dentistry, Department of Prosthodontics, Catholic University of the Sacred Heart, Rome, Italy

Correspondence should be addressed to Paolo Francesco Manicone; pfrancesco.manicone@rm.unicatt.it

Academic Editor: Konstantinos Michalakis

Treatment of complex perioprosthetic cases is one of the clinical challenges of everyday practice. Only a complete and thorough diagnostic setup may allow the clinician to formulate a realistic prognosis to select the abutments to support prosthetic rehabilitation. Clinical, radiographic, or laboratory parameters used separately are useless to correctly assign a reliable prognosis to single teeth except in the case of a clearly hopeless tooth. Therefore, it is crucial to gather the greatest quantity of data to determine the role that every single element can play in the prosthetic rehabilitation of the case. The following report deals with the management of a multidisciplinary periodontally compromised case in which a treatment strategy and chronology were designed to reach clinical predictability while reducing the duration of the therapy.

1. Introduction

The treatment planning approach and prosthetic abutment selection have been severely affected by the introduction of end osseous dental implants in daily practice. Implant success has been well documented in fully edentulous [1] and partially edentulous patients [2, 3]. Parallel to the introduction and evolution of osseointegrated implants, all other dental disciplines have evolved both clinically and technologically by significantly raising their level of predictability and success. Therefore, the following question is still to be answered: should we treat periodontally or endodontically compromised teeth or should we extract them and replace them with dental implants?

Despite the efforts of clinicians and researchers, there is still scarce evidence in the literature supporting this choice [4]. Dental implants may be successfully placed in a periodontally compromised patient once periodontitis has been treated and controlled [5, 6], even though this group of patients seems to be more exposed to the risk of developing peri-implantitis compared to a nonperiodontitis group over the long term [6]. Controlling periodontal disease may be

achieved only by a strict application of clinical protocols and by placing patients on a strict regimen of maintenance. Due to the chronic nature of the disease, only long-term follow-up may be able to determine the real treatment success [7].

Whenever dental implants are integrated into a complex perioprosthetic rehabilitation, it is critical for the final and long-term success of the therapy to design a treatment strategy in order to monitor the effect of the treatment delivered while shortening the treatment length. The following report deals with the management of a multidisciplinary periodontally compromised case in which a treatment strategy and chronology were designed to reach clinical predictability while reducing the duration of the therapy.

2. Case Presentation

A 56-year-old female patient presented in May 2000 in our clinic complaining of functional and esthetic alterations and reporting the progressive migration of several teeth. Her medical history included myocardial infarction about one year earlier. The patient was under pharmacological control

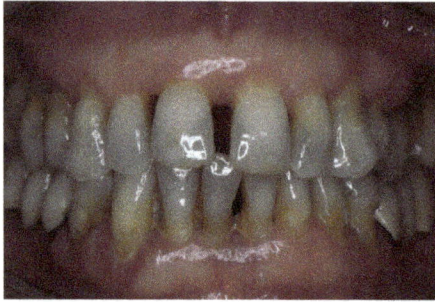

FIGURE 1: Initial case: clinical frontal view of the patient as she presented in May 2000.

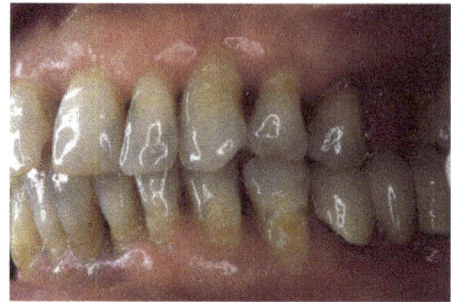

FIGURE 2: Initial case: lateral view, right side.

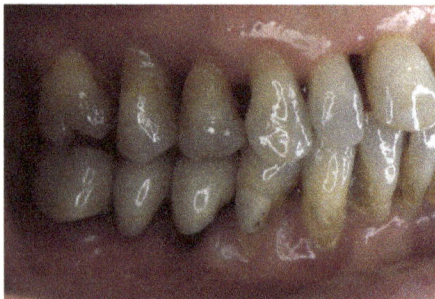

FIGURE 3: Initial case: lateral view, left side.

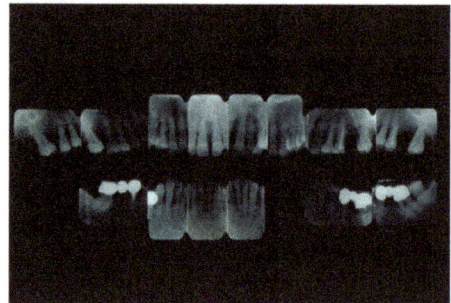

FIGURE 4: Initial case: full-mouth intraoral radiographic exam (May 2000).

for taking antihypertensive, anticlotting, and antiarrhythmic drugs. She used to be a smoker and quit after the heart attack.

3. Clinical Exam

Periodontally, the patient presented with clear signs of gingival inflammation with abundant plaque and calculus accumulation in both supra- and subgingival ways and with probing depth ranging from 1 to 10 mm. Teeth migration due to secondary occlusal trauma was evident, and diastema was present between teeth 11 and 12, 11 and 21, and 13 and 14. There was mesial inclination of teeth 11, 15, 17, and 23, and supereruption and buccal inclination of teeth 31, 32, 41, and 42. There was also a faulty restoration (46-x-44, 35-x-37) and carious lesions on several teeth (13–17).

The smile line was altered with a buccal inclination of the incisors in relation to the upper lip (Figures 1–3). The clinical frame was therefore characterized by a reduction of function determined by periodontal disease and occlusal instability. Chewing activity was severely compromised and limited by the presence of several mobile and tender teeth.

4. Radiographic Examination

A radiographic loss of about 50% of the alveolar bone was detectable. Teeth 14, 15, 24, and 25 were affected by a circumferential type of defect reaching the apical third of the root. Teeth 17 and 27 had unfavorable root anatomy with an associated vertical alveolar defect leaving only 30–40% of periodontal support. Teeth 21, 34, 35, 43, and 44 presented

shallow infrabony defects, and teeth 31 and 41 completely lost the interdental septum (Figure 4).

5. Diagnosis

The clinical and radiographic data collected led us to formulate the following diagnosis:

(1) Generalized chronic moderate to severe periodontitis (according to the 1999 AAP)

(2) Secondary occlusal trauma

(3) Caries in teeth 13 and 17

(4) Occlusal instability

(5) Incompetent lips

6. Prognosis

The first step to come up with a complete treatment plan was to formulate a general prognosis and then determine a tooth-by-tooth prognosis in order to select the abutments that could be used for occlusal rehabilitation [8]. From a periodontal standpoint, the general prognosis was good in both the short and long terms.

Due to loss of periodontal support and unfavorable root anatomy, the teeth located in the posterior sextants (17, 27, 37, 38), except tooth 47, had a poor prognosis. The same prognosis was assigned to teeth 14, 15, 24, 25, 31, 32, 41, and 42 for anatomical, periodontal, and endodontic limitations.

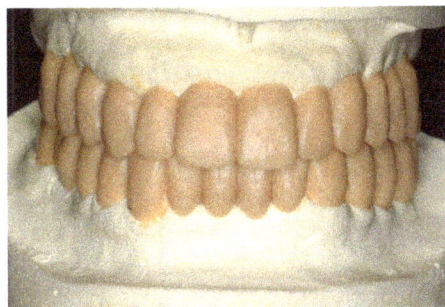

FIGURE 5: A diagnostic wax-up was made on casts mounted on a semi-individual articulator.

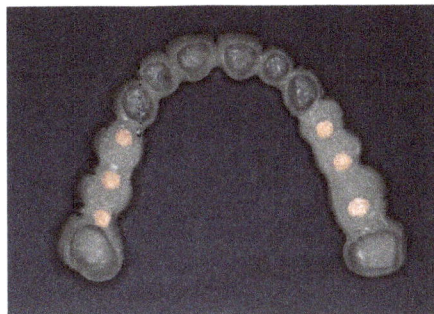

FIGURE 6: A first set of temporary restorations was developed. The wax-up included implant restorations and radiopaque landmarks embedded in the temporary crowns.

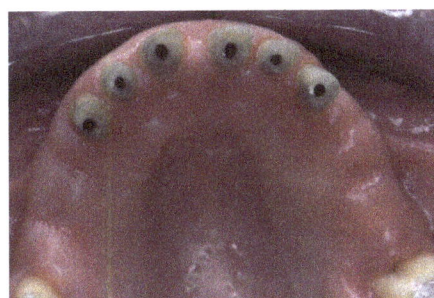

FIGURE 7: The abutment preparations were done in one appointment with a feather-edge finishing line.

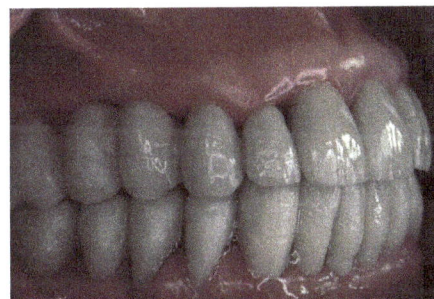

FIGURE 8: First set of temporary restorations relined and occlusally adjusted.

7. Treatment Goals

Treatment objectives included the reestablishment of periodontal health through the elimination of etiological factors, the creation of a stable occlusal scheme for function, and the enhancement of the esthetic appearance by closing the diastema between teeth 11 and 21 according to the patient's chief complaint.

Periodontal stability may be achieved by bringing probing depth within normal range, reducing inflammatory indices below 10%, as this is a good parameter to prevent disease progression [9] and achieve good plaque control.

In order to maximize patient acceptance and comfort during the treatment, teeth 17 and 27, which were judged hopeless, were scheduled to be used to support a fixed temporary full arch restoration until implant integration would be completed and the case would be ready to be finalized and then extracted. The treatment plan was outlined while taking into consideration the patient's desire to have a normal social and professional life during the treatment and trying to address the patient's chief complaint.

8. Phase I

Oral hygiene instructions and motivation combined with several appointments for supra- and subgingival scaling were useful to improve periodontal conditions and test the patient's compliance. Teeth 37 and 38 were extracted due to their hopeless prognosis, whereas the other teeth scheduled for extraction were extracted at the time of temporary restoration. Root canal therapy was done on all the abutment teeth, forecasting an aggressive type of prosthetic preparation at the time of periodontal surgery. A Lucia jig type of appliance was used to occlusally decondition the patient so that, using a bimanual manipulation of the mandible, we were able to accurately detect a centric relation.

Three months after initial consultation and once the patient was considered compliant with the prescribed oral hygiene regimen, the rehabilitation of the case started with the fabrication and delivery of the temporary restorations and the extraction of teeth 14, 15, 24, 25, 31, 32, 41, and 42. Teeth 17 and 27 were used as distal abutments of the cross-arch fixed temporary restoration.

A diagnostic wax-up was made on casts mounted on a semi-individual articulator (Figure 5), and a first set of

temporary restorations was developed. The wax-up included implant restorations, and a radiopaque landmark was embedded in the temporary crowns not in relation to the provisional crown but in relation to the final prosthesis (Figure 6). This was done in order to maintain the two maxillary second molars, which were mesially inclined, during the whole treatment. Another advantage of having the radiopaque marking embedded in the temporary crowns was that the patient was able to have a CT scan taken without removing the provisional restorations.

The abutment preparations were done in one appointment with a feather-edge finishing line (Figure 7). The temporary crowns were relined and occlusally adjusted, achieving a coincidence between centric occlusion and maximum intercuspation and carefully controlling the incisal plane (Figures 8 and 9).

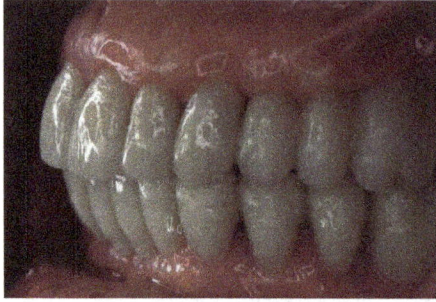

FIGURE 9: Coincidence between centric occlusion and maximum intercuspation and determination of the incisal plane.

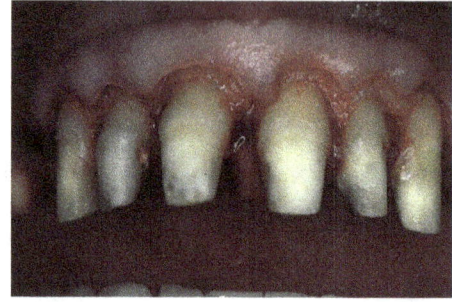

FIGURE 10: Osseous resective surgery in the maxillary anterior sextant.

9. Periodontal Surgery

After nonsurgical periodontal therapy, a periodontal reevaluation was carried out and residual probing depth ranging from 5 to 7 mm was still present particularly in the maxillary anterior sextant. Four months from the beginning of the treatment, osseous resective surgeries were carried out in both the maxillary anterior sextant and the bilaterally posterior mandibular sextants. Main surgical goals were to (1) eliminate periodontal pockets; (2) eliminate infrabony osseous defects; (3) establish a positive bone architecture. In all instances, the intraoperatory abutment preparation according to DiFebo et al. [10] was used in order to achieve better maintenance of the abutments and better tissue healing and to eliminate anatomical root alterations. A brief description of the surgical procedures is reported. Both surgical sessions were conducted under local anesthesia with ultracain supplemented with epinephrine 1:100,000 to ensure good hemostasis.

9.1. Maxillary Arch.
Buccally, after crestal probing and considering the abundant presence of keratinized gingival, a 2 mm scalloped incision was outlined with a blade number 15 (BD, Bard Parker). A mucoperiosteal flap was raised from teeth 13 to 23 up to the mucogingival line. Palatally, a submarginal beveled incision for crestal anticipation was carried out. The secondary flap and the interproximal tissue were completely removed, and the bone crest was exposed (Figure 10). The deepest part of the intrabony defects was used as a reference to perform osseous resective surgery [11]. Osteoplasty was done using a diamond coarse round bur mounted on a high-speed hand piece under abundant cooling. Ostectomy was achieved mainly using hand-bone chisels. Alveolar bone removal was done until a positive architecture was reached. At this point, a feather-edge preparation was used for the abutment teeth, deeply modifying the root anatomy and opening the interproximal spaces (Figures 11 and 12). Sling vertical mattress sutures were used to achieve passive flap adaptation to the bone crest (Figure 13).

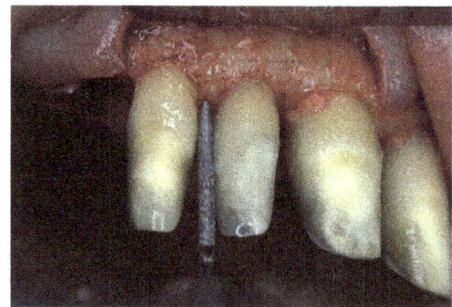

FIGURE 11: A feather-edge preparation was used for the abutment teeth, deeply modifying the root anatomy and opening the interproximal spaces.

9.2. Mandibular Arch.
The mandibular left and right sextants were treated simultaneously. Briefly, intrasulcular beveled incisions were outlined, and a split thickness flap was raised in order to preserve the minimal keratinized tissue present in the area. Lingually, a scalloped submarginal full-thickness flap was outlined according to the osseous crest anatomy. Once the interproximal tissue was removed, osseous recontouring was done, and the teeth were prepared as in the maxillary arch. Flaps were moved apically to the bone crest using sling horizontal mattress sutures, trying to increase the amount of keratinized tissue around the abutment teeth.

In both cases, temporaries were cemented back at the end of the surgery. The patient was instructed to refrain from brushing the surgical area, to follow a soft diet, and to use a mouthwash (CHX 0.2 twice a day) until mechanical home-care could be resumed. A nonsteroidal anti-inflammatory drug was prescribed (Nimesulide 100 mg,) for the first two days and then only when needed. Healing of the surgical areas was uneventful, with minimal patient discomfort. Once the initial healing was completed, 3 months later (Figure 14), the temporaries were relined, and a new set of precision impressions was taken to fabricate and deliver a second set of temporaries. At this point, the patient was sent for a CT scan for evaluation of the implant sites. Based upon this information and using the diagnostic wax-up, surgical stents were fabricated (Figures 15 and 16).

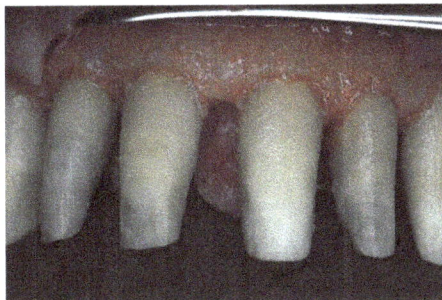

FIGURE 12: Alveolar bone removal was done until a positive architecture was reached.

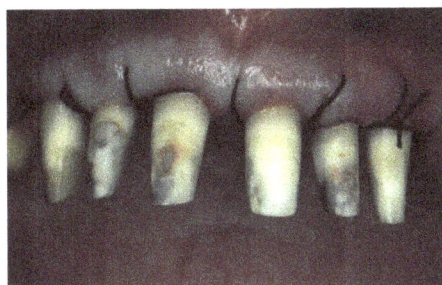

FIGURE 13: Sling vertical mattress sutures were used to achieve passive flap adaptation to the bone crest.

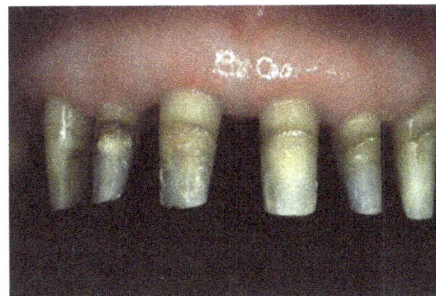

FIGURE 14: Once the initial healing was completed, 3 months later, the temporaries were relined.

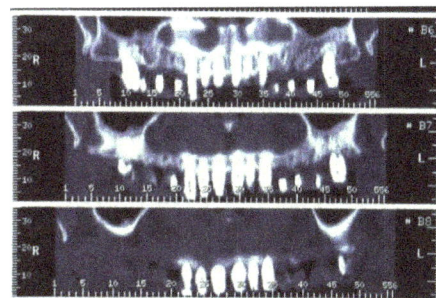

FIGURE 15: CT scan for evaluation of implant sites.

10. Implant Surgery and Temporary Prosthetic Treatment

One month after periodontal surgical therapy was completed, implant surgery was carried out. Implants insertion was completed in one surgical session under local anesthesia. Paracrestal full-thickness flaps were elevated (Figure 17). Alveolar bone crests were adequate except in two sites where bone defects had to be managed during implant insertion. In implant position 26, there was an adjacent vertical defect mesial to tooth 27. This defect was managed by distally inclining the implant in order to avoid thread exposure distally. The second site was a vertical defect mesial to tooth 17 influencing the insertion of implant 16 (Figure 18). Odontoplasty mesial to tooth 17 was then performed to allocate implant 16 in a prosthetically proper position. Once the osteotomy was completed following the surgical stent (Figure 19), threaded self-tapping 3.75×13 mm implants (Twist max Zimmer dental) were screwed into positions 14, 15, 16, 24, 25, 26, and 36. All implants achieved good primary stability with an insertion torque of at least 35 N/cm. At the time of the insertion, buccal fenestration appeared on implant 14 that required an autologous bone chips graft covered by a resorbable collagen membrane (Biomend, Zimmer) (Figure 20). During the surgery, a pick-up impression was taken by connecting the implant mounts to the modified surgical stents with a self-polymerizing acrylic resin (Duralay, Reliance Dental MFG Inc.) (Figure 21).

In the radiographic postoperative control, there was a coincidence of radiopaque landmarks embedded in the temporary crowns and the implant positions 14, 15, 16, 24, 25, and 26 (Figures 22 and 23). In the lab, on the casts used to fabricate the surgical stents, the implant position was transferred. The impression copings used as temporary abutments were milled down according to the prosthetic need, and a second set of temporary restorations was fabricated (Figures 24–26).

Five months after implant surgery, a second stage was conducted. During the healing phase, a spontaneous exposure occurred to some of the implants, requiring a conservative type of uncovering to preserve and augment the KG tissue present (Figure 27). Using the technique described by Palacci [12], the implants were exposed. Provisional abutments were tightened down, and after abutment teeth repreparation the second set of temporaries was delivered (Figures 28–30), thus allowing extractions of teeth 17 and 27 according to the treatment plan (Figure 31).

11. Final Restoration

At this point, the patient could be considered stable from a perioprosthetic point of view, and we waited 6 more months for a final reevaluation (Figure 32). Periodontal probing was within normal limits, and no inflammation was recorded around the abutment teeth and implants. Thus, a final impression was performed using a single-phase technique with double components polyether and individual tray (Figures 33 and 34). A transferring face-bow with new occlusal registrations was used to mount the casts on a semi-individual articulator. UCLA abutments were used for abutment casting. Final framework and ceramization were performed with the cross-mounting technique: the occlusal scheme was designed with anterior guidance allowing complete disclusion in both

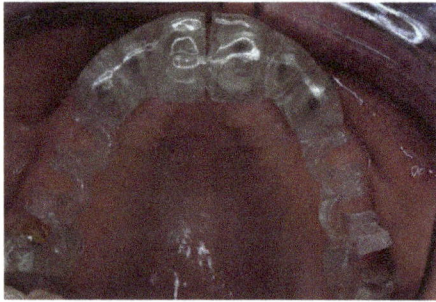

FIGURE 16: Surgical stents were fabricated based upon the information from the CT scan and using the diagnostic wax-up.

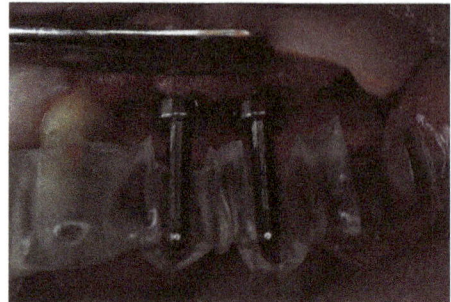

FIGURE 17: Implant insertion was completed in one surgical session under local anesthesia. Paracrestal full-thickness flaps were elevated.

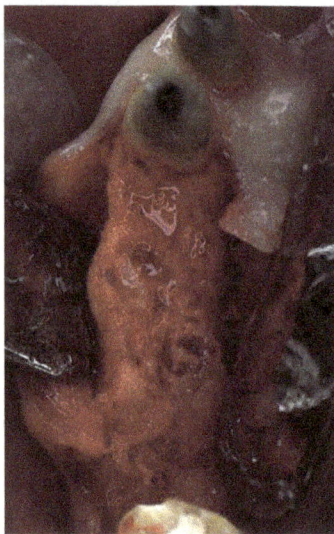

FIGURE 18: An odontoplasty mesial to tooth 17 was then performed to allocate implant 16 in a prosthetically proper position.

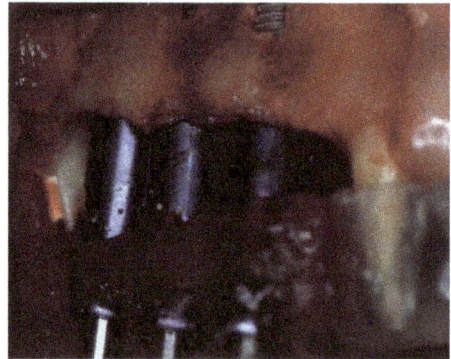

FIGURE 19: The osteotomy was completed following the surgical stent.

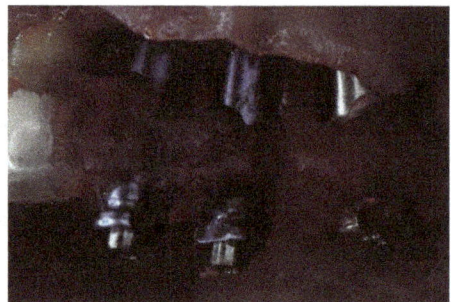

FIGURE 20: At the time of the insertion, buccal fenestration appeared on implant 14 that required an autologous bone chips graft covered by a resorbable collagen membrane (Biomend).

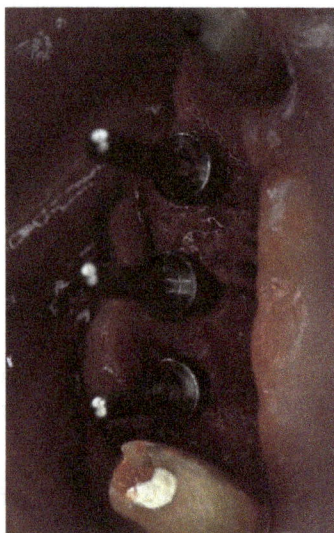

FIGURE 21: During the surgery, pick-up impression was taken by connecting the implant mounts to the modified surgical stents with a self-polymerizing acrylic resin (Duralay).

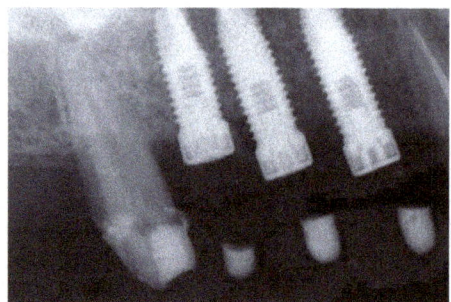

FIGURE 22: Radiographic postoperative control: coincidence of radiopaque landmarks embedded in the temporary crowns and the implant position of 14, 15, and 16.

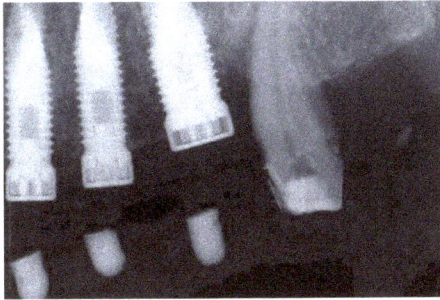

FIGURE 23: Radiographic postoperative control: coincidence of radiopaque landmarks embedded in the temporary crowns and the implant position of 24, 25, and 26.

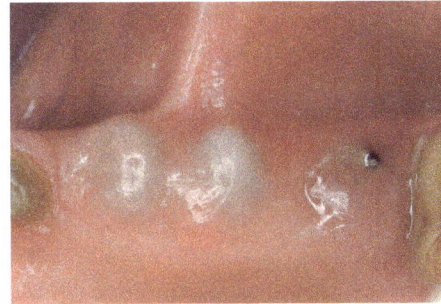

FIGURE 27: A second stage was performed 5 months after implant surgery.

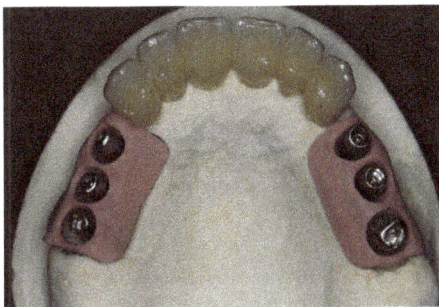

FIGURE 24: The position of the implants was transferred on the casts used to fabricate the surgical stents.

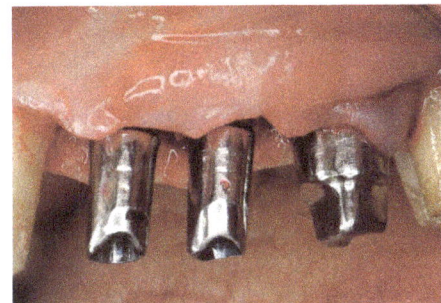

FIGURE 28: Tightening of the provisional abutments.

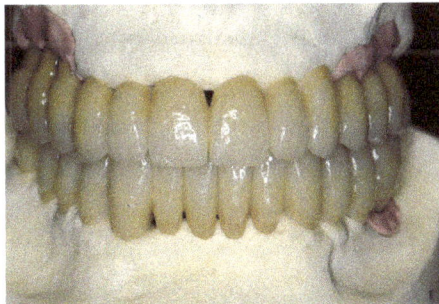

FIGURE 25: Second set of temporaries: frontal view.

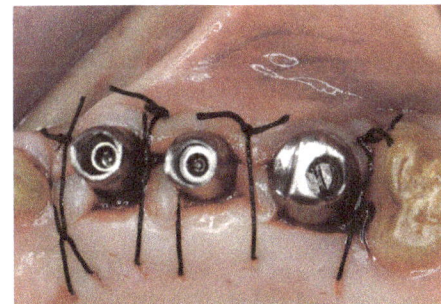

FIGURE 29: A conservative type of uncovering to preserve and augment the KG tissue present was required.

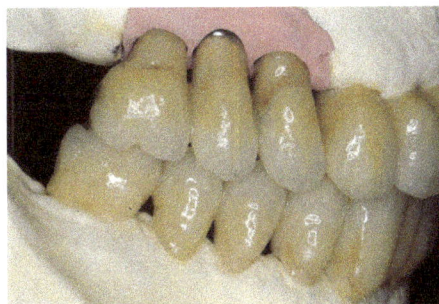

FIGURE 26: The impression copings used as temporary abutments were milled down according to the prosthetic need, and a second set of temporary restorations was fabricated.

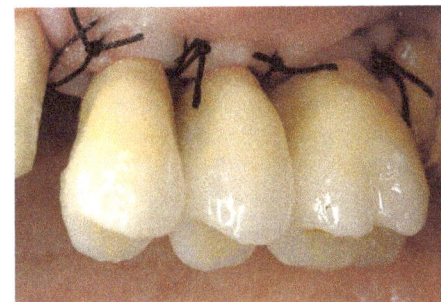

FIGURE 30: Delivery of the second set of temporaries.

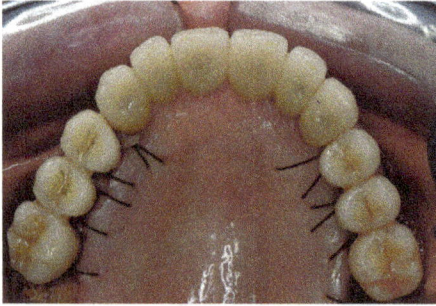

FIGURE 31: Delivery of the second set of temporaries and extractions of teeth 17 and 27 according to the treatment plan.

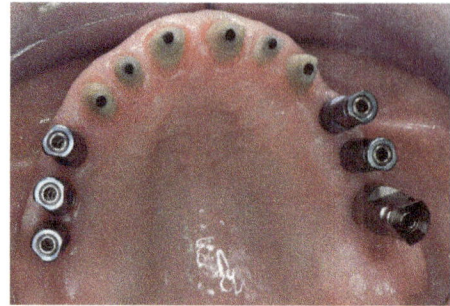

FIGURE 33: Final preparations from teeth 13 to 23 and positioning of the impression copings for a pick-up impression.

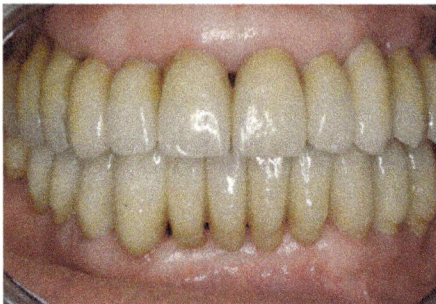

FIGURE 32: At this point, the patient could be considered stable from a perioprosthetic point of view, waiting 6 more months for a final reevaluation.

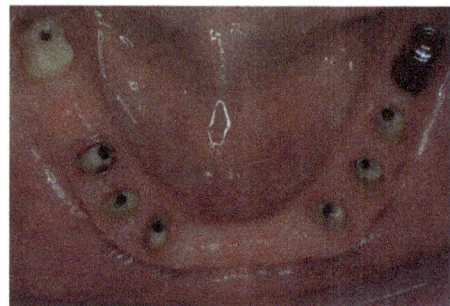

FIGURE 34: The final impression was performed using a single-phase technique with double components polyether and individual tray.

the lateral and protrusive excursions. The final restoration included a tooth-borne fixed partial denture from teeth 13 to 23 and two implant-supported fixed partial dentures, one from implant 16 to 14 and the other from implant 24 to 26. In the mandible, a one-piece framework was fabricated splinting teeth 35 to 47, and a single implant supported the PFM crown on 36 (Figures 35–38). Prosthetic bridgeworks were delivered two years after initial diagnosis in May 2002.

At the completion of the treatment, a maxillary retained night guard was provided to prevent any possible negative effect of parafunctional habits. This is in accordance with what has been presented in the literature by Brägger et al. [13] on the incidence of complications in prosthetic success due to parafunctions. From a functional and esthetic standpoint, the objectives were achieved of restoring good occlusal stability and a pleasant and harmonious smile line (Figures 39–41).

The patient was placed on 3 months of supportive periodontal treatment. Periodontal goals were achieved at the end of treatment. Adequate plaque control, low inflammatory indices, and physiologic probing ranging from 1 to 4 mm around all the abutment teeth and implants were recorded at the end of treatment.

12. Discussion

Treatment of complex perioprosthetic cases is one of the clinical challenges of everyday practice. Only a complete and thorough diagnostic setup may allow the clinician to formulate a realistic prognosis to select the abutments to

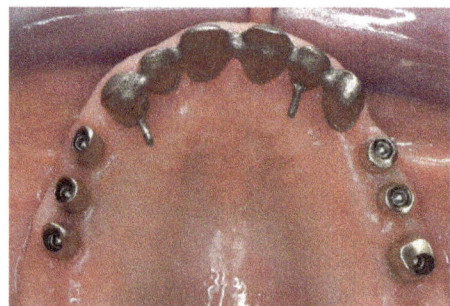

FIGURE 35: The final restoration included a tooth-borne fixed partial denture from teeth 13 to 23 and two implant-supported fixed partial dentures, one from implant 16 to 14 and the other from implant 24 to 26.

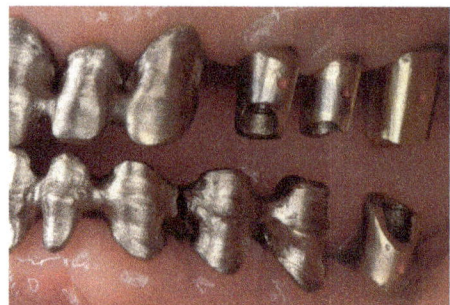

FIGURE 36: Final framework and ceramization were performed with the cross-mounting technique.

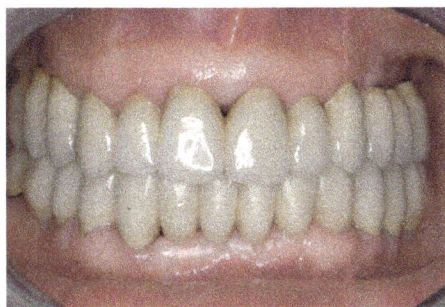

FIGURE 37: Final delivery of the prosthetic reconstruction (May 2002). From a functional standpoint, the objective of restoring good occlusal stability was achieved.

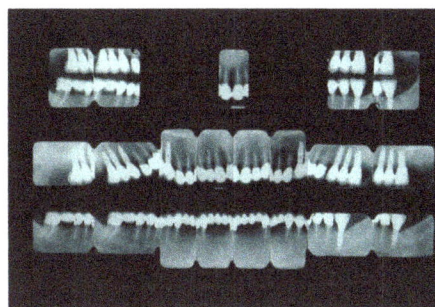

FIGURE 41: Final case: full-mouth intraoral radiographic exam (May 2002).

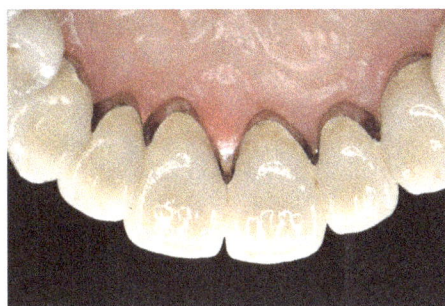

FIGURE 38: The occlusal scheme was designed with anterior guidance allowing a complete disclusion in both the lateral and protrusive excursions.

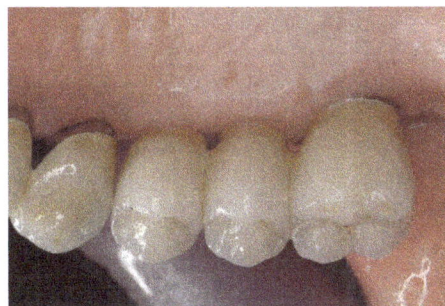

FIGURE 39: Adequate plaque control, low inflammatory indices, and physiologic probing ranging from 1 to 4 mm around all the abutment teeth and implants were recorded at the end of treatment.

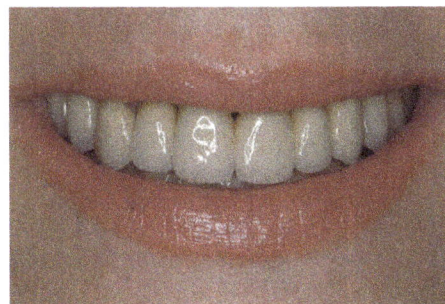

FIGURE 40: From an esthetic standpoint, the objective of restoring a pleasant and harmonious smile line was achieved.

support occlusal rehabilitation. According to McGuire and Nunn [8], clinical, radiographic, or laboratory parameters used separately are useless to correctly assign a reliable prognosis to single teeth except in the case of a clearly hopeless tooth. Therefore, it is extremely important to gather the greatest quantity of data, such as probing depth, attachment level, mobility, root anatomy, furcation involvement, inflammatory and hygiene indices, crown-to-root ration, and strategic value, to determine the role that every single element can play in the prosthetic rehabilitation of the case.

The effect of periodontal therapy to preserve compromised and mobile teeth as abutments for complex prosthetic rehabilitation has been widely documented [14]. Those restorations included extensive cantilever in the case of missing molars. Recently, Brägger et al. [13] reported that extensive cantilever should be considered as a true risk factor for failure of fixed partial denture implants or supported teeth. The introduction of oral implants greatly simplified the design of the prosthetic rehabilitation, eliminating the need for a cantilever. However, careful patient selection should be done before implant insertion. Periodontally compromised patients may be eligible for implant therapy only after periodontitis is under control to reduce the risk of developing peri-implantitis [5, 6, 15]. Periodontal control may be achieved by reducing probing within physiologic range, controlling inflammatory indices and plaque scores, and eliminating other potential noxious behaviors such as smoking. In the present case, molars have a negative prognosis due to severe periodontal destruction and poor root anatomy. On the other hand, the anterior maxillary teeth could be treated periodontally. Despite the work of Badersten et al. [16], who were able to manage pockets up to 7 mm in depth with a nonsurgical approach, it is quite clear that, in the case of extensive prosthetic rehabilitation, a more definitive approach should be used. Whenever there is prosthetic commitment in the esthetic zone, the principles of osseous resective surgery may be applied [11, 17]. This treatment modality has been shown to reduce probing for a longer period of time compared to other treatment modalities [18]. The reduction of probing depths has a tremendous impact to shift the periodontal microflora to a nonpathogenic population, thus reducing the risk of peri-implant infection [19].

In the reported case, the use of osseous resective surgery combined with an intrasurgical root preparation [10] resulted in the development of a physiologic hard and soft tissue anatomy compatible with optimal maintenance. Throughout the 24 months of treatment, the patient showed a high level of compliance and good functional and esthetic comfort. Such an extended time frame allowed us to evaluate the patient's response to the treatment and ensure periodontal tissue maturation and stability before the final restorations [20, 21].

The presence of distal teeth allowed us to use those abutments to support conventional temporary cross-arch splinted restorations. Despite the introduction of advanced protocols for implant immediate loading [22] and the use of an enhanced implant surface that may allow healing time reduction [23], we believe it may still be useful to consider hopeless teeth as temporary abutments for extended restorations, provided the teeth can be maintained throughout the treatment free of complications. However, even in a conventional approach, strategies can be implemented to speed up the treatment, such as a pick-up impression of the implant at the time of the surgery. This may also permit the early and progressive functional loading of the implants and the development of a more physiologic soft tissue profile.

13. Conclusions

We have reported an advanced periodontally compromised case treated with a multidisciplinary approach. The treatment strategies, rationale, and timing have been presented and explained in detail. Periodontal and prosthetic control of the case and good patient compliance are the key factors for success.

Competing Interests

The authors declare that there is no conflict of interests regarding the publication of this paper.

References

[1] R. Adell, U. Lekholm, B. Rockler, and P. I. Branemark, "A 15-year study of osseointegrated implants in the treatment of the edentulous jaw," *International Journal of Oral Surgery*, vol. 10, no. 6, pp. 387–416, 1981.

[2] G. A. Zarb and A. Schmitt, "The longitudinal clinical effectiveness of osseointegrated dental implants in anterior partially edentulous patients," *The International Journal of Prosthodontics*, vol. 6, no. 2, pp. 180–188, 1993.

[3] G. A. Zarb and A. Schmitt, "The longitudinal clinical effectiveness of osseointegrated dental implants in posterior partially edentulous patients," *The International Journal of Prosthodontics*, vol. 6, no. 2, pp. 189–196, 1993.

[4] M. Esposito, P. Coulthard, H. V. Worthington, and A. Jokstad, "Quality assessment of randomized controlled trials of oral implants," *International Journal of Oral and Maxillofacial Implants*, vol. 16, no. 6, pp. 783–792, 2001.

[5] M. Quirynen, W. Peeters, D. van Steenberghe, I. Naert, W. Coucke, and D. van Steenberghe, "Peri-implant health around screw-shaped c.p. titanium machined implants in partially edentulous patients with or without ongoing periodontitis," *Clinical Oral Implants Research*, vol. 12, no. 6, pp. 589–594, 2001.

[6] B. Ellegaard, V. Baelum, and T. Karring, "Implant therapy in periodontally compromised patients," *Clinical Oral Implants Research*, vol. 8, no. 3, pp. 180–188, 1997.

[7] G. C. Armitage, "Periodontal disease: diagnosis," *Annals of Periodontology*, vol. 1, pp. 37–215, 1997.

[8] M. K. McGuire and M. E. Nunn, "Prognosis versus actual outcome. II. The effectiveness of clinical parameters in developing an accurate prognosis," *Journal of Periodontology*, vol. 67, no. 7, pp. 658–665, 1996.

[9] P. P. Cortellini, M. Tonetti, and G. P. Pini Prato, "Periodontal regeneration of human infrabony defects. V. Effect of oral hygiene on long-term stability," *Journal of Clinical Periodontology*, vol. 21, pp. 606–610, 1994.

[10] G. DiFebo, G. Carnevale, and S. F. Sterrantino, "Treatment of a case of advanced periodontitis: clinical procedures utilizing the 'combined preparation' technique," *The International Journal of Periodontics & Restorative Dentistry*, vol. 5, no. 1, pp. 52–62, 1985.

[11] C. Ochsenbein, "Osseous resective surgery: a primer," *International Journal of Periodontics and Restorative Dentistry*, vol. 6, pp. 8–47, 1986.

[12] P. Palacci, *Optimal implant positioning & soft tissue management for the Branemark system*, Quintessence Publishing, Chicago, Ill, USA, 1995.

[13] U. Brägger, S. Aeschlimann, W. Bürgin, C. H. F. Hämmerle, and N. P. Lang, "Biological and technical complications and failures with fixed partial dentures (FPD) on implants and teeth after four to five years of function," *Clinical Oral Implants Research*, vol. 12, no. 1, pp. 26–34, 2001.

[14] J. Lindhe and S. Nyman, "Long-term maintenance of patients treated for advanced periodontal disease," *Journal of Clinical Periodontology*, vol. 11, no. 8, pp. 504–514, 1984.

[15] A. Mombelli, "Microbiology and antimicrobial therapy of peri-implantitis," *Periodontology 2000*, vol. 28, no. 1, pp. 177–189, 2002.

[16] A. Badersten, R. Nilveus, and J. Egelberg, "Effect of nonsurgical periodontal therapy II. Severely advanced periodontitis," *Journal of Clinical Periodontology*, vol. 11, no. 1, pp. 63–76, 1984.

[17] E. P. Barrington, "An overview of periodontal surgical procedures," *Journal of Periodontology*, vol. 52, no. 9, pp. 518–528, 1981.

[18] W. B. Kaldahl, K. L. Kalkwarf, K. D. Patil, M. P. Molvar, and J. K. Dyer, "Long-term evaluation of periodontal therapy: I. Response to 4 therapeutic modalities," *Journal of Periodontology*, vol. 67, no. 2, pp. 93–102, 1996.

[19] M.-C. Tuan, H. Nowzari, and J. Slots, "Clinical and microbiological study of periodontal surgery by means of apically positioned flaps with and without osseous recontouring," *The International Journal of Periodontics and Restorative Dentistry*, vol. 20, pp. 469–475, 2000.

[20] R. Pontoriero and G. Carnevale, "Surgical crown lengthening: a 12-month clinical wound healing study," *Journal of Periodontology*, vol. 72, no. 7, pp. 841–848, 2001.

[21] H. Smukler and M. Chaibi, "Periodontal and dental considerations in clinical crown extension: a rational basis for treatment," *International Journal of Periodontics and Restorative Dentistry*, vol. 17, no. 5, pp. 465–477, 1997.

[22] M. Degidi and A. Piattelli, "Comparative analysis study of 702 dental implants subjected to immediate functional loading and immediate non-functional loading to traditional healing period

with a follow-up up to 24 months," *The International Journal of Oral & Maxillofacial Implants*, vol. 20, pp. 99–107, 2005.

[23] M. K. Jeffcoat, E. A. McGlumphy, M. S. Reddy, N. C. Geurs, and H. M. Proskin, "A comparison of hydroxypataite (HA)-coated threaded, HA-coated cylindric and titanium threaded endosseous dental implants," *The International Journal of Oral & Maxillofacial Implants*, vol. 18, pp. 406–410, 2003.

16

Excision of Mucocele Using Diode Laser in Lower Lip

Subramaniam Ramkumar,[1] Lakshmi Ramkumar,[2] Narasimhan Malathi,[3] and Ramalingam Suganya[3]

[1]*Department of Oral & Maxillofacial Surgery, Faculty of Dental Sciences, Sri Ramachandra University, Chennai, India*
[2]*Dr. Ram's Dental Care & Maxillofacial Center, Chennai, India*
[3]*Department of Oral Pathology and Microbiology, Faculty of Dental Sciences, Sri Ramachandra University, Chennai, India*

Correspondence should be addressed to Ramalingam Suganya; drsuganyapavendhan@yahoo.com

Academic Editor: Tommaso Lombardi

Mucoceles are nonneoplastic cystic lesions of major and minor salivary glands which result from the accumulation of mucus. These lesions are most commonly seen in children. Though usually these lesions can be treated by local surgical excision, in our case, to avoid intraoperative surgical complications like bleeding and edema and to enable better healing, excision was done using a diode laser in the wavelength of 940 nm.

1. Introduction

Mucoceles are known as "mucus filled cavities" usually present in the oral cavity, lacrimal sac, and paranasal sinuses [1]. Mucus extravasation and mucus retention are the two most frequently occurring primary mechanical obstructive diseases of salivary glands [2]. Formation of mucus extravasation cyst is mainly due to mechanical trauma causing rupture of ductal system of salivary gland and mucin spills into adjacent soft tissues [3, 4]. Mucus retention cyst is formed markedly by obstruction of salivary ductal walls causing dilatation of ducts without spillage of mucin [5, 6].

2. Case Report

A 16-year-old female presented with a swelling in the lower left labial mucosal region for the past few months. She complained of intermittent swelling which often bursts and disappears for a few days. On clinical examination, lesion was soft, painless, fluid-filled, and approximately 1×1 cm in size (Figure 1). The history and clinical presentations were consistent with mucocele. Various treatment modalities such as surgical incision, cauterization, and laser excision were explained to the patient's guardian and obtained willingness to perform the most recent treatment option of laser excision.

Following minimal infiltration of 1 : 2,00,000 Xylocaine, the lesion was excised using soft diode laser in wavelength of 940 nm, 400 μm diameter tip at 1.5 W in continuous mode. The incision was placed on the uppermost site of the lesion and complete excision was performed (Figures 2, 3(a), and 3(b)). The specimen (Figure 4) was subjected to histopathological examination and showed cystic cavity lined by thick fibrous capsule. Cystic lumen contains mucin, foamy macrophages, and chronic inflammatory cells. Areas of coagulation necrosis surrounding the intended biopsy material were also evident. Adjacent mucous salivary gland was also seen. With all these histopathological features, diagnosis of mucous extravasation cyst was given (Figures 5 and 6). Patient was prescribed analgesics. There was uneventful healing on 45 days of follow-up (Figures 7, 8, 9, 10, and 11).

3. Discussion

Mucocele is the second most common lesion in the oral cavity followed by irritational fibroma. Incidence of this lesion occurs in the age group between 10 and 29 years with equal gender distribution [7]. Mucoceles appear as dome-shaped mucosal swellings with the characteristic accumulation of

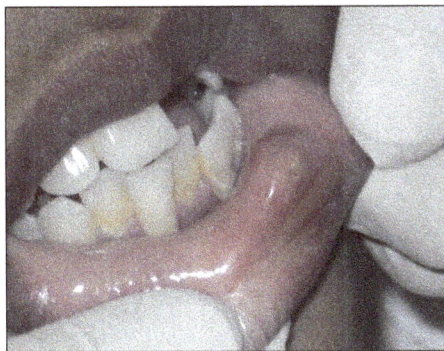

FIGURE 1: Swelling in the left labial mucosal region.

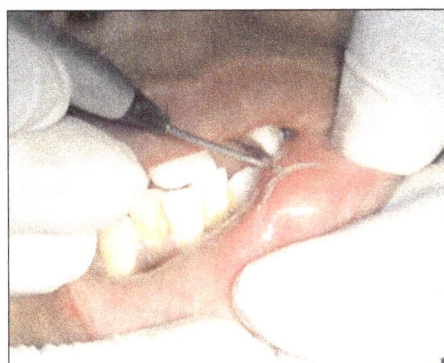

FIGURE 2: Application of laser: parameters, 940 nm and 1.5 W; continuous mode, 400 microns.

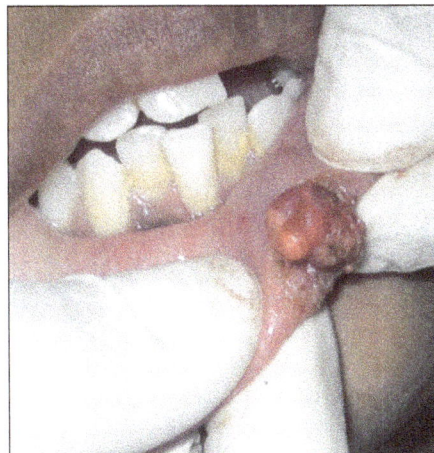

(a)

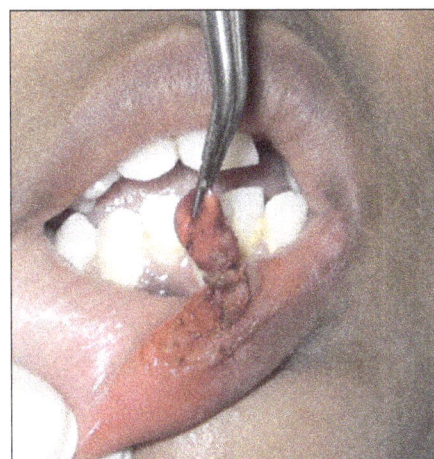

(b)

FIGURE 3: Intraoperative photograph.

mucin. These lesions usually impart bluish, transparent hue of variable size from 1-2 mm to several centimetres in dimension [3, 8]. Lower lip is the most common site of occurrence of mucocele followed by the buccal mucosa and floor of mouth [9]. Depending upon the size and location of mucoceles, the various clinical features include external swelling and interference with mastication, swallowing, and speech and discomfort might occur [7]. Histopathologic examination of mucocele often reveals formation of well-circumscribed, cyst-like space surrounded by granulation tissue and the presence of mucinophages in the collapsed wall of granulation tissue [10]. The adjacent salivary gland tissue should also be present because mucocele should always be removed along with feeder glands/ducts which minimize recurrence of the lesion.

There are various treatment aspects available for the management of mucocele early: scalpel incision, complete surgical excision, marsupialization, micromarsupialization, intralesional injections of corticosteroids, cryosurgery, laser ablation, sclerosing agent, and electrocautery methods [8].

The main advantages of soft tissue laser applications are minimal intraoperative bleeding and swelling and postoperative pain and very less surgical time, scarring, and coagulation, without any need of suturing after excision because of natural wound dressing due to denatured proteins. Various procedures like minor and major soft tissue surgery, bone cutting, and implant exposure with bone removal can be

performed in patients with bleeding disorders by using soft tissue lasers [11, 12].

The semiconductor diode lasers are available in different wavelengths such as 810–830 nm, 940 nm, and 980 nm [13]. The present case was performed by using 940 nm in which excellent hemostasis can be achieved due to good affinity for pigments like haemoglobin [14].

Diode lasers can be a useful alternative to larger surgical lasers such Er:YAG and CO2 lasers. Their small size and low cost are distinct advantages. They can give a well-defined cutting edge, as well as coagulation and hemostasis during excisions [12].

Absorption of laser energy into the target tissue releases heat by photothermal process which further causes intra- and extracellular vaporization of cells with resultant cellular explosion and tissue ablation. Adjacent lateral tissues will also absorb heat, on enough time of laser application. This will occur in concentric serial circles around the homogeneous target tissue. Reversible or irreversible damage of areas surrounding the target tissue by the thermal effects of laser results in zone of coagulation necrosis. Delayed healing and

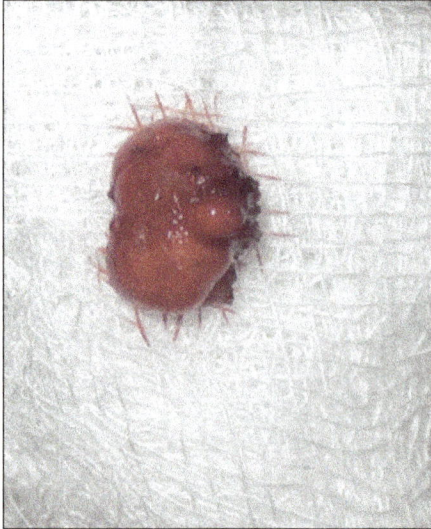

FIGURE 4: Excised specimen.

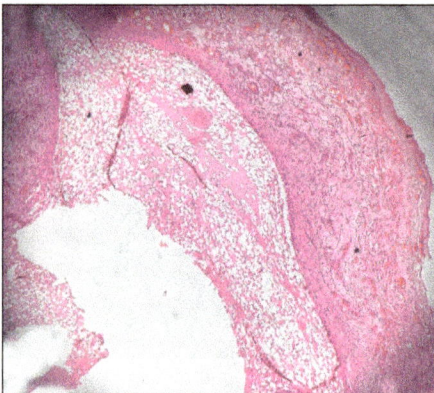

FIGURE 5: Photomicrograph showing H&E 40x view cystic cavity lined by thick fibrous capsule. Cystic lumen contains mucin, foamy macrophages, and chronic inflammatory cells.

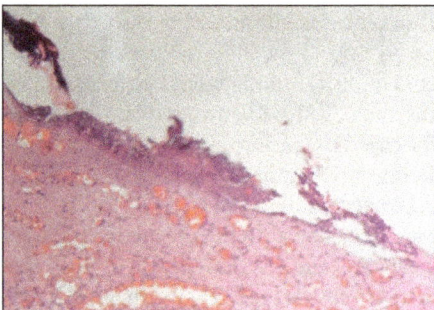

FIGURE 6: Photomicrograph showing H&E 40x view zone of coagulation necrosis surrounding the intended biopsy material.

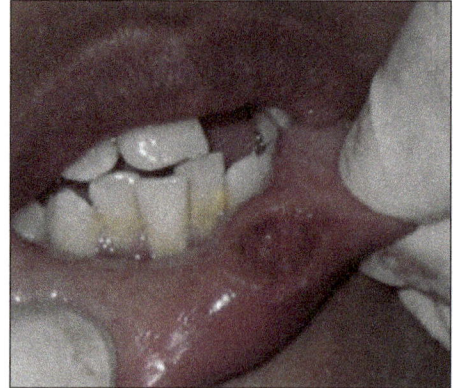

FIGURE 7: Photograph showing immediate postoperative day.

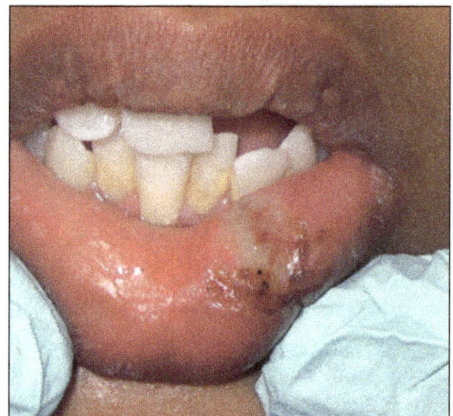

FIGURE 8: Photograph showing postoperative view: Day 1.

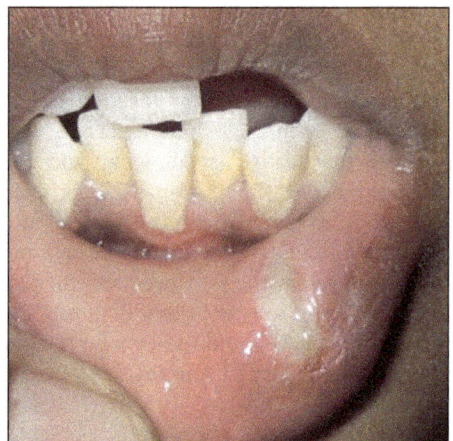

FIGURE 9: Photograph showing postoperative view: Day 4.

a larger wound site may occur on increased time of laser application. On the other hand, sealing of small diameter of vessels rather than the area of coagulation necrosis provides advantages like hemostasis during laser surgery. Area of adjacent coagulation ends with less bleeding at surgical site. The presence of border of necrotic and coagulated tissue in an incisional or excisional biopsy may result in intricacy of histopathological identification [15].

Histological examination of laser excised tissue shows improved epithelization and lesser inflammation. Intact basement membrane and connective tissue matrix can also be observed. Matrix proteins initiate reparative synthesis on these tissues. Resistance of matrix proteins against laser

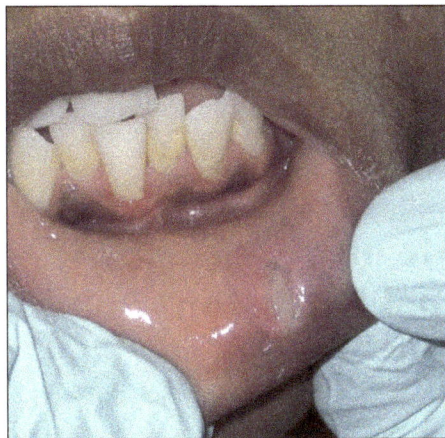

FIGURE 10: Photograph showing postoperative view: Day 8.

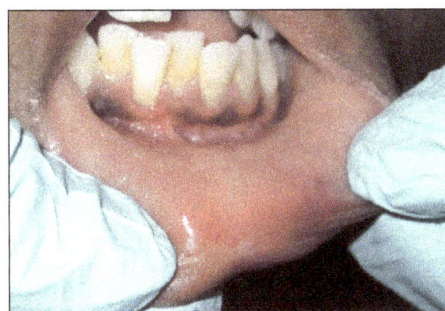

FIGURE 11: Photograph showing postoperative view: Day 45.

application and replacement as well as removal of residual matrix is responsible for reduced scarring and contraction [16].

4. Conclusion

Our present case report reveals knowledge about using diode laser for the treatment of mucocele with a variety of beneficial effects such as minimal anesthesia, less procedural timings, good surgical site visualization, hemostasis, and minimal carbonization in 45 days of periodical follow-up. Laser application makes it possible to reduce apprehension and fear in pediatric and geriatric patients.

Competing Interests

The authors declare that there is no conflict of interests regarding the publication of this paper.

References

[1] A. Qafmolla, M. Bardhoshi, N. Gutknecht, and E. Bardhoshi, "Evaluation of early and long term results of the treatment of mucocele of the lip using 980 nm diode laser ," *European Scientific Journal*, vol. 10, no. 6, 2014.

[2] G. L. Ellis, P. L. Auclair, and D. R. Gnepp, *Surgical Pathology of the Salivary Glands*, Saunders, Philadelphia, Pa, USA, 1991.

[3] B. W. Neville, D. D. Damm, M. Allen, and J. E. Bouqot, Eds., *Oral and Maxillofacial Pathology*, Saunders, Philadelphia, Pa, USA, 2nd edition, 2002.

[4] N. Madan, "Excision of mucocele: a surgical case report," *Biological and Biomedical Reports*, vol. 2, no. 2, 2012.

[5] J. Ata-Ali, C. Carrillo, C. Bonet, J. Balaguer, M. Peñarrocha Diago, and M. Peñarrocha, "Oral mucocele: review of the literature," *Journal of Clinical and Experimental Dentistry*, vol. 2, no. 1, pp. e18–e21, 2010.

[6] M. Shear and P. Speight, *Cyst of the Oral and Maxillofacial Region*, Blackwell Munksgaard, New York, NY, USA, 4th edition, 2007.

[7] D. Re Cecconi, A. Achilli, M. Tarozzi et al., "Mucoceles of the oral cavity: a large case series (1994–2008) and a literature review," *Medicina Oral, Patologia Oral y Cirugia Bucal*, vol. 15, no. 4, pp. e551–e556, 2010.

[8] J. Yagüe-García, A.-J. España-Tost, L. Berini-Aytés, and C. Gay-Escoda, "Treatment of oral mucocele-scalpel versus CO2 laser," *Medicina Oral, Patologia Oral y Cirugia Bucal*, vol. 14, no. 9, pp. e469–e474, 2009.

[9] K. Chawla, A. K. Lamba, F. Faraz, S. Tandon, S. Arora, and M. Gupta, "Treatment of lower lip mucocele with Er, Cr: YSGG laser—a case report," *The Journal of Oral Laser Applications*, vol. 10, no. 4, pp. 181–185, 2010.

[10] E. Lee, S. H. Cho, and C. J. Park, "Clinical and immunehisto-chemical characteristics of mucoceles," *Annals of Dermatology*, vol. 21, no. 4, pp. 345–351, 2009.

[11] L. J. Walsh, "The current status of laser applications in dentistry," *Australian Dental Journal*, vol. 48, no. 3, pp. 146–155, 2003.

[12] E. Azma and N. Safavi, "Diode laser application in soft tissue oral surgery," *Journal of Lasers in Medical Sciences*, vol. 4, no. 4, pp. 206–211, 2013.

[13] A. C. Robert, *Principles and Practice of Laser Dentistry*, Mosby Elsevier, Maryland Heights, Mo, USA, 2010.

[14] G. Agarwal, A. Mehra, and A. Agarwal, "Laser vaporization of extravasation type of mucocele of the lower lip with 940-nm diode laser," *Indian Journal of Dental Research*, vol. 24, no. 2, p. 278, 2013.

[15] G. A. Catone, C. C. Ailing, and B. M. Smith, "Laser Applications in Oral and Maxillofacial Surgery," *Implant Dentistry*, vol. 6, no. 3, p. 238, 1997.

[16] M. Luomanen, J. H. Meurman, and V. P. Lehto, "Extracellular matrix in healing CO_2 laser incision wound," *Journal of Oral Pathology & Medicine*, vol. 16, no. 6, pp. 322–331, 1987.

17

The Effect of Mineral Trioxide Aggregate on the Periapical Tissues after Unintentional Extrusion beyond the Apical Foramen

Pradnya S. Nagmode, Archana B. Satpute, Ankit V. Patel, and Pushpak L. Ladhe

Department of Conservative Dentistry and Endodontics, SMBT Dental College & Hospital, Sangamner, India

Correspondence should be addressed to Archana B. Satpute; archana.satpute5@gmail.com

Academic Editor: Sonja Pezelj Ribarić

Introduction. Single-step apexification procedures using mineral trioxide aggregate (MTA) have been reported as favorable treatment options for teeth with an open apex, posing greater benefits compared to the other available medicaments. However, controlled apical placement of MTA is a challenging procedure to perform using orthograde approach. This case series describes the outcome of the unintentional extrusion of MTA into periradicular tissues during apexification, in three separate cases. *Methods.* Three adult patients reported to the Department of Conservative Dentistry and Endodontics for the management of maxillary incisors with open apices. After isolation, conventional access, and cleaning and shaping procedures, one-step MTA apexification was performed. On subsequent radiographs, a considerable amount of MTA was seen to be extruded in all the three cases. *Results.* During follow-up examination the teeth were seen to be asymptomatic in all cases and radiographically demonstrated repair of the periapical lesion. *Conclusion.* The results of these cases suggest that extrusion of MTA into the periapical tissues does not cause any detrimental effect, which could be attributed to the biologic properties of MTA.

1. Introduction

The conventional school of thought regarding the clinical treatment of a traumatized or an infected immature vital tooth is preserving the vitality by apexogenesis or revascularization so as to allow complete root formation. However, such teeth with nonvital pulps require a hard-tissue apical barrier for the completion of the root filling [1, 2].

Earlier, intracanal medicaments were used over several appointments to treat cases with open apices, with the hope of creating a barrier over which gutta-percha could eventually be placed. The treatment could be prolonged to a year, with little evidence of an apical barrier, resulting in thinner and brittle roots which are more susceptible to fracture [3].

Mineral trioxide aggregate (MTA) has evolved as a material of choice for apexification owing to its properties of better biocompatibility, good sealability, ability to promote dental pulp, and periradicular tissue regeneration. Moreover, it can also harden in the presence of moisture [4]. Apexification

with MTA can be performed as a one- or two-visit procedure, eliminating the need for extended periods of dressing with calcium hydroxide. It also allows for immediate restoration, which further reduces the potential of catastrophic, vertical, or oblique root fractures of such teeth [5].

However, MTA has been known to exhibit certain shortcomings, which include long setting time, the potential to discolour teeth, technique sensitivity, and high cost [6, 7]. Also, any variation in pH as a result of inflammatory changes in periradicular lesions may adversely affect the physical, chemical, and hydration properties of MTA [8].

The lack of normal apical constriction of the root canal in teeth with open apices complicates the procedures for apexification. The wide apical foramen requires a large volume of filling material that may extrude into the periradicular tissues. This produces undesirable tissue inflammation, neurotoxic effects, and foreign body reaction [1]. Overfillings have a deleterious effect on the prognosis of root canal treatments; the teeth obturated within 0–2 mm from the apex have a

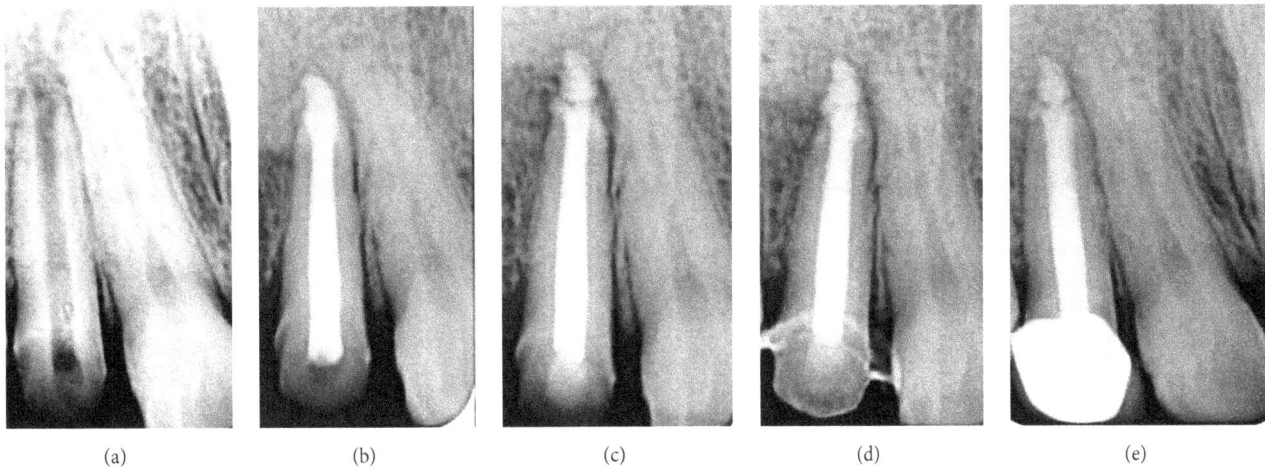

FIGURE 1: (a) Preoperative IOPA, (b) unintentional extrusion of MTA from apical foramen, (c) 1-month follow-up, (d) 3-month follow-up, and (e) 6-month follow-up.

success rate of 94%, which drops down to 76% if the teeth are overfilled [9]. The response of periapical tissues to the root filling material, as a consequence of the complex and dubious interaction between the materials and the host defences, determines the prognosis for an endodontically treated tooth which has been overfilled [10].

This case series describes the outcomes of unintentional extrusion of MTA into the periradicular tissues during apexification, in three separate cases.

2. Case Reports

2.1. Case 1. A 29-year-old female patient reported to the Department of Conservative Dentistry and Endodontics for endodontic retreatment of the right maxillary lateral incisor. The chief complaint was pain with tooth #12. She presented with a history of root canal treatment with the same tooth 2 years back. Medical history was not contributory. On clinical examination, the tooth was tender to percussion. A localized, erythematous swelling could be appreciated on the buccal mucosa surrounding the tooth. Radiographically, tooth #12 showed periapical rarefaction measuring approximately 2 mm (width) × 4 mm (height), with a resorbed apex (Figure 1(a)). A diagnosis of chronic apical abscess was made, and endodontic retreatment was planned.

Following placement of the rubber dam, endodontic access cavity was modified and the gutta-percha was removed using xylene (RC Solve; Prime Dental Products Pvt. Ltd., Thane, India) and ProFile rotary instruments. The canal was instrumented with K-files up to size #50, irrigated with 5.25% NaOCl (Prime Dental Products Pvt. Ltd., Thane, India), and dressed with calcium hydroxide (RC Cal; Prime Dental Products Pvt. Ltd., Thane, India). The entire length of a size #40 Lentulo spiral (Maillefer, Ballaigues, Switzerland) was coated with the paste, introduced into the canal to the working length, and then rotated at 500 rpm using a handpiece mounted on a speed and torque control machine (X-smart, Dentsply, Tulsa Dental, Tulsa, OK, USA). After ten days, the tenderness had disappeared, and no soft tissue swelling, erythema, or canal exudate were seen. The temporary restoration was then removed under rubber dam isolation and local anaesthesia, and the calcium hydroxide dressing was flushed out using alternating irrigation with 5.25% NaOCl and 17% EDTA (Prime Dental Products Pvt. Ltd., Thane, India) together with gentle filing with a size of 50 K file. Since no exudate was found on the blotted paper points test, a one-step apexification procedure with MTA was performed. MTA (ProRoot MTA; Dentsply Tulsa Dental Specialties, Johnson City, TN, USA) was manipulated according to the manufacturer's instructions, carried to the apical 4 mm of the canal using an MTA carrier, and then condensed with measured endodontic pluggers under an operating dental microscope (Seiler IQ: St. Louis, MO). Radiograph taken during the procedure displayed considerable extrusion of the MTA into the periradicular tissues (Figure 1(b)). No attempt was made to remove the extruded MTA, and the access cavity was sealed with sterile cotton pellets and temporary restorative material (Cavit, 3M/ESPE, Seefeld, Germany). The patient was kept under observation.

At the following appointment the cotton pellet was removed; the setting of MTA and other clinical signs and symptoms were verified. The remaining pulp space was back-filled with thermoplasticized gutta-percha (E and Q Plus-Meta Biomed Co., Ltd.) and AH Plus sealer (Dentsply; Detrey, Konstanz) by using warm vertical condensation technique. The tooth was restored with a composite resin (Z250; 3M ESPE, St. Paul, MN) and the patient was informed regarding the possible need for surgical intervention. On the 1-month recall visit, the patient reported no episodes of discomfort and/or swelling (Figure 1(c)). Periapical radiographs taken at 3- and 6-month recall visits to evaluate the periapical condition showed slight resorption of the MTA which was

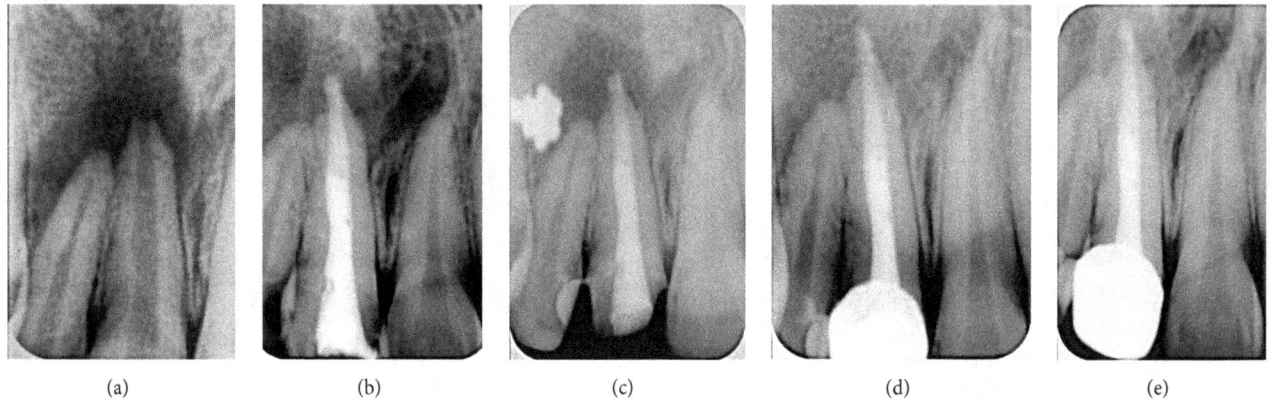

FIGURE 2: (a) Preoperative IOPA, (b) unintentional extrusion of MTA from apical foramen, (c) 1-month follow-up, (d) 3-month follow-up, and (e) 6-month follow-up.

extruded into periapical area (Figures 1(d) and 1(e)). Clinical examination revealed the absence of any signs and symptoms, with adequate function.

2.2. Case 2. A 30-year-old female patient reported to the Department of Conservative Dentistry and Endodontics with the complaint of pain associated with the left maxillary central incisor (tooth #21). She presented with a history of trauma to tooth #21, about 18–20 years ago. Tenderness on palpation was noted in the vestibule area. Radiographic examination revealed open apex of tooth #21 associated with a large periapical lesion of about 8 mm in diameter (Figure 2(a)). The tooth #22 was found to be vital on electric pulp testing and cold test. A diagnosis of chronic apical abscess with incompletely formed apex of tooth #21 was made, and nonsurgical endodontic treatment was planned. Access cavity and cleaning and shaping procedures were performed as described earlier. A calcium hydroxide paste (RC Cal; Prime Dental Products Pvt. Ltd., Thane, India) was placed using a size #40 Lentulo spiral (Maillefer, Ballaigues, Switzerland) to the working length and rotated at 500 rpm using a handpiece mounted on a speed and torque control machine (X-smart, Dentsply, Tulsa Dental, Tulsa, OK, USA), as an intracanal medicament for a week.

One week later, the canal of tooth #21 was irrigated alternately with 5.25% NaOCl (Prime Dental Products Pvt. Ltd., Thane, India) and 17% EDTA (Prime Dental Products Pvt. Ltd., Thane, India) and dried with sterile paper points. A one-step MTA (ProRoot MTA; Dentsply Tulsa Dental Specialities, Johnson City, TN, USA) apexification was performed as described in Case 1. Despite adequate precautions ensured during MTA placement, there was some extrusion of MTA (Figure 2(b)) into the periapical tissues. The patient was kept under observation for any signs or symptoms of clinical discomfort. After 15 days, the patient was recalled and assessed. No history of discomfort was reported. The root canal was then backfilled with thermoplasticized gutta-percha (E and Q Plus-Meta Biomed Co., Ltd.) and the access cavity was restored with a composite resin. The patient was scheduled for follow-up at 1- and 3-month intervals (Figures

2(c) and 2(d)). The patient was seen to be asymptomatic. Thereafter, at 6-month recall, a decrease in size of the periapical radiolucency was noted on periapical radiograph (Figure 2(e)).

2.3. Case 3. A 17-year-old male patient reported to the Department of Conservative Dentistry and Endodontics with aesthetic concerns resulting from the discolouration of the maxillary right central incisor. The medical history was non-contributory. The patient's history included a traumatic injury in that region 5-6 years back. Extraoral examination revealed normal soft tissue structures with no apparent pathosis. On intraoral examination, a sinus tract was located in association with the maxillary right anterior region. Evaluation of periapical radiographs showed a large radiolucent lesion with well-defined margins around the root of tooth #11 along with an open apex and root resorption (Figure 3(a)). The tooth was tender to percussion. Electronic pulp testing (Electric Pulp Tester; Parkell, Farmingdale, NY) and cold application with a carbon dioxide snow (Odontotest; Moyco Union Broach, York, PA) were negative. On the basis of these findings, the patient was diagnosed as having a large periradicular lesion in the left maxillary incisor with a necrosed pulp and an open apex.

At the first visit, root canal treatment was initiated on tooth #11 under rubber dam isolation, and the access cavity was prepared. Necrotic pulp tissue was extirpated, and the working length was estimated as being 1 mm short of the radiographic apex. The drainage of pus was noted. The cleaning shaping procedures were performed as described earlier. A calcium hydroxide paste (RC Cal; Prime Dental Products Pvt. Ltd., Thane, India) was placed using a size #40 Lentulo spiral (Maillefer, Ballaigues, Switzerland) to the working length and then rotated at 500 rpm using a hand-piece mounted on a speed and torque control machine (X-Smart, Dentsply, Tulsa Dental, Tulsa, OK, USA), as an intra-canal medicament for one week. Sterile cotton pellets were placed into the access cavity before sealing it with temporary filling material (Cavit, 3M/ESPE, Seefeld, Germany). When the patient reported back after 1 week, the tooth was seen

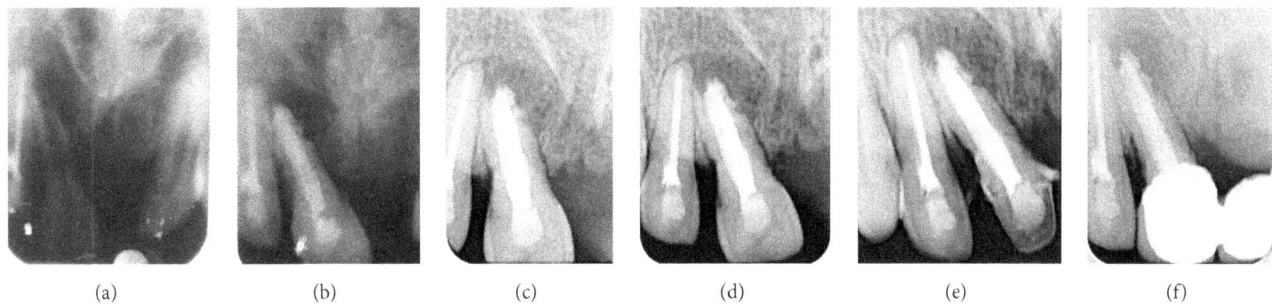

FIGURE 3: (a) Preoperative IOPA, (b) unintentional extrusion of MTA from apical foramen, (c) 1-month follow-up, (d) 2-month follow-up, (e) 3-month follow-up, and (f) 6-month follow-up.

to be asymptomatic. The tooth was reopened, and calcium hydroxide paste was removed. The canals were irrigated alternately with 5.25% NaOCl (Prime Dental Products Pvt. Ltd., Thane, India) and 17% EDTA (Prime Dental Products Pvt. Ltd., Thane, India) with a final rinse with normal saline solution and dried with sterile paper points. MTA apexification was performed as described earlier, but unintentionally a considerable amount of MTA was seen to have extruded into the periapical region, when checked on periapical radiograph (Figure 3(b)). A moistened cotton pellet was placed in the root canal and the patient was kept under observation for 15 days. The access cavity was sealed with temporary filling material (Cavit, 3M/ESPE, Seefeld, Germany). At the subsequent appointment, the cotton pellet was removed, and after verifying the clinical signs and symptoms and the set of the MTA, the remaining pulp space was obturated with gutta-percha (Dentsply Maillefer, Dentsply India Pvt. Ltd., Haryana) and AH Plus sealer (Dentsply; Detrey, Konstanz) by using the lateral condensation technique. The tooth was restored with a composite resin.

At the one-month follow-up appointment (Figure 3(c)), the tooth was asymptomatic. The 3- and 6-month follow-up periapical radiographs showed gradual healing of the periapical lesion along with resorption of the MTA (Figures 3(e) and 3(f)).

3. Discussion

The low cytotoxic potential of MTA explains its wide range of applications in endodontics [4]. It has been shown that the human osteoblasts were able to attach and proliferate on MTA surfaces, suggesting the suitable use of this material adjacent to bone [11]. In addition, MTA is responsible for induction of hydroxyapatite crystal on its surface on contact with tissue fluids, which makes it a bioactive material [12]. The material derives its biocompatibility, potential for hard-tissue induction and sealing ability from this phenomenon. Also, these characteristics make MTA a suitable material to be used for apexification.

For the present case series, undesirably so, during apexification procedure, an appreciable amount of MTA was extruded into the apical lesion. It may be contemplated that the wide apical foramen might have resulted in the dislodgement of MTA through it, or it might have been pushed

actively beyond apical foramen as a result of condensation pressure during placement. The healing outcomes of these three cases were very similar and favorable as compared to the materials that contain paraformaldehyde, calcium hydroxide, and/or eugenol. The outcomes of these present cases mirrored the results from animal studies as well [13].

In this case series, calcium hydroxide was used as an intracanal medicament before MTA placement to allow adequate disinfection of the root canal without the risk of compromised root strength. Researchers have proved that calcium hydroxide pastes do not significantly affect the seal-ability of MTA [14]. In contrast, other authors have suggested that the remnants of calcium hydroxide on the canal walls react to form calcium carbonate that can interfere with the seal [15]. The acidic pH has a negative influence on the setting characteristics of MTA [4]. In fact, the combination of MTA and calcium hydroxide in apexification procedures has been shown to favorably influence the regeneration of the periodontium [14].

The studies on the effectiveness of intracanal placement techniques of calcium hydroxide state that the most effective delivery of calcium hydroxide was achieved when the paste carriers were introduced to working length [16]. Therefore, in all the three cases described here, Lentulo spiral was used to deliver the intracanal medicament to the working length. The use of a Lentulo spiral in cases of large periapical lesions especially associated with teeth having wide apical diameters carries a risk of medicament extrusion. To avoid this, the rotation speed during the spiral filling technique was limited to 500 rpm. Hence, in none of the cases described here, calcium hydroxide was seen to be extruded, which was confirmed radiographically.

On the other hand, the use of calcium hydroxide as an intracanal medicament prior to MTA apexification has been related to the extrusion of the MTA material [15]. Therefore, use of calcium hydroxide might have resulted in the apical extrusion of the MTA material. Witherspoon and Ham [17] have reported successful and clinically effective one-visit MTA apexification procedures when MTA apical plug was placed with an orthograde approach, irrespective of the application of any internal matrix or intracanal medicament.

Although MTA is a nontoxic material, it should be restricted to the root canal space, and the condensation pressure is required to be considerably reduced in order to prevent MTA from being pushed beyond the apex [18]. A resorbable matrix has been suggested for the easy length control and for prevention of overfilling [19]. Calcium sulfate has been used as an internal matrix. However, the use of CollaPlug (Zimmer Dental, Warsaw, In, USA) as an apical matrix did not significantly prevent extrusion or improve the sealing ability of MTA [20].

It was demonstrated in this case series that there were no undue complications when MTA was applied as a root canal filling and extruded into the periradicular lesion associated with necrotic pulps. The teeth were continuously asymptomatic for the entire duration after the MTA filling was extruded. There was no complete resorption of the filling material, although gradual periradicular healing and slight resorption of extruded material were observed. Osseous repair was also noted. Indeed, the absence of clinical and radiographic symptoms justified the initial nonsurgical approach.

4. Conclusion

The clinical findings of the present cases imply evidence that MTA favors the apexification and periapical healing, even though a considerable amount of this material had unintentionally been extruded. The follow-up observations at 3- and 6-month intervals support the fact that the extruded material does not act as a hindrance for the healing of periapical tissues. The present case series also reinforces the importance of cautious placement of MTA apical plugs and does not recommend intentional overfilling of MTA into the periapical lesion in any clinical scenario. Revascularization procedures can be considered for such cases to obtain biological healing of the periradicular tissues, which would thereby eliminate the likelihood of material extrusion.

Competing Interests

The authors declare that there is no conflict of interests regarding the publication of this paper.

References

[1] M. Rafter, "Apexification: a review," Dental Traumatology, vol. 21, no. 1, pp. 1–8, 2005.

[2] R. Y. Ding, G. S.-P. Cheung, J. Chen, X. Z. Yin, Q. Q. Wang, and C. F. Zhang, "Pulp revascularization of immature teeth with apical periodontitis: a clinical study," Journal of Endodontics, vol. 35, no. 5, pp. 745–749, 2009.

[3] E. C. Sheehy and O. J. Roberts, "Use of calcium hydroxide for apical barrier formation and healing in non-vital immature permanent teeth: a review," British Dental Journal, vol. 183, no. 7, pp. 241–246, 1997.

[4] M. Torabinejad and N. Chivian, "Clinical applications of mineral trioxide aggregate," Journal of Endodontics, vol. 25, no. 3, pp. 197–205, 1999.

[5] S. Hatibovic-Kofman, L. Raimundo, L. Chong, J. Moreno, and L. Zheng, "Mineral trioxide aggregate in endodontic treatment for immature teeth," in Proceedings of the 28th Annual International Conference of the IEEE Engineering in Medicine and Biology Society (EMBS '06), pp. 2094–2097, 2006.

[6] H. Chng, I. Islam, A. Yap, Y. Tong, and E. Koh, "Properties of a new root-end filling material," Journal of Endodontics, vol. 31, no. 9, pp. 665–668, 2005.

[7] Y.-L. Lee, B.-S. Lee, F.-H. Lin, A. Yun Lin, W.-H. Lan, and C.-P. Lin, "Effects of physiological environments on the hydration behavior of mineral trioxide aggregate," Biomaterials, vol. 25, no. 5, pp. 787–793, 2004.

[8] M. S. Namazikhah, M. H. Nekoofar, M. S. Sheykhrezae et al., "The effect of pH on surface hardness and microstructure of mineral trioxide aggregate," International Endodontic Journal, vol. 41, no. 2, pp. 108–116, 2008.

[9] U. Sjögren, B. Hägglund, G. Sundqvist, and K. Wing, "Factors affecting the long-term results of endodontic treatment," Journal of Endodontics, vol. 16, no. 10, pp. 498–504, 1990.

[10] U. Sjögren, D. Figdor, S. Persson, and G. Sundqvist, "Influence of infection at the time of root filling on the outcome of endodontic treatment of teeth with apical periodontitis," International Endodontic Journal, vol. 30, no. 5, pp. 297–306, 1997.

[11] E. AL-Rabeah, H. Perinpanayagam, and D. MacFarland, "Human alveolar bone cells interact with ProRoot and tooth-colored MTA," Journal of Endodontics, vol. 32, no. 9, pp. 872–875, 2006.

[12] M. G. Gandolfi, P. Taddei, A. Tinti, and C. Prati, "Apatite-forming ability (bioactivity) of ProRoot MTA," International Endodontic Journal, vol. 43, no. 10, pp. 917–929, 2010.

[13] Y. M. Masuda, X. Wang, M. Hossain et al., "Evaluation of biocompatibility of mineral trioxide aggregate with an improved rabbit ear chamber," Journal of Oral Rehabilitation, vol. 32, no. 2, pp. 145–150, 2005.

[14] S. Asgary and S. Ehsani, "MTA resorption and periradicular healing in an open-apex incisor: a case report," The Saudi Dental Journal, vol. 24, no. 1, pp. 55–59, 2012.

[15] S. Stefopoulos, D. V. Tsatsas, N. P. Kerezoudis, and G. Eliades, "Comparative in vitro study of the sealing efficiency of white vs grey ProRoot mineral trioxide aggregate formulas as apical barriers," Dental Traumatology, vol. 24, no. 2, pp. 207–213, 2008.

[16] T. Zarra, T. Lambrianidis, and E. Kosti, "Comparative study of calcium hydroxide extrusion with different techniques of intracanal placement," Balkan Journal of Stomatology, vol. 15, no. 01, pp. 5–10, 2011.

[17] D. E. Witherspoon and K. Ham, "One-visit apexification: technique for inducing root-end barrier formation in apical closures," Practical Procedures & Aesthetic Dentistry, vol. 13, no. 6, pp. 455–462, 2001.

[18] M. H. Nekoofar, G. Adusei, M. S. Sheykhrezae, S. J. Hayes, S. T. Bryant, and P. M. H. Dummer, "The effect of condensation pressure on selected physical properties of mineral trioxide aggregate," International Endodontic Journal, vol. 40, no. 6, pp. 453–461, 2007.

[19] R. R. Lemon, "Nonsurgical repair of perforation defects. Internal matrix concept," Dental Clinics of North America, vol. 36, no. 2, pp. 439–457, 1992.

[20] L. Zou, J. Liu, S. Yin, W. Li, and J. Xie, "In vitro evaluation of the sealing ability of MTA used for the repair of furcation perforations with and without the use of an internal matrix," Oral Surgery, Oral Medicine, Oral Pathology, Oral Radiology, and Endodontology, vol. 105, no. 6, pp. e61–e65, 2008.

18

The Case for Improved Interprofessional Care: Fatal Analgesic Overdose Secondary to Acute Dental Pain during Pregnancy

Sarah K. Y. Lee,[1] **Rocio B. Quinonez,**[2] **Alice Chuang,**[3] **Stephanie M. Munz,**[4] **and Darya Dabiri**[4]

[1]*Department of Prosthodontics, School of Dentistry, University of North Carolina at Chapel Hill, Chapel Hill, NC, USA*
[2]*Department of Pediatric Dentistry and Pediatrics, Schools of Dentistry and Medicine, University of North Carolina at Chapel Hill, Chapel Hill, NC, USA*
[3]*Department of Obstetrics and Gynecology, School of Medicine, University of North Carolina at Chapel Hill, Chapel Hill, NC, USA*
[4]*Department of Oral and Maxillofacial Surgery/Hospital Dentistry, School of Dentistry, University of Michigan, Ann Arbor, MI, USA*

Correspondence should be addressed to Sarah K. Y. Lee; sarah_lee@unc.edu

Academic Editor: Asja Celebić

Prenatal oral health extends beyond the oral cavity, impacting the general well-being of the pregnant patient and her fetus. This case report follows a 19-year-old pregnant female presenting with acute liver failure secondary to acetaminophen overdose for management of dental pain following extensive dental procedures. Through the course of her illness, the patient suffered adverse outcomes including fetal demise, acute kidney injury, spontaneous bacterial peritonitis, and septic shock before eventual death from multiple organ failure. In managing the pregnant patient, healthcare providers, including physicians and dentists, must recognize and optimize the interconnected relationships shared by the health disciplines. An interdisciplinary approach of collaborative and coordinated care, the timing, sequence, and treatment for the pregnant patient can be improved and thereby maximize overall quality of health. Continued efforts toward integrating oral health into general healthcare education through interprofessional education and practice are necessary to enhance the quality of care that will benefit all patients.

1. Introduction

The pregnant dental patient exemplifies the need for collaborative practices between health disciplines. The latest national consensus statement regarding oral healthcare during pregnancy indicates patients can and should undergo routine dental treatment during all stages of pregnancy as "oral health care, including use of radiographs, pain medication, and local anesthesia, is safe throughout pregnancy" [1]. While treatment rendered during the second trimester provides the greatest comfort, pregnancy alone is not a contraindication to receiving dental treatment [1]. For some women, pregnancy may in fact provide the opportunity to pursue their oral healthcare needs [2, 3]. For example, some states' government assistance programs include dental care as a covered pregnancy-related service [4]. In 2000, the Children's Health Insurance Program extended coverage to include pregnant women who do not qualify for Medicaid [3].

Despite these progressive efforts to provide prenatal oral healthcare, inconsistencies between the knowledge and practices of dental and medical providers regarding prenatal oral healthcare remain. Pregnant patients continue to encounter barriers that may adversely affect their oral health and negatively impact their pregnancy [1–11]. This case report describes a sequence of events, precipitated by dental pain, in which lapses in patient oral health literacy, the rendering of dental treatment, and coordination of interprofessional collaborative treatment within the healthcare system culminated in the demise of both the fetus and pregnant patient.

2. Case Presentation

A 19-year-old at 17-week gestation presented to her local hospital's emergency department (ED) complaining of abdominal pain and nausea. She was diagnosed with acute liver failure secondary to acetaminophen overdose for dental pain management. The admission record indicated, as per patient report, that she had received dental treatment 2 weeks earlier, with the dentist reportedly prescribing 20 tablets of Tylenol #3 (acetaminophen with codeine) for postoperative pain. The patient initially took 1-2 tablets per day, but due to persisting symptoms, she communicated with her obstetrician who recommended over-the-counter Tylenol for pain management. The patient obtained Extra Strength Tylenol (500 mg acetaminophen/tablet) and for a 10-day period reported taking 2-3 tablets of Extra Strength Tylenol, 10 times per day, approximating 20–30 tablets daily or 10,000–15,000 mg daily. Preliminary ED laboratory studies indicated acute liver injury consisting of coagulopathy and abnormal transaminases with significantly elevated acetaminophen levels. To address the liver toxicity, N-acetylcysteine (NAC) protocol was initiated at the local ED and continued when the patient was transferred to a larger academic center's pediatric intensive care unit (ICU) (Table 1).

When transferred, a consultation with obstetrics and gynecology (ObGyn) was completed. A live singleton fetus had been initially confirmed by ultrasound; however, on reevaluation on her second day of hospitalization, no fetal cardiac activity was detected and fetal demise was diagnosed. The following day, a dental consultation was initiated due to the patient's complaint of pain on mastication of the right mandibular dentition. Clinical and radiographic examination initially revealed no emergent dental needs, and occlusal adjustments to alleviate symptoms were performed as the first course of action (Figure 1).

While undergoing care the patient was diagnosed with Wilson's disease, an autosomal recessive genetic disorder causing copper accumulation in tissues that can lead to further liver complications [12]. Her laboratory findings confirmed the abnormally elevated copper levels, which in addition to her acute liver injury from toxicity resulted in the recommendation for liver transplant. On day 9 of hospitalization, the delivery of the nonviable fetus was completed, and the patient's condition was reported as stable. At this time, a second dental consultation was ordered following the patient's report of a "bubble on [the] gum that popped."

The dental assessment revealed that tooth #30 (permanent right mandibular first molar) had a draining sinus tract. Two days following the diagnosis, prophylactic antibiotic management was initiated and a pulpectomy was scheduled and completed in the hospital's dental clinic under local anesthesia. On the scheduled treatment date, the patient reported not feeling well as she had not ingested solid food or substantial liquids for more than 12 hours, due to her *nil per os* (NPO) status as ordered by her medical care team. While this action resulted in delay of treatment, the pulpectomy was completed without complication that same afternoon. At this time, the dental team overseeing the patient's care discussed the previously rendered treatment with the patient's general dentist via telephone. The following dental treatment had been reportedly completed in a single appointment by the general dentist and was documented in the patient's electronic record: dental restorations on 7 teeth (#12, 13, 16,

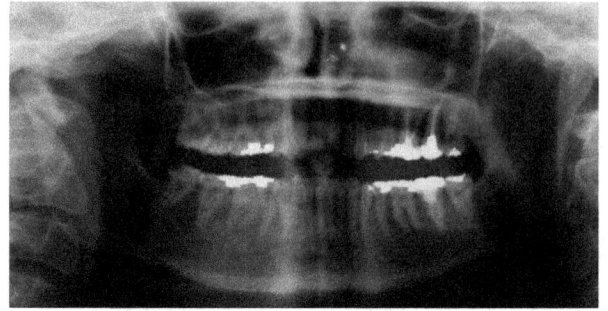

FIGURE 1: Panoramic radiograph of the patient's dental condition on day 15 of first hospitalization.

17, 19, 20, and 21), 3 root canal therapies (#14, 15, and 18), and placement of 2 stainless steel crowns. Further requests were made to the dentist to share treatment records with the hospital dentistry team. To date, these records have not been received.

Dental clearance evaluation and any necessary treatment in preparation for a liver transplant were requested by the patient's medical team. The following treatment was then recommended: endodontic therapy of pulpal necrosis with sinus tract of tooth #30, extraction of tooth #14 (permanent left maxillary molar) due to nonrestorability, and extraction of maxillary and mandibular third molars (teeth #1, 16, 17, and 32) due to impaction causing operculi and periodontal complications. The patient was subsequently discharged from the hospital with plans to address dental treatment needs and management of liver failure by the respective care teams on an outpatient basis.

One week after discharge, the patient was readmitted to the ED for pelvic pain that had been worsening for 3 days. She disclosed, as documented on her electronic record, a lack of compliance with the prescribed medication regimen "as she does not know what these medications do." Treatment for spontaneous bacterial peritonitis (SBP) was initiated by the gastroenterology (GE) team but was discontinued after 2 days due to lack of correlation of signs and symptoms observed from laboratory studies and patient history. During this stay, a dental follow-up evaluation was completed. The patient reported being asymptomatic for any oral pain and, upon clinical examination, the draining sinus tract adjacent to tooth #30 had resolved. No emergent needs were evident. The patient was discharged after a 4-day hospitalization.

Three days after her second hospitalization, the patient presented to the dental outpatient clinic for completion of endodontic therapy for tooth #30 and consultation with the oral and maxillofacial surgery (OMFS) service for extractions of third molars and tooth #14 under general anesthesia. Endodontic therapy was completed in the dental clinic without complication and the patient was scheduled to return to complete other indicated restorative treatments. The extractions were completed in the operating room under general anesthesia by the OMFS service the same week without complications.

TABLE 1: Summary of the patient's course of illness.

Date		Event
2 weeks before hospitalization		Patient obtains dental care. Her dental provider prescribed 20 tabs of Tylenol 3 for pain management. Patient takes 1-2 tabs/day but pain persists. She contacts her obstetrician who advises OTC acetaminophen for pain management. Patient obtains Extra Strength Tylenol (500 mg acetaminophen/tab) and takes 2-3 tabs, 10 times/day for last 10 days (20–30 tabs/day).
	Day 1	Patient presents to local emergency department (ED) for abdominal pain and nausea. Diagnosis of acute liver injury is assessed. N-Acetylcysteine (NAC) treatment is initiated.
	Day 2	Patient transferred to pediatric ICU and liver management continued via NAC protocol. Obstetrics and gynecology (ObGyn) team identifies live singleton fetus via ultrasound.
	Day 3	Undetectable fetal heart sounds or fetal movement by ObGyn. Fetal demise diagnosis is made.
	Day 4	Patient reports pain on mastication of right posterior dentition. Hospital dentistry (HD) consult is requested by patient's care team.
	Day 5	HD consultation completed. Clinical examination reveals no indication for emergent interventional dental treatment. Palliative treatment is rendered via occlusal adjustment.
First hospitalization	Day 7	Wilson's disease diagnosis made. The patient continues undergoing management of acute liver injury.
	Day 10	Delivery of nonviable fetus performed.
	Day 13	Patient reports "bubble on gum that popped" but is asymptomatic. HD consultation completed and reveals tooth #30 (right mandibular molar) has draining sinus tract. Pulpectomy performed on tooth #30 in hospital dental clinic. Dental needs for liver transplant clearance are assessed and scheduled for treatment on an outpatient basis.
	Day 15	Patient's original dentist is contacted via telephone and relays that patient received dental treatment of 10 left posterior teeth, including root canal therapy on 3 molars in 1 visit. Patient discharged from hospital.
6 days after hospitalization		
	Day 1	Patient presents to ED for worsening and persistent pelvic pain. Patient admitted for management with Gastroenterology (GE) team and spontaneous bacterial peritonitis (SBP) treatment is initiated and paracentesis completed.
Second hospitalization	Day 2	HD consultation for post-pulpectomy follow-up. Patient's dental condition is stable and patient is scheduled for further dental management on an outpatient basis.
	Day 3	SBP treatment discontinued.
	Day 5	Patient discharged from hospital.
13 days after hospitalization	Day 3	Oral maxillofacial surgery (OMFS) consultation is completed for extractions under general anesthesia.
	Day 6	OMFS completes dental treatment under general anesthesia (teeth 1, 14, 16, 17, and 32 extracted).
Third hospitalization	Day 1	Patient presents to ED for abdominal pain, nausea, and diarrhea. Patient admitted to adult ICU.
	Day 2	Patient's condition deteriorates and patient is intubated. Patient diagnosed with portal hypertensive gastropathy and ascites.
	Day 3	Continued management of liver complications including paracentesis and esophagogastroduodenoscopy (diagnostic endoscopic procedure for visualization of upper portion of GI tract).
	Day 5	Patient's condition stabilizes and patient is extubated.
	Day 9	Paracentesis completed with 4 L of fluid removal.
	Day 10	Patient has an episode of unresponsiveness to sternal rub, requiring 1.2 IV Narcan administration before patient's mental status returns. This incident is attributed to Phenergan sedation.
	Day 17	Patient discharged from hospital.

TABLE 1: Continued.

Date	Event
6 days after hospitalization	Patient admitted to local ED after found unresponsive at home.
Day 1	Patient transferred to adult ICU and is intubated.
	Patient diagnosed for septic shock secondary to SBP.
	Patient diagnosed for cardiac ischemia with development of nonsustained ventricular tachycardia. Multiorgan failure is observed.
Fourth hospitalization	
Day 3	Patient shows intermittent prolonged unstable arrhythmia with ventricular fibrillation and hypotension.
	Patient's care team discusses poor prognosis with family.
Day 4	Patient dies.

Three days following the extractions, the patient reported a three-day history of abdominal pain, nausea, and diarrhea. Laboratory studies indicated evidence of leukocytosis, resulting in admission to the hospital's adult ICU. The patient was newly diagnosed with portal hypertensive gastropathy with ascites, due to portal hypertension with SBP. Complications led to degradation of her condition requiring intubation and broad-spectrum antibiotic therapy. After one week, her condition stabilized and she was extubated. Paracentesis was completed to remove 4 liters of fluid. An isolated episode of unresponsiveness to sternal rubbing occurred. This was managed by administration of 1.2 mg IV Narcan and later attributed to Phenergan sedation. After 2.5-week hospitalization, the patient was discharged.

The following week, the patient was found to be unresponsive at her home and was readmitted to the ICU. She was observed to be significantly obtunded and jaundiced with distended abdomen and remained minimally responsive. She was eventually diagnosed with septic shock secondary to SBP with new onset of acute kidney injury and hypotension. The option to use continuous renal replacement therapy was declined by the patient's family. On day 2 of her ICU stay, cardiac ischemia was evident with development of nonsustained ventricular tachycardia. She developed intermittent prolonged unstable arrhythmia with ventricular fibrillation and hypotension. The maximum amount of norepinephrine was administered to counter hypotension and heart failure. After the care team discussed the patient's poor prognosis, her family decided to halt further life-sustaining measures. After a 3-day ICU course, the patient died.

3. Discussion

Consolidated guidelines have been established by both separate and collaborative medical and dental organizations to foster and support care integration, particularly for pregnant patients [1, 5]. Provision of prenatal oral healthcare must be managed in a safe and appropriate manner. The quantity of rendered treatment and the postoperative complications prompted the initiation of this patient's course of illness and may have contributed to exacerbation of liver symptoms in conjunction with her unknown, preexisting condition of Wilson's disease. Dentists provide expertise and means for diagnosing, planning, treating, and educating the patient to optimize oral health. With the provision of dental care, the health risks and benefits of providing an extensive amount of invasive treatment, regardless of the patient's pregnancy status, must be considered. For the pregnant patient, it is critical to assess the impact of dental treatment during pregnancy in terms of priority (emergent versus routine), quantity, timeliness, medications involved in rendering treatment, ergonomics while undergoing treatment, and management of posttreatment complications, including pain. It is especially critical that the pregnant patient obtains treatment when she presents with an acute odontogenic infection, as delays can carry greater risks than those associated with exposure to treatment and medications required for management. The use of local anesthetic, modalities of sedation, and analgesia in the pregnant patient has been complex and controversial

[9]. National consensus statements and recent studies have rendered many of these modalities safe when used properly, in consultation with the prenatal provider when needed [1, 5, 9, 13].

Medical providers also contribute expertise to the pregnant patient's oral healthcare. Just as dental providers must take the modifications and potential complications associated with rendering dental care of any patient into consideration, medical providers must also address the oral health needs that may arise in their own patient management. As a provider who also consistently manages the patient throughout her pregnancy, the medical provider is able to identify the need for the patient to be referred for dental care [1, 5, 7, 8, 10]. The medical provider serves as a source of disseminated information that may encourage prevention and early intervention of oral health problems such that these problems and their consequences can be better managed [1, 5]. This provider can also communicate with the dental provider on systemic health considerations such that care can be rendered safely [1, 5].

Evidence-based dental management of the pregnant patient continues to be practiced inconsistently [1, 7, 8, 10, 11, 14–16]. Many pregnant patients are still unable to find a dental provider willing to treat them due to remaining misconceptions regarding oral healthcare. Concerns of unfounded risks to the fetus with dental treatment heighten issues of premature induction labor, lack of knowledge in the safety of treatment, and potential legal risks if negative birth outcomes occur [4, 6, 8, 10, 11]. These are commonly perceived deterrents [8, 10]. Limitations based on incorrect or insufficient knowledge of perinatal oral healthcare by the treating dentist have been shown to have the strongest direct effect on preventing pregnant patients from obtaining dental care [11]. Dentist-imposed barriers to accessing reasonable care can lead to deleterious effects and create greater risk management issues.

Medical professionals have similar hesitations when addressing their pregnant patients' dental status. General health practitioners, midwives, and obstetricians reported their lack of knowledge in understanding the safety of prenatal dental treatment as the most significant limitation [10]. These providers also reported feeling unqualified to address dental issues due to insufficient familiarity and knowledge on oral health topics [8], highlighting the importance of proper training and the need to address these topics in medical and dental curricula. Many educational institutions among the health disciplines exhibit organizational infrastructure, logistical barriers, and isolated education that continue to support a discord at odds with current recommendations [13–15, 17].

While each profession maintains management practices specific to its discipline, it is significant to acknowledge the interrelatedness of the health professions and how care coordination impacts the pregnant patient's overall health. Pregnancy, as a sensitive period in which compromises in oral-systemic health can readily occur, typifies the importance of establishing and maintaining coordination between medicine and dentistry as well as other healthcare professions. Adverse outcomes occur as a result of discordant care among the health disciplines. Pregnant patients and their fetuses are placed at greater risks when preventive and intervening therapies are not provided in a timely and appropriate manner [1, 4]. In this case, for example, the patient's unnecessary placement on NPO status revealed a misunderstanding and lack of communication between the teams coordinating her care. As a result, the patient's treatment was delayed due to her poor disposition. Additionally, missed opportunities for collaboration reinforced the separation of health disciplines and the notion of integrated general health in the mindsets of both providers and patients.

It is important to recognize that while healthcare providers carry many responsibilities in managing a patient's health, the patient is also an active participant in the outcomes that emerge from care. Acetaminophen, a perinatal-appropriate pain medication with a recommended maximum dosage of 4 g in a 24-hour period [18], was independently prescribed by her medical and dental providers, but misused by the patient. This misuse led to an overdose that precipitated the adverse chain of events. As a first-time pregnant, low-income adolescent, this patient belonged to a population that is more susceptible to adverse health outcomes resulting from low health literacy, defined as the "degree to which people have the capacity to obtain, process, and understand basic health information and services that are needed to make appropriate health decisions" [6, 7]. Low health literacy has been associated with poorer health knowledge that can be attributed to poorer health behaviors and outcomes [6, 7, 19]. While undergoing care to manage complications that resulted from the overdose, this patient exhibited noncompliant behavior that further compromised treatment. These key instances reflect a misunderstanding and misuse on the patient's part of the information and resources available to her.

Health literacy is not wholly dictated by the patient's individual characteristics such as socioeconomic status and level of education; the degree of literacy is influenced by established systems of communication for information dissemination and patient education [19, 20]. Social and cultural misconceptions about undergoing care during pregnancy [13] and the lack of awareness of their oral health status and its impact on their pregnancy and general health [4, 8] are contributing barriers that prevent patients from accessing and utilizing care.

Healthcare entails the overall management of the well-being of a patient in aspects of education, treatment, and maintenance. Historically, dentistry has been a very separate branch of healthcare [13–17, 21], practiced on different educational infrastructure, clinical management, and financial models more than medicine [16]. Unfortunately, the disparities in care that have resulted from persisting separation of disciplines are still evident in modern day healthcare practices.

Efforts to integrate dentistry with other health professions have increased with recognition of oral health implications in general health by the medical community, development of collaborative medical-dental training, and incorporation of oral health in medical settings. Unfortunately these efforts remain limited in the educational arena, in part because of the segmented and isolated educational systems between the health branches that have fostered gaps in knowledge and clinical practice between oral and general health [22, 23].

A survey of US dental school indicated a willingness by educators to incorporate prenatal oral health, but clinical experiences remain limited. Barriers included lack of pregnant patients and faculty expertise [24]. Similarly in Canadian dental schools, only 40% of schools report having designated time in their curriculum to cover this topic [25]. Initiatives such as the Prenatal Oral Health Program (pOHP) at the University of North Carolina show promise in helping educate the next generation of providers in a collaborative approach in practice and thereby, improve the quality of rendered care and patient outcomes [26, 27].

Standardization of coordinated care within clinical and educational institutions is likely to be a prolonged process where results may not be rapidly realized. Attitudinal and behavioral practice changes of dental providers to address the needs of high risk populations for adverse health outcomes, as well as prioritizing collaborative efforts with healthcare colleagues and educational initiatives across health professional schools, are essential for tangible, meaningful progress in oral health disparities to occur.

4. Conclusion

This case highlights how practice misconceptions, barriers in collaborative care and communication, and insufficient health literacy are interconnected and complicated by one another. Though specific to the pregnant dental patient, this case offers lessons that can be readily translated to any type of patient, especially other susceptible populations, including the frail elderly, patients with medical complexity, and those with disabilities. Oral health is one part that contributes to overall health. As such, it is important to recognize that a patient's well-being relies on the coordinated efforts of all the health disciplines. This case report highlights some of the challenges of incorporating dental and medical practices within the current healthcare environment. Most prevalent of these issues were the dental and medical providers' inconsistencies in patient management, the segmented, noncollaborative infrastructure of communication and care coordination between these providers, and the patient's lack of knowledge and understanding of her health status. The coordinated efforts between specialties made in the latter part of this patient's care are evidence that collaboration, albeit challenging, is readily possible and critically necessary. Greater emphases on interprofessional education, practice, and systems changes are needed to help address some of the current clinical challenges and disconnects among healthcare professions.

Abbreviations

ED: Emergency department
NAC: N-Acetylcysteine
ICU: Intensive care unit
ObGyn: Obstetrics and gynecology
NPO: Nil per os

SBP: Spontaneous bacterial peritonitis
GE: Gastroenterology
OMFS: Oral and maxillofacial surgery.

Competing Interests

The authors declare that there is no conflict of interests regarding the publication of this paper.

Acknowledgments

The authors gratefully acknowledge Rachel Tambunan Chu, DDS, Si On Lim, DDS, Jayashree Srinivasan, DMD, and Carol Wiese, DDS for their clinical contributions.

References

[1] Oral Health Care During Pregnancy Expert Workgroup, *Oral Health Care During Pregnancy: A National Consensus Statement—Summary of an Expert Workgroup Meeting*, National Maternal and Child Oral Health Resource Center, Washington, DC, USA, 2012.

[2] M. L. Gaffield, B. J. Colley Gilbert, D. M. Malvitz, and R. Romaguera, "Oral health during pregnancy: an analysis of information collected by the pregnancy risk assessment monitoring system," *Journal of the American Dental Association*, vol. 132, no. 7, pp. 1009–1016, 2001.

[3] National Health Law Program, "Dental Coverage for Low-Income Pregnant Women," http://www.healthlaw.org/publications/dental-coverage-for-low-income-pregnant-women#VNje11XF-1A.

[4] K. A. Boggess and B. L. Edelstein, "Oral health in women during preconception and pregnancy: implications for birth outcomes and infant oral health," *Maternal and Child Health Journal*, vol. 10, supplement 1, pp. 169–174, 2006.

[5] American Academy of Pediatric Dentistry Guidelines on Perinatal Oral Health Care, "Academy of pediatric dentistry council on clinical affairs. Adopted 2009," *Journal of Pediatric Dentistry*, vol. 35, no. 6, pp. 131–136, 2013.

[6] J. M. Horn, J. Y. Lee, K. Divaris, A. D. Baker, and W. F. Vann Jr., "Oral health literacy and knowledge among patients who are pregnant for the first time," *Journal of the American Dental Association*, vol. 143, no. 9, pp. 972–980, 2012.

[7] US Department of Health and Human Services (USDHHS), *Healthy People 2010: Understanding and Improving Health*, US Department of Health and Human Services (USDHHS), Washington, DC, USA, 2000.

[8] A. George, S. Shamim, M. Johnson et al., "How do dental and prenatal care practitioners perceive dental care during pregnancy? Current evidence and implications," *Birth*, vol. 39, no. 3, pp. 238–247, 2012.

[9] M. Turner and S. R. Aziz, "Management of the pregnant oral and maxillofacial surgery patient," *Journal of Oral and Maxillofacial Surgery*, vol. 60, no. 12, pp. 1479–1488, 2002.

[10] K. E. Strafford, C. Shellhaas, and E. M. Hade, "Provider and patient perceptions about dental care during pregnancy," *The Journal of Maternal-Fetal & Neonatal Medicine*, vol. 21, no. 1, pp. 63–71, 2008.

[11] M. Le, C. Riedy, P. Weinstein, and P. Milgrom, "Barriers to utilization of dental services during pregnancy: a qualitative analysis," *Journal of Dentistry for Children*, vol. 76, no. 1, pp. 46–52, 2009.

[12] National Digestive Diseases Information Clearinghouse (US) and National Institute of Diabetes and Digestive and Kidney Diseases (US), *Wilson Disease*, US Department of Health and Human Services, National Institutes of Health, National Institute of Diabetes and Digestive and Kidney Diseases, Bethesda, Md, USA, 2009.

[13] A. Hagai, O. Diav-Citrin, S. Shechtman, and A. Ornoy, "Pregnancy outcome after in utero exposure to local anesthetics as part of dental treatment: a prospective comparative cohort study," *Journal of the American Dental Association*, vol. 146, no. 8, pp. 572–580, 2015.

[14] R. S. Gambhir, "Primary care in dentistry—an untapped potential," *Journal of Family Medicine and Primary Care*, vol. 4, no. 1, pp. 13–18, 2015.

[15] Institute of Medicine (U.S.), *Committee on an Oral Health Initiative. Institute of Medicine (U.S.). Board on Health Care Services. Advancing Oral Health in America*, National Academies Press, Washington, DC, USA, 2011.

[16] J. H. Berg and W. E. Mouradian, "Integration of dentistry and medicine and the dentist of the future: changes in dental education," *Journal of the California Dental Association*, vol. 42, no. 10, pp. 697–700, 2014.

[17] Interprofessional Education Collaborative Expert Panel, *Core Competencies for Interprofessional Collaborative Practice: Report of an Expert Panel*, Interprofessional Education Collaborative Expert Panel, Washington, DC, USA, 2011.

[18] D. W. Kaufman, J. P. Kelly, J. M. Rohay, M. K. Malone, R. B. Weinstein, and S. Shiffman, "Prevalence and correlates of exceeding the labeled maximum dose of acetaminophen among adults in a U.S.-based internet survey," *Pharmacoepidemiology and Drug Safety*, vol. 21, no. 12, pp. 1280–1288, 2012.

[19] A. M. Horowitz and D. V. Kleinman, "Oral health literacy: a pathway to reducing oral health disparities in Maryland," *Journal of Public Health Dentistry*, vol. 72, no. 1, pp. S26–S30, 2012.

[20] Y. Guo, H. L. Logan, V. J. Dodd, K. E. Muller, J. G. Marks, and J. L. Riley III, "Health literacy: a pathway to better oral health," *American Journal of Public Health*, vol. 104, no. 7, pp. e85–e91, 2014.

[21] U.S. Department of Health and Human Services Health Resources and Services Administration, "Integration of Oral Health and Primary Care Practice," http://www.hrsa.gov/publichealth/clinical/oralhealth/primarycare/.

[22] R. S. Wilder, J. A. O'Donnell, J. M. Barry et al., "Is dentistry at risk? A case for interprofessional education," *Journal of Dental Education*, vol. 72, no. 11, pp. 1231–1237, 2008.

[23] D. W. Paquette, K. P. Bell, C. Phillips, S. Offenbacher, and R. S. Wilder, "Dentists' knowledge and opinions of oral-systemic disease relationships: relevance to patient care and education," *Journal of Dental Education*, vol. 79, no. 6, pp. 626–635, 2015.

[24] M. Curtis, H. J. Silk, and J. A. Savageau, "Prenatal oral health education in U.S. dental schools and obstetrics and gynecology residencies," *Journal of Dental Education*, vol. 77, no. 11, pp. 1461–1468, 2013.

[25] R. J. Schroth, R. B. Quiñonez, A. B. Yaffe, M. F. Bertone, F. K. Hardwick, and R. L. Harrison, "What are Canadian dental professional students taught about infant, toddler and prenatal oral health," *Journal of the Canadian Dental Association*, vol. 81, p. f15, 2015.

[26] R. B. Quinonez and K. Boggess, "Virtual Prenatal Oral Health
     Program Website," University of North Carolina at Chapel Hill,
     2013, http://www.prenataloralhealth.org/.

[27] J. T. Jackson, R. B. Quinonez, A. K. Kerns et al., "Implementing a
     prenatal oral health program through interprofessional collab-
     oration," *Journal of Dental Education*, vol. 79, no. 3, pp. 241–248,
     2015.

19

Simplifying the Treatment of Bone Atrophy in the Posterior Regions: Combination of Zygomatic and Wide-Short Implants—A Case Report with 2 Years of Follow-Up

Fernanda Faot,[1] Geninho Thomé,[2] Amália Machado Bielemann,[3] Caio Hermann,[2] Ana Cláudia Moreira Melo,[2] Luis Eduardo Marques Padovan,[2] and Ivete Aparecida de Mattias Sartori[2]

[1]School of Dentistry, Federal University of Pelotas (UFPEL), Pelotas, RS, Brazil
[2]Implantology Team, Latin American Institute of Dental Research and Education (ILAPEO), Curitiba, PR, Brazil
[3]Graduate Program in Dentistry, School of Dentistry, Federal University of Pelotas, Pelotas, RS, Brazil

Correspondence should be addressed to Fernanda Faot; fernanda.faot@gmail.com

Academic Editor: Gerardo Gómez-Moreno

The rehabilitation of maxillary and mandibular bone atrophy represents one of the main challenges of modern oral implantology because it requires a variety of procedures, which not only differ technically, but also differ in their results. In the face of limitations such as deficiencies in the height and thickness of the alveolar structure, prosthetic rehabilitation has sought to avoid large bone reconstruction through bone grafting; this clinical behavior has become a treatment system based on evidence from clinical scientific research. In the treatment of atrophic maxilla, the use of zygomatic implants has been safely applied as a result of extreme technical rigor and mastery of this surgical skill. For cases of posterior mandibular atrophy, short implants with a large diameter and a combination of short and long implants have been recommended to improve biomechanical resistance. These surgical alternatives have demonstrated a success rate similar to that of oral rehabilitation with the placing of conventional implants, allowing the adoption of immediate loading protocol, a decrease in morbidity, simplification and speed of the treatment, and cost reduction. This case report presents complete oral rehabilitation in a patient with bilateral bone atrophy in the posterior regions of the maxilla and mandible with the goal of developing and increasing posterior occlusal stability during immediate loading.

1. Introduction

The osseointegrated implants to support fixed prostheses revolutionized the rehabilitation treatment of totally and partially edentulous patients. However, in clinical situations where there is limited bone availability, the surgeon must often resort to bone grafting procedures, which prolong treatment time and increase cost and morbidity [1–3].

Bone graft reconstruction techniques inevitably present a component of risk because they require a precise surgical technique, a good quality of soft tissues that overlie the graft, patient cooperation, and general good health that favors recovery [4]. As these conditions are not always present in a single patient, complications such as graft contamination or exposure can lead to partial or total loss of the graft, resulting

in an unsuccessful treatment that may include deleterious effects [5]. Even in cases where the treatment evolves without major complications and the possibility of installing a fixed prosthesis is given a favorable prognosis, doubts still remain in relation to both the stability of the results and the maintenance of the bone structure and soft tissues [6].

With regard to these problems, clinical strategies have been proposed to increase the success rate of implants installed in critical sites of bone atrophy that include the use of short implants with a wide diameter [7, 8], implants with a rough surface that increases the contact between the bone and the implant [9, 10], an increase in the number of implants [11–13], and even a combination of short and long implants to improve the biomechanical resistance to tension and occlusal forces [14–16].

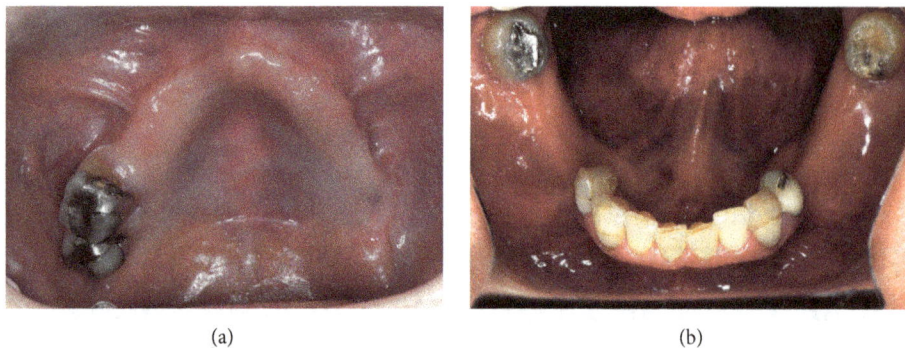

(a)   (b)

FIGURE 1: Clinical view at the initial appointment. Occlusal view of maxillary (a) and mandibular arch (b).

Especially for posterior maxilla atrophy rehabilitation, the development and use of zygomatic implant [17–21] in conjunction with conventional accessory implants on the anterior region has proven a viable alternative [22–24] because it simplifies treatment by using less invasive surgeries and reduces the cost and time of treatment. In addition, this treatment has demonstrated a favorable prognosis and a success rate similar to that of conventional implants [25, 26].

Regarding this scenario, the purpose of this clinical case report is to present and discuss the biomechanical aspects related to oral rehabilitation in a patient with bilateral bone atrophy in the posterior regions of the maxilla and mandible with the goal of developing and increasing posterior occlusal stability during immediate loading.

2. Case Report

Patient I.M.S. (female, 50 years old) checked into ILAPEO (*Latin American Institute of Research and Education in Dentistry*) to undergo oral rehabilitation treatment. The patient presented with a good state of general health with partial edentulism of the upper and lower jaw (Figure 1(a)) and with removable partial prostheses. In the upper jaw, she had a provisional partial prosthesis and, in the lower jaw, a class III removable partial denture was seated on the third molars in an unfavorable position by distal retainers. The patient's main complaint was the lack of stability, retention of the upper removable partial denture, the positioning of the lower third molars, the sensitivity of element 34 due to little bone support, and the difficulty of using the inferior prosthesis, which frequently injured the adjacent soft tissues. After clinical and radiographic analysis by panoramic radiography (Figure 2), poor bone availability in the maxilla and posterior mandible was observed and additionally a computed tomography was requested to plan the case in greater detail (Figure 3). Due to the extreme maxillary atrophy in the right side (including a radiographic image suggesting oral-antral communication), the indication for reconstructive procedures did not have a favorable prognosis as it can be also observed in the 3D reconstruction image (Figure 4). For this case, an anchoring technique combining conventional and zygomatic implants could be an alternative solution for rehabilitation; extraction of elements 25 and 26 was suggested and was subsequently accepted by the patient. In the lower arch, the extraction of

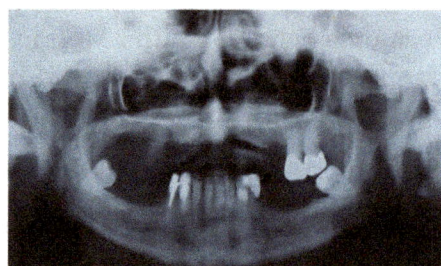

FIGURE 2: Panoramic radiograph from the initial examination.

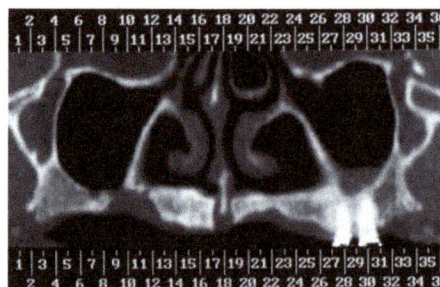

FIGURE 3: Computed tomography of maxilla. Distance between reconstructions: 3 mm.

elements 38, 34, and 48 was also indicated together with a combination of screw retained fixed partial dentures (FPDs).

Prior to the installation of the implants, a prosthetic preparation was performed and included the recording and assembly of the upper teeth performed on a trial basis without anterior vestibular coverage to diagnose the lip support that the FPD would provide. With the patient's approval, this diagnostic assemblage was duplicated, and a multifunctional guide was obtained.

In the atrophic maxilla, to install the zygomatic implants, an intravenous general anesthesia was induced along with preparation for surgery using a local anesthetic based on 2% lidocaine hydrochloride with adrenaline at 1:100,000. Two zygomatic implants (Neodent Implante Osseointegrável, Curitiba, PR, Brazil) of 45 mm were installed with rotation around 800 rpm and their respective prosthetic abutments of 3.0 mm were installed and tightened using a mechanical

(a)

(b)

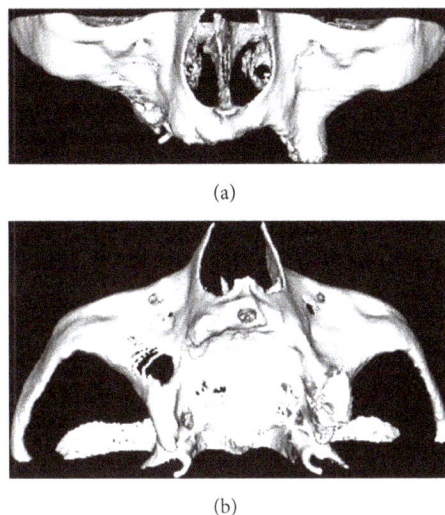

FIGURE 4: Maxilla 3D reconstruction in frontal (a) and occlusal view (b).

FIGURE 5: Wide-short implants installed at the bone level.

torque limiter with 20 N/cm. In addition, to guarantee the Roy Polygon creation orientating the force distribution in the maxilla, four cylindrical implants (Titamax Cone Morse, Neodent Implante Osteointegrável, Curitiba, PR, Brazil) were also installed with diameter of 3.75 mm and a length of 9 mm for elements 11 and 21, 11 mm for element 22, and 13 mm for element 13. The clamping obtained a torque greater than 45 N/cm, showing primary stability that was sufficient for the use of immediate load in the maxilla. Besides, the impression was performed using the multifunctional guide technique, which consists of joining the guide to the impression posts that were previously splinted using self-curing acrylic resin (Pattern Resin, GC America, IL, USA). Afterwards, the interocclusal record was refined by using three points of self-curing acrylic resin after confirming the vertical occlusal dimensions provided by the multifunctional guide record and the material injected between the transferors by a molding syringe. After polymerization of the materials, the screws of the impression posts were loosened, and the multifunctional guide, which had functioned as a molding tray and an interocclusal record, was renewed and taken to the prosthetic laboratory to manufacture a full arch fixed implant-supported prosthesis. Afterwards, the prosthesis was installed with immediate load protocol.

Within the lower posterior edentulous spaces on both sides, cylindrical implants were installed (Titamax CM, Neodent Implante Osteointegrável, Curitiba, PR, Brazil) combined with shorter and wider implants (Titamax WS, Neodent Implante Osseointegrável, Curitiba, PR, Brazil) in the distal ends because of mandibular bone atrophy in these areas. In this case, they were installed with the goal of increasing posterior occlusal stability, avoiding the use of distal cantilevers, and favoring a more uniform distribution of occlusal charges during chewing. These short implants with wide diameter platforms for the cortical bone have the advantage that their cervical diameters correspond to the diameter of the implant's body, favoring the uniform distribution of occlusal charges during chewing. Moreover,

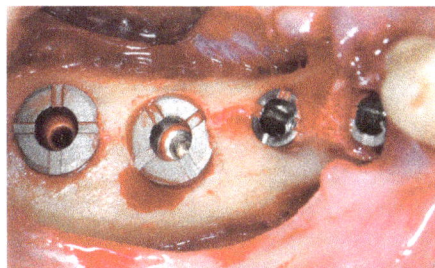

the high cutting power of their angled tips follows the exact same path as that of the pilot drill tip, providing a perfectly fitted installation at the site of the implant and avoiding empty spaces. Specifically, these implants were maintained around 2 mm under the future gingival margin towards the cement enamel junction.

The surgical sequences for perforation to install the conventional implants followed the conventional protocol of progressive diameters with rotation around 1500 rpm and 300 rpm for short implants under abundant irrigation, paying attention to the mesiodistal and buccolingual position of the implant. The conventional cylindrical implants installed had a diameter of 3.75 mm and a width ranging from 7 to 17 mm: 7 mm for elements 36 and 45, 15 mm for element 44, and 17 mm for element 35. Due to a limitation of bone height in the posterior extremity, short implants were installed with a length of 5 mm and a diameter of 5 mm for the region corresponding to element 36 and of 6 mm for the 37 and 47 regions (Figure 5).

Primary stability was also obtained in the mandibular arch and the heights of the mini conical pillars were selected (WS CM, Neodent Implante Osseointegrável, Curitiba, PR, Brazil) and installed (Figure 6) using a torque of 32 N·cm. Afterwards, the impression of the lower arch was made using a perforating tray after installing the square impression posts for mini conical pillars that were splinted using self-curing acrylic resin.

After obtaining the impression (Speedex Light Body, Coltene, Vigodent SA Indústria e Comércio, RJ, Brazil) two provisional partial lower fixed dentures in acrylic resin were constructed. During the installation of the fixed dentures, periapical radiographs were performed in both sides and an occlusal adjustment was performed to establish simultaneous bilateral occlusal contacts in relation to the centric occlusion and the anterior guide. Procedures for the definitive lower prostheses were performed at the same time in both sides after three months and consisted of the following: obtaining a new impression, performing a radiographic test and evaluation of the metallic infrastructures, and registering the interocclusal record. Subsequently, a ceramic trial was performed and partial fixed denture prostheses (FDPs) were installed using a torque of 10 N·cm in the prosthetic screws (Figures 7 and 8). The occlusal adjustment also aimed to establish a mutually protected occlusion. The final periapical radiographic preservation (Figure 9) and 2 years of follow-up can be observed in the panoramic radiographic (Figure 10).

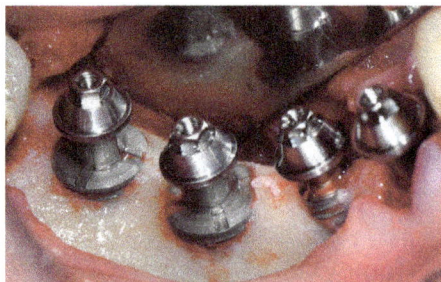

FIGURE 6: Abutments for multiple prosthesis installed during the surgery.

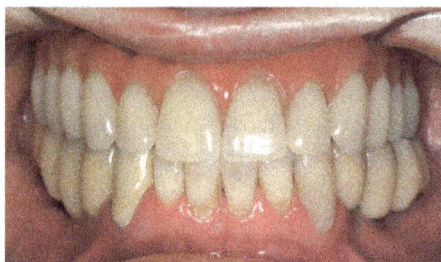

FIGURE 7: Frontal view of final restoration.

3. Discussion

The implants used in this clinical study have a morse taper connection. These implants have prosthetic abutments with a concave format design, associated with various biological advantages such as the preservation of the peri-implant bone and improved soft tissue quality [27]. The concave part of the prosthetic abutment allows the collagen fibers to fill the created space, resulting in a fabric necklace that will act as an effective attachment for connective tissue.

Prosthetic advantages ensure better stability of the prosthetic component and improvement in the biological aspect to reduce bone loss. The better mechanical stability and fixation of the prosthesis reduce rotational movement, resulting in higher resistance to screw loosening. It also reduces the clearance between the implant and the middle pillar and improves the junction and the implant abutment's bacterial seal [27]. However, this system also has some disadvantages. It demands greater accuracy in the preparation of the surgical bed and larger surgical care and there is less versatility with respect to prosthetic components for external hexagon connections [28].

Although the zygomatic implant technique is not considered a simple and common procedure in the clinical practice [17, 18, 20], it could be considered as an alternative to bone reconstructive procedures (grafts) and moreover as an excellent option of rehabilitation treatment for maxillary atrophy when combined with implants placed in the premaxilla [25, 26] to complete the biomechanical polygon. This biomechanical set will promote stability by allowing the vector cancellation of lateral forces considered deleterious to the zygomatic implants, since they are long and have a sharp lever arm due to the inclination of 45° between the platform

and the body of anchorage [29, 30]. In addition, the choice from conventional, transepithelial, or tapered mini-pillar abutments is crucial, because of its position at the head of the implant, which will depend on the prosthetic connection and its respective prosthetic cylinders. Thus, it is preferable to use lower prosthetic abutments, thereby facilitating sculpturing of the metal structure and reducing the total volume of the final prosthesis.

The acceptance of the zygomatic implant technique by patients has increased because the need for grafts is eliminated, and there is a possibility of combining zygomatic implants with immediate loading [31]. In addition, factors such as the age of the patient, the time, the cost, and the morbidity may also guarantee predictability [32]. The failures indices reported in previous clinical studies are low, and most were detected at the abutment connection phase (6 months after the surgery of implant placement) or before [33]. It is also important to remember that the success rate is directly related to the experience and technical skills of the surgical team.

The patient's satisfaction with fixed prostheses supported by zygomatic implants in relation to comfort, stability, ability to talk, easiness to clean, aesthetics, and functionality has been similar to that related by patients rehabilitated using fixed prostheses with conventional implant [34, 35]. Another important issue is that, due to the anatomical limitations of the patient, this technique should be recommended to treat patients with maxillary bone atrophy who accept the rehabilitation required by the degree of atrophy because this procedure can result in metal-plastic prostheses with pink acrylic resin (flange exposition) in order to compensate horizontal and vertical discrepancies. As many patients expect to receive fixed prostheses with naturally sized teeth and with an emergence of gingival tissue, it is fundamental to the treatment's success that cases should start with prior prosthetic preparation. This would allow the surgeon to diagnose the degree of absorption and assess the relation of the interarches and would allow the patient to visualize these factors. The various therapeutic possibilities for resolving these cases should be weighed by the professional, emphasizing to the patient their advantages and limitations.

Implants of larger diameter are recommended in the posterior region of the mandible and in bones with lower quality or reduced volumes. The latter aims to increase the tolerance to occlusal force, preventing initial instability and promoting a more favorable tension balance around the bone [36]. Theoretically, wide diameter implants anchored in cortical bones can achieve an increase in stability proportional to its diameter [37] because of the anchorage in the lingual or the buccal cortical bone. The reduced height would then be partially compensated by an increase in the implant diameter, producing a larger superficial contact area between the bone and the titanium and resulting in a lower failure rate for short implants, mainly in the posterior atrophic mandible region [38].

The main downside of the larger diameter is a larger volume of bone substituted by titanium, which can induce bone loss around the implant. In addition, the posterior region of the mandible typically has dense cortical tissue with low vascularization and remodeling/formation. The latter

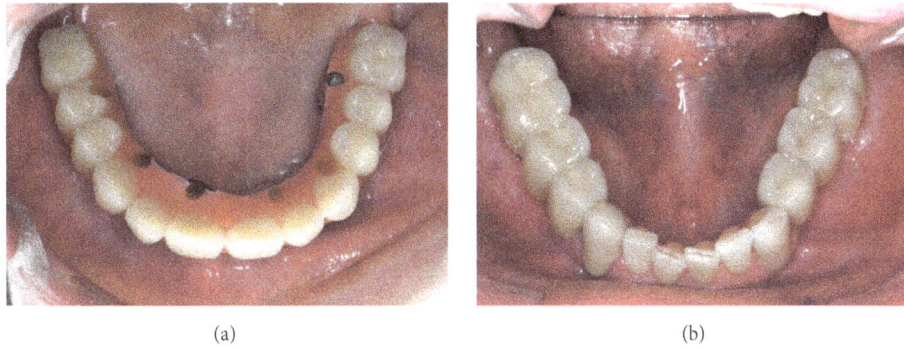

FIGURE 8: Occlusal view of final restoration: (a) maxilla and (b) mandible.

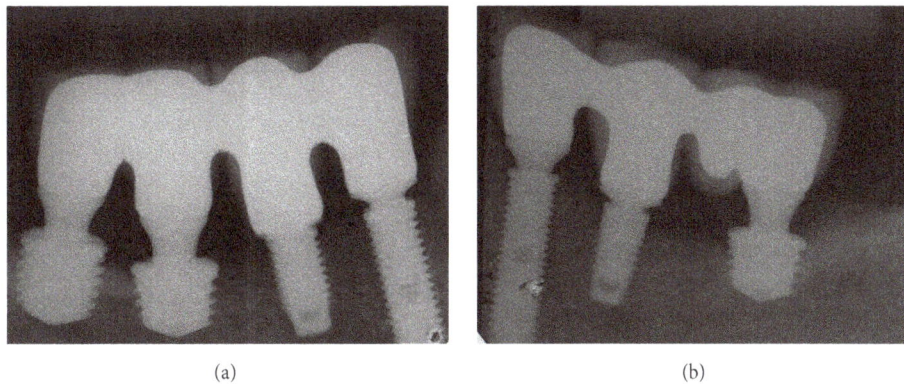

FIGURE 9: Periapical radiographs at the prosthesis installation session in the mandibular arch: (a) right and (b) left side.

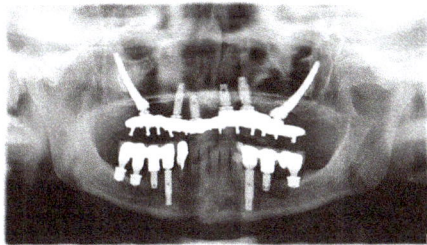

FIGURE 10: Panoramic radiograph at 2 years of follow-up.

suggests that the risk of initial stability loss can be reduced during the remodeling phase [39]. Finally, the available surface area for implants in most systems is limited, reducing its applicability and such systems have lower resistance to occlusal forces.

Concerning the treatment of atrophy of the posterior mandible with short implants, a high clinical success rate (ranging from 80 to 100%) has been reported in prospective, retrospective, and case report follow-up studies [40–45]. Furthermore, differences have not been observed between short implants and other modalities of prosthetic rehabilitation of severe resorptive mandibles [40–42]. Thus, these studies are providing reason for the reevaluation of the results of previous studies that indicate that short implants can properly support most of prosthetic restorations.

The longevity of short implants relies on prosthetic factors such as crown, implant ratio, occlusal table width, occlusion with normal maxillomandibular relationship towards buccolingual orientation, rigid union of the implants through metal structures, and antagonist dentition [12]. Occlusal and anatomic factors in relation to the quality and quantity of the remaining bone, the length of the mesiodistal edentulous space, and the maxillomandibular relationship should also be carefully evaluated [16]. The complications observed in this kind of treatment can be related to the increase of the crown height, a higher bite force in the posterior regions, and low bone density [12]. Furthermore, literature has shown that most of the cases recording a loss of these implants occur in the first year before the patient receives the prosthetic loading [40–42] and one factor that directly influences the osseointegration and survival rate of these types of implants is their rigid union through a metallic infrastructure when the prostheses are installed [9, 46].

Therefore, based on the scientific literature, we infer that the prognosis of the clinical case reported herein, referring to the rehabilitation of the posterior mandible region, can be considered favorable and well established because in the right free end it was combined with implants of 3.75×17 mm, 3.75×7 mm, and 6.0×5 mm, which resulted in a bone contact area of approximately 572.42 mm^2 while in the left free end there were implants of 3.75×15 mm, 3.75×7 mm, 5.0×5 mm, and 6.0×5 mm, and the bone contact area was 509.32 mm^2. Moreover, the rigid union through a metallic infrastructure with immediate function was considered a positive factor during the osseointegration period.

4. Conclusion

Zygomatic and short implants are a reality and make the rehabilitation of areas with severely low bone availability possible. These treatment options offer the possibility of reducing surgical procedures such as sinus lifting, bone grafts, transposition of the mandibular nerve, and positioning in areas of reduced prosthetic space and the possibility of avoiding cantilever in posterior regions.

Competing Interests

The authors declare that there is no conflict of interests regarding the publication of this paper.

References

[1] U. Lekholm, K. Wannfors, S. Isaksson, and B. Adielsson, "Oral implants in combination with bone grafts. A 3-year retrospective multicenter study using the Brånemark implant system," *International Journal of Oral and Maxillofacial Surgery*, vol. 28, no. 3, pp. 181–187, 1999.

[2] K.-E. Kahnberg, A. Ekestubbe, K. Gröndahl, P. Nilsson, and J.-M. Hirsch, "Sinus lifting procedure. I. One-stage surgery with bone transplant and implants," *Clinical Oral Implants Research*, vol. 12, no. 5, pp. 479–487, 2001.

[3] R. G. Triplett, S. R. Schow, and D. M. Laskin, "Oral and maxillofacial surgery advances in implant dentistry," *The International Journal of Oral & Maxillofacial Implants*, vol. 15, no. 1, pp. 47–55, 2000.

[4] T. L. Aghaloo and P. K. Moy, "Which hard tissue augmentation techniques are the most successful in furnishing bony support for implant placement?" *The International Journal of Oral & Maxillofacial Implants*, vol. 22, supplement, pp. 49–70, 2007.

[5] M. Hallman, A. Mordenfeld, and T. Strandkvist, "A retrospective 5-year follow-up study of two different titanium implant surfaces used after interpositional bone grafting for reconstruction of the atrophic edentulous maxilla," *Clinical Implant Dentistry and Related Research*, vol. 7, no. 3, pp. 121–126, 2005.

[6] O. Mardinger, J. Nissan, and G. Chaushu, "Sinus floor augmentation with simultaneous implant placement in the severely atrophic maxilla: technical problems and complications," *Journal of Periodontology*, vol. 78, no. 10, pp. 1872–1877, 2007.

[7] O. Bahat and M. Handelsman, "Use of wide implants and double implants in the posterior jaw: a clinical report," *The International Journal of Oral & Maxillofacial Implants*, vol. 11, no. 3, pp. 379–386, 1996.

[8] T. J. Griffin and W. S. Cheung, "The use of short, wide implants in posterior areas with reduced bone height: a retrospective investigation," *The Journal of Prosthetic Dentistry*, vol. 92, no. 2, pp. 139–144, 2004.

[9] R. Goene, C. Bianchesi, M. Huerzeler et al., "Performance of short implants in partial restorations: 3-year follow-up of Osseotite implants," *Implant Dentistry*, vol. 14, no. 3, pp. 274–280, 2005.

[10] A. Jokstad, U. Braegger, J. B. Brunski, A. B. Carr, I. Naert, and A. Wennerberg, "Quality of dental implants," *International Dental Journal*, vol. 53, supplement 6, pp. 409–443, 2003.

[11] A. Rosén and G. Gynther, "Implant treatment without bone grafting in edentulous severely resorbed maxillas: a long-term follow-up study," *Journal of Oral and Maxillofacial Surgery*, vol. 65, no. 5, pp. 1010–1016, 2007.

[12] C. E. Misch, "Implant design considerations for the posterior regions of the mouth," *Implant Dentistry*, vol. 8, no. 4, pp. 376–386, 1999.

[13] C. E. Misch, J. Steigenga, E. Barboza, F. Misch-Dietsh, and L. J. Cianciola, "Short dental implants in posterior partial edentulism: a multicenter retrospective 6-year case series study," *Journal of Periodontology*, vol. 77, no. 8, pp. 1340–1347, 2006.

[14] C. M. ten Bruggenkate, P. Asikainen, C. Foitzik, G. Krekeler, and F. Sutter, "Short (6-mm) nonsubmerged dental implants: results of a multicenter clinical trial of 1 to 7 years," *The International Journal of Oral & Maxillofacial Implants*, vol. 13, no. 6, pp. 791–798, 1998.

[15] D. Deporter, R. M. Pilliar, R. Todescan, P. Watson, and M. Pharoah, "Managing the posterior mandible of partially edentulous patients with short, porous-surfaced dental implants: early data from a clinical trial," *International Journal of Oral & Maxillofacial Implants*, vol. 16, no. 5, pp. 653–658, 2001.

[16] G. Tawil and R. Younan, "Clinical evaluation of short, machined-surface implants followed for 12 to 92 months," *The International Journal of Oral & Maxillofacial Implants*, vol. 18, no. 6, pp. 894–901, 2003.

[17] B. R. Chrcanovic, T. Albrektsson, and A. Wennerberg, "Survival and complications of zygomatic implants: an updated systematic review," *Journal of Oral and Maxillofacial Surgery*, vol. 74, no. 10, pp. 1949–1964, 2016.

[18] L. E. M. Padovan, P. D. Ribeiro-Júnior, I. A. de Mattias Sartori, G. Thomé, E. M. Sartori, and J. Uhlendorf, "Multiple zygomatic implants as an alternative for rehabilitation of the extremely atrophic maxilla: a case letter with 55 months of follow-up," *The Journal of Oral Implantology*, vol. 41, no. 1, pp. 97–100, 2015.

[19] P. Maló and M. de Araújo Nobre, "A new approach for maxilla reconstruction," *European Journal of Oral Implantology*, vol. 2, no. 2, pp. 101–114, 2009.

[20] P. H. O. Rossetti, W. C. Bonachela, and L. M. N. Rossetti, "Relevant anatomic and biomechanical studies for implant possibilities on the atrophic maxilla: critical appraisal and literature review," *Journal of Prosthodontics*, vol. 19, no. 6, pp. 449–457, 2010.

[21] C. Aparicio, W. Ouazzani, and N. Hatano, "The use of zygomatic implants for prosthetic rehabilitation of the severely resorbed maxilla," *Periodontology 2000*, vol. 47, no. 1, pp. 162–171, 2008.

[22] C. Aparicio, W. Ouazzani, A. Aparicio et al., "Immediate/early loading of zygomatic implants: clinical experiences after 2 to 5 years of follow-up," *Clinical Implant Dentistry and Related Research*, vol. 12, no. 1, supplement, pp. e77–e82, 2010.

[23] E. J. Ferreira, M. R. Kuabara, and J. L. Gulinelli, "'All-on-four' concept and immediate loading for simultaneous rehabilitation of the atrophic maxilla and mandible with conventional and zygomatic implants," *The British Journal of Oral & Maxillofacial Surgery*, vol. 48, no. 3, pp. 218–220, 2010.

[24] M. Mozzati, S. B. Monfrin, G. Pedretti, G. Schierano, and F. Bassi, "Immediate loading of maxillary fixed prostheses retained by zygomatic and conventional implants: 24-month preliminary data for a series of clinical case reports," *The International Journal of Oral & Maxillofacial Implants*, vol. 23, no. 2, pp. 308–314, 2008.

[25] C. Aparicio, C. Manresa, K. Francisco et al., "The long-term use of zygomatic implants: a 10-year clinical and radiographic

report," *Clinical Implant Dentistry and Related Research*, vol. 16, no. 3, pp. 447–459, 2014.

[26] M. Degidi, D. Nardi, A. Piattelli, and C. Malevez, "Immediate loading of zygomatic implants using the intraoral welding technique: a 12-month case series," *The International Journal of Periodontics & Restorative Dentistry*, vol. 32, no. 5, pp. e154–e161, 2012.

[27] C. M. Schmitt, G. Nogueira-Filho, H. C. Tenenbaum et al., "Performance of conical abutment (Morse Taper) connection implants: a systematic review," *Journal of Biomedical Materials Research—Part A*, vol. 102, no. 2, pp. 552–574, 2014.

[28] F. Faot, D. Suzuki, P. M. Senna, W. J. da Silva, and I. A. de Mattias Sartori, "Discrepancies in marginal and internal fits for different metal and alumina infrastructures cemented on implant abutments," *European Journal of Oral Sciences*, vol. 123, no. 3, pp. 215–219, 2015.

[29] S. A. Romeed, R. Malik, and S. M. Dunne, "Zygomatic implants: the impact of zygoma bone support on biomechanics," *The Journal of Oral Implantology*, vol. 40, no. 3, pp. 231–237, 2014.

[30] M. I. Ishak, M. R. Abdul Kadir, E. Sulaiman, and N. H. Abu Kasim, "Finite element analysis of different surgical approaches in various occlusal loading locations for zygomatic implant placement for the treatment of atrophic maxillae," *International Journal of Oral and Maxillofacial Surgery*, vol. 41, no. 9, pp. 1077–1089, 2012.

[31] R. M. Migliorana, B. S. Sotto-Maior, P. M. Senna, C. E. Francischone, and A. A. D. B. Cury, "Immediate occlusal loading of extrasinus zygomatic implants: a prospective cohort study with a follow-up period of 8 years," *International Journal of Oral and Maxillofacial Surgery*, vol. 41, no. 9, pp. 1072–1076, 2012.

[32] E. Bedrossian, "Rescue implant concept: the expanded use of the zygoma implant in the graftless solutions," *Dental Clinics of North America*, vol. 55, no. 4, pp. 745–777, 2011.

[33] B. R. Chrcanovic and M. H. N. G. Abreu, "Survival and complications of zygomatic implants: a systematic review," *Oral and Maxillofacial Surgery*, vol. 17, no. 2, pp. 81–93, 2013.

[34] M. Peñarrocha, C. Carrillo, A. Boronat, and E. Martí, "Level of satisfaction in patients with maxillary full-arch fixed prostheses: zygomatic versus conventional implants," *International Journal of Oral and Maxillofacial Implants*, vol. 22, no. 5, pp. 769–773, 2007.

[35] E. M. Sartori, L. E. M. Padovan, I. A. De Mattias Sartori, P. D. Ribeiro Jr., A. C. Gomes De Souza Carvalho, and M. C. Goiato, "Evaluation of satisfaction of patients rehabilitated with zygomatic fixtures," *Journal of Oral and Maxillofacial Surgery*, vol. 70, no. 2, pp. 314–319, 2012.

[36] H. Kido, E. E. Schulz, A. Kumar, J. Lozada, and S. Saha, "Implant diameter and bone density: effect on initial stability and pull-out resistance," *The Journal of Oral Implantology*, vol. 23, no. 4, pp. 163–169, 1997.

[37] C. J. Ivanoff, K. Grondahl, L. Sennerby, C. Bergstrom, and U. Lekholm, "Influence of variations in implant diameters: a 3- to 5-year retrospective clinical report," *The International Journal of Oral & Maxillofacial Implants*, vol. 14, no. 2, pp. 173–180, 1999.

[38] B. Langer, L. Langer, I. Herrmann, and L. Jorneus, "The wide fixture: a solution for special bone situations and a rescue for the compromised implant. Part 1," *The International Journal of Oral & Maxillofacial Implants*, vol. 8, no. 4, pp. 400–408, 1993.

[39] N. Von Wowern, "Variation in bone mass in the trabecular bone within the mandible," *Calcified Tissue Research*, vol. 22, no. 1, supplement, pp. 517–520, 1976.

[40] A. Monje, J.-H. Fu, H.-L. Chan et al., "Do implant length and width matter for short dental implants (<10 mm) a meta-analysis of prospective studies," *Journal of Periodontology*, vol. 84, no. 12, pp. 1783–1791, 2013.

[41] M. Srinivasan, L. Vazquez, P. Rieder, O. Moraguez, J.-P. Bernard, and U. C. Belser, "Survival rates of short (6 mm) micro-rough surface implants: a review of literature and meta-analysis," *Clinical Oral Implants Research*, vol. 25, no. 5, pp. 539–545, 2014.

[42] B. Balevi, "In selected sites, short, rough-surfaced dental implants are as successful as long dental implants: a critical summary of Pommer B, Frantal S, Willer J, Posch M, Watzek G, Tepper G. Impact of dental implant length on early failure rates: a meta-analysis of observational studies. J Clin Periodontol 2011;38(9):856–863," *The Journal of the American Dental Association*, vol. 144, no. 2, pp. 195–196, 2013.

[43] S. Gray, "Success of short implants in patients who are partially edentulous," *Journal of the American Dental Association*, vol. 144, no. 1, pp. 59–60, 2013.

[44] M. A. Atieh, H. Zadeh, C. M. Stanford, and L. F. Cooper, "Survival of short dental implants for treatment of posterior partial edentulism: a systematic review," *The International Journal of Oral & Maxillofacial Implants*, vol. 27, no. 6, pp. 1323–1331, 2012.

[45] S. Annibali, M. P. Cristalli, D. Dell'Aquila, I. Bignozzi, G. La Monaca, and A. Pilloni, "Short dental implants: a systematic review," *Journal of Dental Research*, vol. 91, no. 1, pp. 25–32, 2012.

[46] M. L. Arlin, "Short dental implants as a treatment option: results from an observational study in a single private practice," *The International Journal of Oral & Maxillofacial Implants*, vol. 21, no. 5, pp. 769–776, 2006.

20

Extramedullary Plasmacytoma Diagnosed in an HIV-Positive Patient by an Unusual Clinical Presentation

Paulo de Camargo Moraes,[1] Luiz Alexandre Thomaz,[2] Victor Angelo Martins Montalli,[3] José Luiz Cintra Junqueira,[2] Camila Maria Beder Ribeiro,[4] and Luciana Butini Oliveira[2]

[1]*Department of Oral Surgery, School of Dentistry, SLMandic, Campinas, SP, Brazil*
[2]*Department of Oral Radiology, School of Dentistry, SLMandic, Campinas, SP, Brazil*
[3]*Department of Oral Pathology, School of Dentistry, SLMandic, Campinas, SP, Brazil*
[4]*Department of Oral Pathology and Stomatology, FOP-UNICAMP, Piracicaba, SP, Brazil*

Correspondence should be addressed to Luciana Butini Oliveira; lubutini@uol.com.br

Academic Editor: Sukumaran Anil

The aim of this paper is to describe a case report of EMP in an HIV-positive patient. A 44-year-old, dark-skinned HIV-infected woman was referred to the Oral Diseases Treatment Center with a swelling at palate and left gingival fornix in the maxilla. Biopsy was taken and the oral lesion was diagnosed as EMP with well-differentiated plasma cells and restriction of the lambda light-chain. Skeletal survey was performed and no radiograph alterations were observed, thus supporting the diagnosis of EMP. Patient was referred to treatment and after two months of chemo and radiotherapy, an expanding lesion was observed in L5/S1 patient's vertebrae. Biopsy of the spinal lesion was consistent with lymphoma with plasmocitary differentiation, supporting the diagnosis of multiple myeloma (MM). Regarding the medical history, the final diagnostic was an oral extramedullary plasmacytoma with rapid progression into multiple myeloma. It is crucial to emphasize the relevance of HIV infection as a risk factor for both aggressive clinical behavior and unusual clinical presentation of extramedullary plasmacytoma cases.

1. Introduction

According to the World Health Organization (WHO), extramedullary plasmacytoma (EMP) is a monoclonal plasmatic soft-tissue proliferation, without bone marrow involvement. It is a tumor composed almost exclusively of plasma cells arranged in clusters or sheets with a scant, delicate, supportive, and connective tissue stroma [1, 2].

Extramedullary plasma cell tumors occur in a wide variety of organs and tissues. However, it has been reported in head and neck of more than 80% of the cases, usually in the nasal cavity with associated bone destruction [3, 4]. Extramedullary plasmacytomas vary considerably in size, the diameter ranging from one to several centimeters. They are usually well limited, firm, and spherical, but they may be lobulated, pedunculated, or polypoid and show evidence of infiltration. The great majority are yellow-gray with a red cut surface, while some of the other tumors have a blue-red appearance. Involved regional lymph nodes are firm, gray white, and may measure up to 3 cm. The symptoms are those due to pressure and obstruction [5]. The tumor is usually highly sensitive to radiotherapy, and most cases do not progress into multiple myeloma [3, 6]. Recently, Ngolet et al. [7] reported that a secondary metastatic cutaneous plasmacytoma is a multiple extramedullary plasma cell proliferation involving skin. Its occurrence was associated with advanced myeloma and a poor prognosis.

Over the last 10 years, it has become apparent that the spectrum of malignant diseases associated with human immunodeficiency virus (HIV) has been expanding [8]. Plasma cell tumors are extremely rare in this group of patients [9] and it has been found that these patients are younger and they present a greater tendency to develop solitary extramedullary plasmacytoma with atypical clinical evolution and greater aggressiveness of the neoplastic process [10]. It has a shorter

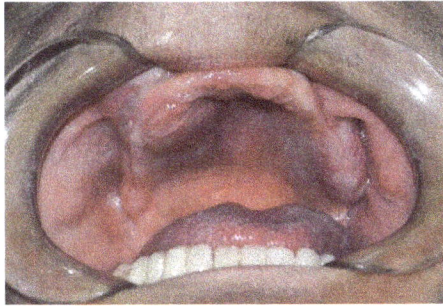

FIGURE 1: Clinical intraoral presentation at time of the first appointment.

latency period and often has extramedullary involvement with unusual clinical presentation [11–13]. There are only few cases of extramedullary plasmacytoma of the head and neck region associated with HIV-positive patients published in the literature. Therefore, the aim of this paper is to present case report of an HIV-positive patient diagnosed for extramedullary plasmacytoma.

2. Case Report

A 44-year-old, dark-skinned woman was referred to the Oral Disease Treatment Center of São Leopoldo Mandic Dental School, Campinas/Brazil, with a complaint of difficulty in wearing her dentures. Her medical history revealed HIV infection, with irregular use of antiretroviral therapy. Patient also reported multiple sexual partners and use of injection drugs, cocaine, crack, and marijuana.

Clinical examination revealed an asymptomatic swelling at right gingival sulcus in the maxilla (Figure 1).

Computed tomography scan revealed a solid tumor mass on the floor of the nasal cavity, measuring 5.6 × 5.2 × 5.2 cm, leading to erosion of the hard palate and of the medial wall of the maxillary sinus, bilaterally (Figure 2). No involvement of cervical lymph nodes was present.

Diagnostic hypotheses were lymphoma, osteosarcoma, and malignant salivary gland neoplasia. Fine needle aspiration and incisional biopsy were performed at the same day of the initial appointment. Microscopic analysis revealed a neoplasm of well-differentiated plasma cells, with restriction of the lambda light-chain (Figure 3). Immunohistochemistry (IHC) showed positivity for CD138 and EMA in the neoplasm; CD79a in a strong and diffuse pattern through the neoplasm; CD56 in the membrane; and lambda in a focal pattern in the neoplasm. IHC was negative for kappa, IgG, and IgM. Bone marrow biopsy revealed reactional lymphoplasmacytic infiltrate and absence of infiltrative neoplastic cells. IHC showed positivity for CD20, CD3, kappa, and lambda (Figure 3).

In addition, total serum proteins, albumin-globulin ratio, and all other laboratory tests were within normal limits. No Bence Jones protein was found. Skeletal survey was performed, with no alterations on plain radiographs. These findings, in association with clinical data, led to the definitive diagnosis of EMP.

After the diagnosis procedure, the tumor was classified as T4N0M0 (Figure 4) and the patient was submitted to chemotherapy with thalidomide, dexamethasone, and pamidronate.

The tumor was also treated by radiation a total dosage of 42 Gy and a fraction size of 200 cGy during 2 months. When examined 3 months later, the nasal obstruction was relieved completely and no residual tumor was observed (Figure 5).

However, two months later, the patient developed sensitive and motor numbness in the lower limbs. Magnetic resonance imaging showed an expanding lesion in L5/S1 vertebrae, presenting medulla compression. Biopsy of the spinal lesion was performed, and microscopic features were consistent with lymphoma with plasmocitary differentiation. IHC was positive for CD20, CD3, and lambda and negative for kappa.

According to World Health Organization Classification of Tumors [1], the diagnosis of a plasmacytoma on biopsy and the presence of lytic bone lesions show multiple myeloma diagnosis (MM). The patient was submitted to chemotherapy with rituximab, cyclophosphamide, doxorubicin, vincristine, and prednisolone but discontinued treatment and quit attending the medical appointments. Information was later obtained that the patient had deceased for unknown causes, probably due to complications of the untreated multiple myeloma.

3. Discussion

The present study reports a case of EMP with atypical features which have been associated with the presence of HIV infection. Such neoplasms in this group of patients are extremely rare [9]. In addition, this tumor shows a different clinical behavior among HIV patients: occurrence in a younger age group, with a shorter latency period, with often extramedullary involvement and in a more aggressive clinical course, with a poor prognosis due to the poor immunity of the patient [9, 11–14]. Indeed, the mean of age of EMP is 60 years in noninfected patients [2], but in HIV-positive patients the mean age is 33 years [15]. In this study, the patient was 44 years-old.

Although a male predominance has been reported for EMP [5], in this study the patient was female. Other characteristics of the case herein reported are consistent with the ones described in the literature. Monoclonal gammopathies have a higher incidence among dark-skinned individuals, and EMP has been reported to occur more frequently in nasal cavity, nasopharyngeal, and paranasal sinus [1, 3, 16, 17]. In this study, the patient was dark skinned, and it is likely that the lesion was originated from the nasal cavity. However, the size of the lesion (bigger than 5 cm), at the time of diagnosis, makes it difficult to define a precise location.

According to Joseph et al. [10], differentiating between plasmablastic lymphoma, plasma cell myeloma, and the solitary EMPs is in itself a diagnostic challenge. EMP has been treated with surgical excision, radiotherapy, chemotherapy, or combined surgery and radiotherapy [9]. EMP is a highly radiosensitive lesion; however, no firmly dose-response relationship has been established due to small patient series and low local failure rates [6]. An optimal radiation dosage

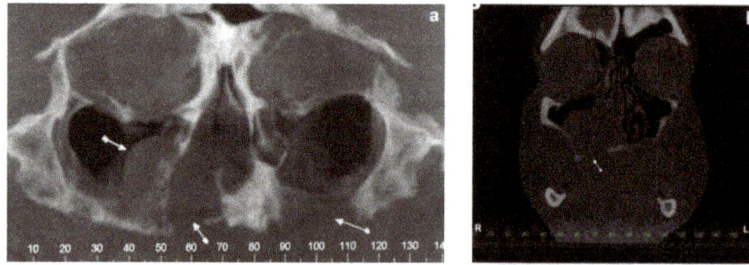

FIGURE 2: Extent of bone destruction seen on CT scans ((a) CT, axial view; (b) CT, coronal view).

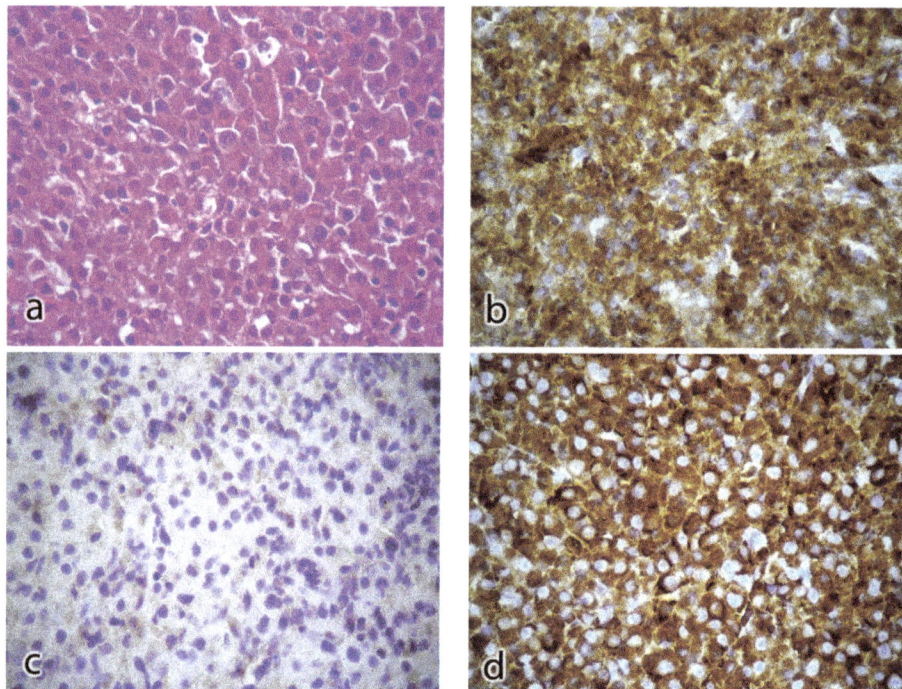

FIGURE 3: Microscopic examination revealed a plasma cell tumor. The histological sections showed lymphoid origin of tumor fragment characterized by the proliferation of atypical plasma cells which are arranged in sheets (a, HE); immunohistochemical reactions were positive for plasm cell (b); negative for kappa (c); and positive for lambda (d).

appears to be in the range of 40–50 Gy [18]. In the present case, a complete regression of the EMP was obtained following a total dosage of 42 Gy of radiotherapy.

The case presented in this study showed a rapid evolution into MM, only 6 months after the initial diagnosis, in an aggressive clinical behavior. It is estimated that 20% to 36% of the cases of EMP can progress into MM [1, 3, 4, 17]. However, in HIV-positive patients, plasma cell tumors may present at unusual sites and progress rapidly to involve multiple sites, including the soft tissues and viscera [19].

Previous studies have investigated the risk factors that would predispose patients with solitary plasmacytoma to disease progression. Thus, in age below 60 years, extramedullary localization and radiotherapy have been related to a 10-year disease-free survival [4]. On the other hand, unfavorable factors for MM development were identified on people older than 60 years and bone localization [4].

The case reported here presented all factors for a favorable outcome and even so showed an aggressive evolution of EMP into MM and eventually death. Such outcome emphasizes the relevance of HIV infection in a more aggressive clinical cause and, eventually, a poor prognosis in patients with EMP [8, 11, 19].

The proposed mechanism for this clinical behavior in HIV-positive patients is related to impaired T-cell function, deregulation, and hyperactivity of B cells. These factors, associated with persistent antigenic stimulation, could encourage transformation of stimulated B cells into malignant plasma cells [15]. However, the final outcome of the case herein reported cannot be adequately discussed since the patient discontinued her treatment after the diagnosis of MM. So far there have been no large studies reporting an optimal therapy for myeloma and other plasma cell dyscrasias in the HIV-positive population [14].

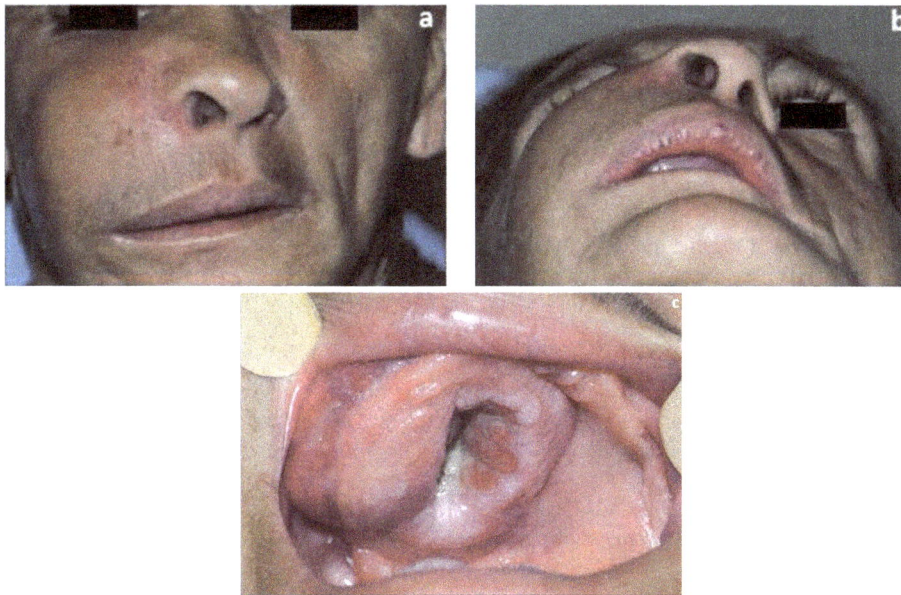

FIGURE 4: Clinical presentation at time of tumor staging ((a) fontal view; (b) coronal view; (c) intraoral view).

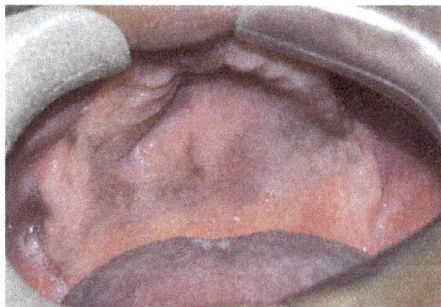

FIGURE 5: Clinical intraoral presentation after two months of chemo-radiotherapy treatment.

Concerning the microscopic features, the WHO diagnostic criteria state that EMP shows identical microscopic and immunophenotype features as those of plasma cell myeloma [1]. Microscopic features frequently show plasma cells morphology, and IHC may show expression of EMA, an epithelial membrane antigen of plasma cells; of CD56/58, a natural killer antigen; of the immunoglobulin-associated antigen CD79a; and of CD138, a reliable marker for identifying and quantifying normal and tumoral plasma cells in paraffin sections [1, 19]. Light-chain immunoglobulins are identified in 11% of the cases of plasma cell tumors, with a higher prevalence of the kappa light-chain [20]. In the case reported here, unusual microscopic features were observed, with a predominance of lambda light-chain among monoclonal gammopathies.

Regarding previous studies there is emphasis on the association of HIV infection, EMP, and MM. Ngolet et al. [7] described a secondary metastatic cutaneous plasmacytoma as a multiple extramedullary plasma cell proliferation involving skin. Its occurrence was associated with advanced myeloma.

According to Hazarika et al. [21], in view of high incidence of progression to MM in due course the patients should be kept under constant surveillance. However, further studies are required to identify risk factors that correlate EMP and its rapid progression into MM.

4. Conclusion

In conclusion, this study reports a case of EMP in an HIV-positive patient. It is important to observe the association of HIV infection and a higher incidence of these lesions, as well as its aggressive clinical behavior and unusual clinical presentation.

Competing Interests

The authors declare that there is no conflict of interests regarding the publication of this work.

References

[1] World Health Organization, *Pathology and Genetics of Tumours of Soft Tissue and Bone*, IARC Press, Lyon, France, 2002.

[2] World Health Organization, *Patology & Genetics—Head and Neck Tumors*, IARC Press, Lyon, France, 2005.

[3] R. H. Liebross, C. S. Ha, J. D. Cox, D. Weber, K. Delasalle, and R. Alexanian, "Clinical course of solitary extramedullary plasmacytoma," *Radiotherapy and Oncology*, vol. 52, no. 3, pp. 245–249, 1999.

[4] M. Ozsahin, R. W. Tsang, P. Poortmans et al., "Outcomes and patterns of failure in solitary plasmacytoma: a multicenter rare cancer network study of 258 patients," *International Journal of Radiation Oncology Biology Physics*, vol. 64, no. 1, pp. 210–217, 2006.

[5] S. Dolin and J. P. Dewar, "Extramedullary Plasmacytoma," *American Journal of Pathology*, vol. 21, no. 1, pp. 83–103, 1956.

[6] R. Soutar, H. Lucraft, G. Jackson et al., "Guidelines on the diagnosis and management of solitary plasmacytoma of bone and solitary extramedullary plasmacytoma," *British Journal of Haematology*, vol. 124, no. 6, pp. 717–726, 2004.

[7] L. O. Ngolet, N. L. N'soundhat, I. Kocko, D. C. N. Kidédé, and H. Ntsiba, "Secondary cutaneous plasmacytoma revealing multiple myeloma: about a case," *The Pan African Medical Journal*, vol. 24, p. 44, 2016.

[8] C. Theodossiou, R. Burroughs, R. Wynn, and P. Schwarzenberger, "Plasmacytoma in HIV disease: two case reports and review of the literature," *The American Journal of the Medical Sciences*, vol. 316, no. 5, pp. 351–353, 1998.

[9] D. Cao, Y. Hu, L. Li, W. Xiao, and Q. Wei, "Retroperitoneal laparoscopic management of a solitary extramedullary plasmacytoma associated with human immunodeficiency virus infection: a case report," *Oncology Letters*, vol. 11, no. 1, pp. 767–769, 2016.

[10] A. A. Joseph, S. Pulimood, M. T. Manipadam, A. Viswabandya, and E. Sigamani, "Extramedullary plasmacytoma: an unusual neoplasm in a HIV-positive patient," *International Journal of STD & AIDS*, vol. 27, no. 10, pp. 909–911, 2016.

[11] L. Feller, J. White, N. H. Wood, M. Bouckaert, J. Lemmer, and E. J. Raubenheimer, "Extramedullary myeloma in an HIV-seropositive subject. literature review and report of an unusual case," *Head and Face Medicine*, vol. 5, no. 1, article 4, 2009.

[12] R. Juglard, V. Vidal, P. Calvet et al., "Plasmacytoma and AIDS: an unusual duodenal manifestation," *Journal de Radiologie*, vol. 82, no. 12, pp. 1729–1731, 2001.

[13] F. Lallemand, L. Fritsch, C. Cywiner-Golenzer, and W. Rozenbaum, "Multiple myeloma in an HIV-positive man presenting with primary cutaneous plasmacytomas and spinal cord compression," *Journal of the American Academy of Dermatology*, vol. 39, no. 3, pp. 506–508, 1998.

[14] L. Pantanowitz, H. P. Schlecht, and B. J. Dezube, "The growing problem of non-AIDS-defining malignancies in HIV," *Current Opinion in Oncology*, vol. 18, no. 5, pp. 469–478, 2006.

[15] S. Herranz, M. Sala, M. Cervantes, M. Sasal, A. Soler, and F. Segura, "Neoplasia of plasma cell with atypical presentation and infection by human immunodeficiency virus presentation of two cases," *American Journal of Haematolology*, vol. 65, pp. 239–242, 2000.

[16] O. Landgren and B. M. Weiss, "Patterns of monoclonal gammopathy of undetermined significance and multiple myeloma in various ethnic/racial groups: support for genetic factors in pathogenesis," *Leukemia*, vol. 23, no. 10, pp. 1691–1697, 2009.

[17] O. Landgren, G. Gridley, I. Turesson et al., "Risk of monoclonal gammopathy of undetermined significance (MGUS) and subsequent multiple myeloma among African American and white veterans in the United States," *Blood*, vol. 107, no. 3, pp. 904–906, 2006.

[18] D. Knobel, A. Zhouhair, R. W. Tsang et al., "Prognostic factors in solitary plasmacytoma of the bone: a multicenter Rare Cancer Network study," *BMC Cancer*, vol. 6, article 118, 2006.

[19] A. Salarieh, C. Rao, S. R. S. Gottesman, O. Alagha, R. Todor, and C. A. Axiotis, "Plasma cell tumors in HIV-positive patients: report of a case and review of the literature," *Leukemia & Lymphoma*, vol. 46, no. 7, pp. 1067–1074, 2005.

[20] R. A. Kyle, T. M. Therneau, S. V. Rajkumar et al., "Prevalence of monoclonal gammopathy of undetermined significance," *The New England Journal of Medicine*, vol. 354, no. 13, pp. 1362–1369, 2006.

[21] P. Hazarika, R. Balakrishnan, R. Singh, K. Pujary, and B. Aziz, "Solitary extramedullary plasmacytoma of the sinonasal region," *Indian Journal of Otolaryngology and Head & Neck Surgery*, vol. 63, supplement 1, pp. 33–35, 2011.

21

Our Experience in the Management of Traumatic Wound Myiasis

Anand Deep Shukla,[1] Abhay T. Kamath,[1] Adarsh Kudva,[1] Deepika Pai,[2] and Nilesh Patel[1]

[1]*Department of Oral and Maxillofacial Surgery, Manipal College of Dental Sciences, Manipal, India*
[2]*Department of Pedodontics, Manipal College of Dental Sciences, Manipal, India*

Correspondence should be addressed to Anand Deep Shukla; drandymanipal@gmail.com

Academic Editor: Yuk-Kwan Chen

Compromised health and hygiene can lead to many complications and one among them is traumatic wound myiasis. Myiasis is the invasion of living tissues by larvae of flies. Three cases of traumatic orofacial wound myiasis and treatment strategies followed for the management of them are reported in this paper.

1. Introduction

Myiasis is a term derived from a Latin word *Muia* which means fly and *iasis* which means disease [1]. The term was christened by Hope in 1849 [2] and explained by Zupmt [3]. It is a pathological condition in which there is growth of dipterous larvae in a living individual which at least for a certain period of time feed on the host's dead or living tissues and develop as parasites [1, 4].

Myiasis is very commonly seen in the rural areas mostly in the animals like cats, dogs, and cows. It is also reported in human beings, especially individuals of low economic status in poor countries [5].

Myiasis can be classified depending on the condition of the tissues that are involved [6]:

Obligatory. It requires the presence of living tissues for larvae development.

Facultative. It requires the presence of dead tissues for laying eggs and incubating.

In the human beings the most common site of myiasis is nose, ear, vagina, and skin [7]. It is not very commonly seen in the oral cavity although we report 3 cases of oral myiasis reported to the Department of Oral and Maxillofacial Surgery, MCODS, Manipal, and the different treatment strategies used for the management of them.

2. Case Series

2.1. Case 1. A 70-year-old male was reported to trauma triage of KMC Manipal with a history of road traffic accident two days back; he was initially admitted in a local hospital for two days, after which he was referred to KMC Manipal. Patient was having a laceration over the chin region which was sutured by the registrar of the Department of Oral and Maxillofacial Surgery. He was admitted under the Department of Neurosurgery as an internal head injury component was present.

A call was given to us the next day saying that worms were coming out of the sutured chin wound (Figure 1). When the wound was inspected small maggots were coming out of the sutured wound. Once the suture was removed and the wound was inspected small maggots were crawling out of the wound. Around 45–50 live maggots were removed in the ward (Figure 2). Once the accessible maggots were removed, turpentine oil was applied over the wound, and the wound was left open. Daily wound debridement was done

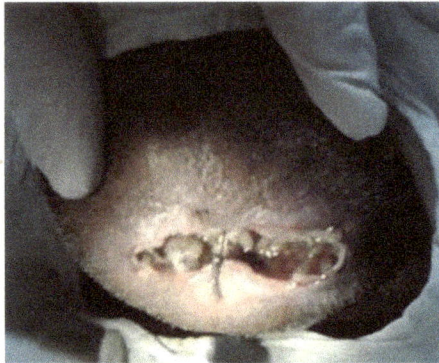

FIGURE 1

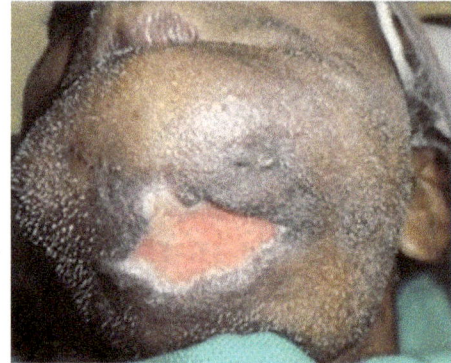

FIGURE 2

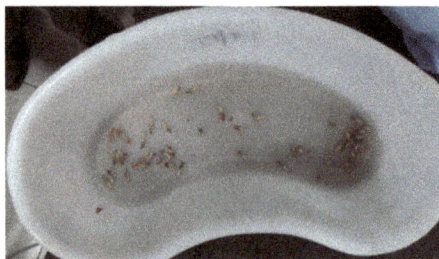

FIGURE 3

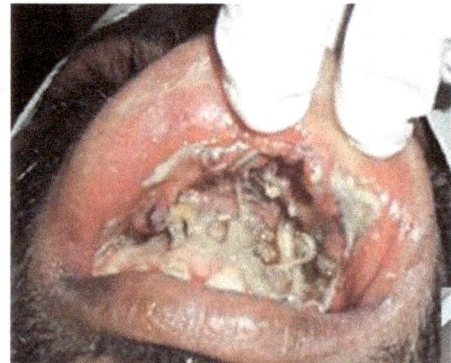

FIGURE 4

and maggots were removed daily over a course of 4-5 days. Topical application of placentrex was also done, which aids in healing of wound. In total 150–200 maggots were removed. Patient also had a left mandibular angle fracture, for which he was taken up for open reduction and internal fixation under general anesthesia. A skin graft was also harvested from the patient's right thigh and secured over the chin wound. Patient recovered well and the wound over the chin region healed without any complications (Figure 3).

2.2. Case 2. The second case that was reported to us was a 30-year-old known alcoholic male with a history of fall from a tree, following which he was lying unattended there for a long time, when the wound over the intraoral region got contaminated with dust. Patient reported to our OPD one day after the fall with the complaint of pain and swelling over the mouth. Once the wounds were inspected intraorally, live maggots were seen crawling in the patient's oral cavity (Figure 4). Around 35–40 maggots were removed in the OPD (Figure 5) and the patient was admitted for further management of the wounds. Turpentine oil was applied topically over the intraoral wound and maggots that had infested the wound were removed. Daily wound debridement was done and it was supplemented by application of placentrex which aids in granulation. Patient's recovery was uneventful and he showed a very good healing of the wound (Figure 6).

2.3. Case 3. The third case is of a 22-year-old female with mental retardation, who was reported to us with a history of fall at home three days back. Accompanying attendant detailed that she had developed pain and swelling over the

mouth since past three days after the fall. On thorough examination she showed presence of live maggots in the oral cavity (Figure 7). The maggots were removed mechanically in the Oral and Maxillofacial Surgery OPD. Around 25–30 maggots were removed, followed by application of turpentine oil. Subsequently patient was admitted for the management of the intraoral wounds and debridement. She was put on IV Antibiotics and analgesics and daily wound debridement was done. She was advised to apply placentrex gel intraorally. Patient recovered well and was discharged after a period of 7 days (Figure 8).

3. Discussion

Oral myiasis is most commonly seen in bed ridden patients and patients with special needs who need a caregiver for the maintenance of their oral hygiene [8]. Substance abusers are more likely to suffer from oral myiasis as they are negligent towards their oral and overall hygiene. As can be observed in the presented cases, patients with history of abuse of drugs and alcoholics and bed ridden patients are more likely to present with oral myiasis [9].

A standard guideline for the management of oral myiasis has not been laid down, but the most commonly followed approach is the mechanical removal of all the larvae followed by daily wound debridement and irrigation [10]. Application of turpentine oil over the wound also helps to remove the maggots as it creates an atmosphere deficit in oxygen which

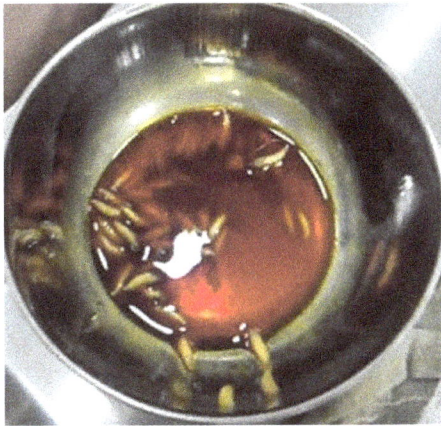

FIGURE 5

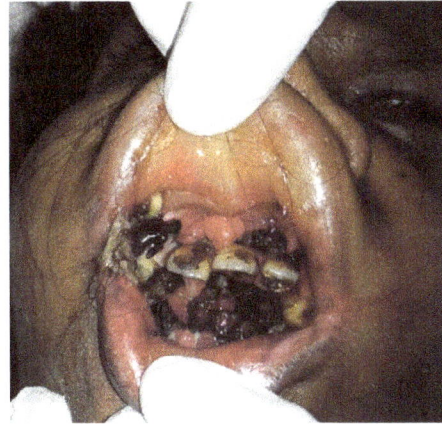

FIGURE 7

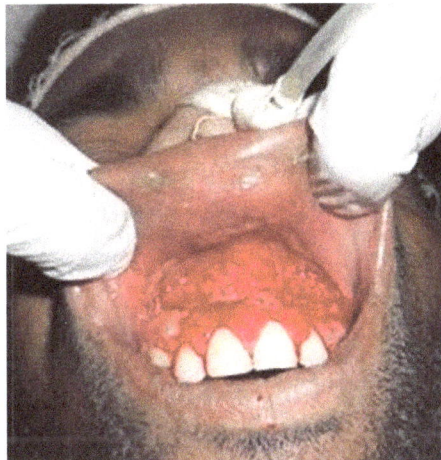

FIGURE 6

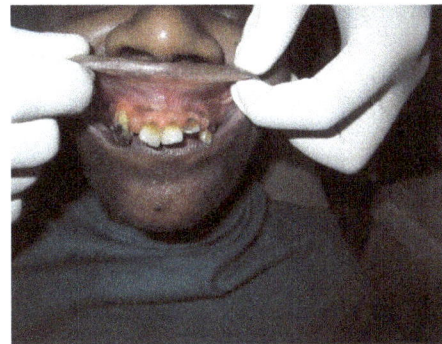

FIGURE 8

forces the maggots to come to the surface, and then they can be mechanically removed [11]. Once the maggots are removed we also subjected the patient to the application of placentrex gel, which aids in faster granulation.

Treatment strategies other than mechanical removal of the maggots include use of larvicidal drugs and occlusion of the area with pressure dressing. Ivermectin has been used to reduce the extent of mechanical debridement of the wound [11]. Occlusion with a pressure dressing reduces the oxygen supply for the maggots causing them to come on the surface, and hence they can be easily removed.

Oral myiasis is more commonly seen in males because of outdoor activities and tendency to neglect the oral hygiene. It is commonly seen in adults, but children can also be affected [12].

In these cases a mechanical removal of the maggots followed by application of turpentine oil was done. Patients were then started on IV Augmentin and Metrogyl. Daily wound debridement was done, supplemented by the application of placentrex gel which aids in faster granulation. In our experience placentrex gel has a very good effect on the

healing of oral wounds and should be used more frequently [13].

4. Conclusion

Oral myiasis is an uncommon condition seen in the oral cavity. Its incidence can be reduced by raising the quality of life and paying attention to oral hygiene. Old and debilitated patients and patients with special needs are more prone for the development of oral myiasis and hence special care should be taken of these patients. As surgeons it is our duty to raise awareness that a special needs patient should be exposed to proper dental checkup so that complications in the form of oral myiasis do not develop.

Competing Interests

The authors declare that there is no conflict of interests regarding the publication of this paper.

References

[1] J. Sharma, G. P. Mamatha, and R. Acharya, "Primary oral myiasis: a case report," *Medicina Oral, Patología Oral y Cirugía Bucal*, vol. 13, no. 11, pp. 714–716, 2008.

[2] R. R. Felices and K. U. Ogbureke, "Oral myiasis: Report of case and review of management," *Journal of Oral and Maxillofacial Surgery*, vol. 54, no. 2, pp. 219–220, 1996.

[3] F. Zupmt, *Myiasis in Man and Animals in the Old World. A Textbook for Physicians, Vetrinarians and Zoologists*, Butterworth and Co Ltd, London, UK, 1965.

[4] F. Hope, "On Insects and their larvae occasionaly found in the human body," *Transactions of the Royal Entomological Society*, vol. 2, pp. 256–271, 1840.

[5] J. G. Gabriel, S. A. Marinho, F. D. Verli, R. G. Krause, L. S. Yurgel, and K. Cherubini, "Extensive myiasis infestation over a squamous cell carcinoma in the face. Case report," *Medicina Oral, Patologia Oral y Cirugia Bucal*, vol. 13, no. 1, pp. E9–E11, 2008.

[6] R. S. Gomez, P. F. Perdigão, F. J. G. S. Pimenta, A. C. Rios Leite, J. C. Tanos de Lacerda, and A. L. Custódio Neto, "Oral myiasis by screwworm *Cochliomyia hominivorax*," *British Journal of Oral and Maxillofacial Surgery*, vol. 41, no. 2, pp. 115–116, 2003.

[7] M. J. R. Hall and R. Wall, "Myiasis of humans and domestic animals," *Advances in Parasitology*, vol. 35, pp. 257–334, 1995.

[8] R. Dandriyal and S. Pant, "Oral myiasis in mentally challenged patient: a case report," *Journal of Clinical and Experimental Dentistry*, vol. 3, no. 2, pp. e155–e157, 2011.

[9] S. Godhi, S. Goyal, and M. Pandit, "Oral myiasis: a case report," *Journal of Maxillofacial Surgery*, vol. 7, pp. 292–293, 2008.

[10] A. P. Bhatt and A. Jayakrishnan, "Oral myiasis: a case report," *International Journal of Paediatric Dentistry*, vol. 10, pp. 67–70, 2000.

[11] W. C. Campbell, "Ivermectin: an update," *Parasitology Today*, vol. 1, no. 1, pp. 10–16, 1985.

[12] E. B. Droma, A. Wilamowski, H. Schnur, N. Yarom, E. Scheuer, and E. Schwartz, "Oral myiasis: a case report and literature review," *Oral Surgery, Oral Medicine, Oral Pathology, Oral Radiology, and Endodontics*, vol. 103, no. 1, pp. 92–96, 2007.

[13] G. Thakur, S. Thomas, D. Bhargava, and A. Pandey, "Does topical application of placental extract gel on postoperative fibrotomy wound improve mouth opening and wound healing in patients with oral submucous fibrosis?" *Journal of Oral and Maxillofacial Surgery*, vol. 73, no. 7, pp. 1439.e1–1439.e10, 2015.

22

Implant-Retained Obturator for an Edentulous Patient with a Hemimaxillectomy Defect Complicated with Microstomia

Pravinkumar G. Patil[1] and Smita Nimbalkar-Patil[2]

[1]Division of Clinical Dentistry, School of Dentistry, International Medical University, Kuala Lumpur, Malaysia
[2]Department of Orthodontics, Faculty of Dentistry, MAHSA University, Kuala Lumpur, Malaysia

Correspondence should be addressed to Pravinkumar G. Patil; pravinandsmita@yahoo.co.in

Academic Editor: Jose López-López

Patient. A 68-year-old man was operated on for squamous cell carcinoma (T3N3M0) of the maxilla creating the hemimaxillary surgical defect on right side. The remaining arch was completely edentulous. There was remarkable limitation in the oral opening with reduced perimeter of the oral cavity due to radiation and surgical scar contracture. This article describes prosthetic rehabilitation by modifying the design of the obturator and achieving the retention with dental implant. *Discussion.* Severe limitation in the oral opening may occur in clinical situations following the postsurgical management of oral and maxillofacial defects. The prosthetic rehabilitation of the surgical defect in such patients becomes a challenging task due to limited access to the oral cavity. This challenge becomes even more difficult if the patient is edentulous and there are no teeth to gain the retention, stability, and support. *Conclusion.* In severe microstomia prosthesis insertion and removal can be achieved with modification of the maximum width of the prosthesis. Dental implant retention is useful treatment option in edentulous patients with maxillary surgical defect provided that sufficient bone volume and accessibility are there for implant placement.

1. Introduction

Microstomia is defined as an abnormally small oral orifice [1]. Head and neck cancer are commonly treated with surgical intervention and radiotherapy [2, 3]. Limited oral opening can be caused by head and neck radiation [3–6], reflex spasm [4], surgically treated head and neck tumors [7], microinvasion of the muscles of mastication [4, 8], connective tissue disease [9], fibrosis of masticatory muscles [10], facial burns [11], and reconstructive lip surgeries [12]. Clinical management of the problems associated with providing dental prostheses for patients with trismus is not well reported [13], although the following management techniques have been described: surgery [4, 14], the use of dynamic opening devices [15], and modification of denture designs [13, 16]. The postsurgical microstomia usually leads to very stiff oral aperture and the stretching of the lips becomes a difficult task during various treatment stages of prosthesis fabrication. To make a primary impression the height of the tray should be smaller than the interarch space and the lips can be stretched to a width

that is equal to or greater than the width of an impression tray. In situations where scar tissue formation has decreased the flexibility of the lips significantly, insertion and removal of stock impression trays become difficult. Maxillofacial prosthesis in completely edentulous patient is a challenging task. This article describes the prosthetic management of a patient with an edentulous maxilla and midfacial defect complicated by severe postsurgical microstomia.

2. Outline of the Case

2.1. Case History. A 68-year-old man was referred postsurgically from the ENT Surgery Department to the Department of Prosthodontics for prosthodontic assessment for hemimaxillectomy defect. The patient was frustrated using a gauze-pack since one month and was keen to use any kind of prosthesis that can facilitate his oral feeding and not really concerned with the esthetics. A detailed medical and dental history revealed that he was operated on for the squamous cell carcinoma (T3N3M0) of the right maxilla 1 month ago.

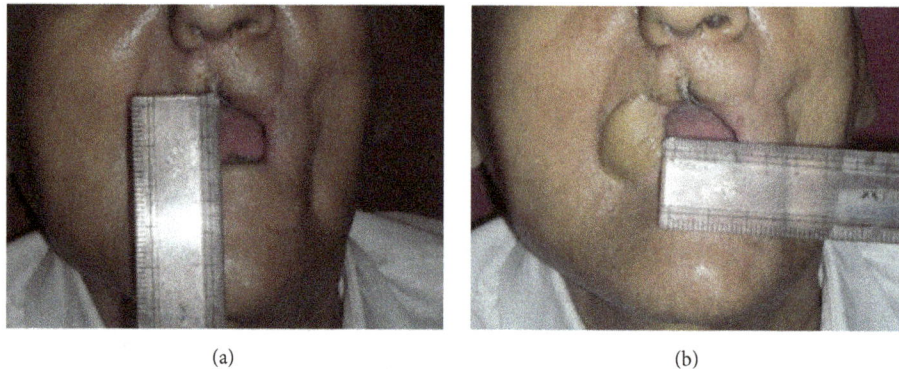

(a)   (b)

FIGURE 1: Extraoral view with maximum oral opening with (a) limited vertical length of oral aperture and (b) limited horizontal length of oral aperture.

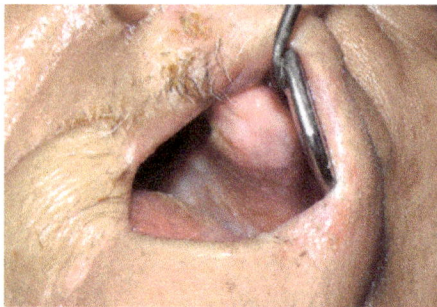

FIGURE 2: Intraoral view with maximum oral opening. Note the reduced aperture in relation to mouth mirror head.

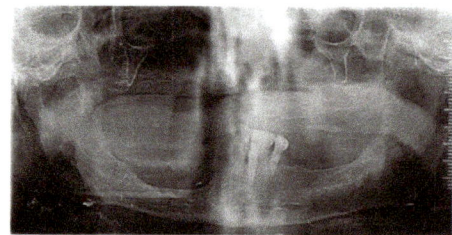

FIGURE 3: Postsurgical orthopantomograph revealing right side hemimaxillectomy.

The right hemimaxillectomy was performed together with removal of his remaining anterior teeth including central incisor, lateral incisor, and canine on right side and left central incisor. The patient received a preoperative course of total dose of 7200 cGy external beam radiation within a period of 6 weeks in fractions (a fraction of 200 cGy/day for 5 days in a week). The patient was restricted to a liquid-diet through a nasogastric tube for initial 2 weeks after surgery followed by oral liquid feeding for next 2 weeks. He was instructed to use the gauze-pack covered with the polymer sheet (to be replaced twice a day) to block the defect area while taking liquid and semisolid food for next 1 month. Clinical examination revealed a partially edentulous maxilla and mandible. There was remarkable limitation in the oral opening with reduced perimeter of the oral cavity (Figures 1(a) and 1(b)). Intraoral examination revealed healthy maxillary edentulous ridge on left side (Figure 2). Reduced oral aperture size made this case difficult to restore with a conventional obturator prosthesis. Clinical examination revealed that remaining left side of the maxillary arch was completely edentulous and the mandibular arch remained only with left lateral incisor, canine, and first premolar. Postoperative OPG revealed removal of all maxillary teeth along with the right half of the maxilla (Figure 3).

2.2. Fabrication of Definitive Obturator. Fabrication of definitive obturator prosthesis was planned. There were three challenges during the obturator fabrication: (1) Remarkable restricted mouth opening and microstomia, which makes standard stock impression trays go inside the mouth; (2) edentulous remaining maxillary arch, which makes the retention of the obturator prosthesis difficult; and (3) difficulty in using mandibular partial denture due to lack of attached mucosa on right side of the mandibular arch. A preoperative diagnostic cast was not available. Due to small aperture size, use of standard sized stock trays was impossible. The plastic perforated stock tray was modified according to the need by trimming the borders and palatal portion of the tray to fit it inside the mouth and the impression was made with irreversible hydrocolloid with the thick mix consistency. The impression was made with the detail records of remaining part of the hard palate and the defect marginal areas along the midpalatine raphe. Remaining portion of the defect area was built up with modelling wax arbitrarily to achieve the natural contour of the palate (Figure 4). The cast was poured in the type III gypsum material (Kalstone; Kalabhai Karson, Mumbai, India). The palatal-obturator-plate was fabricated covering unresected portion and contoured resected portion of the cast in heat polymerized acrylic resin (Heat Cure Acrylic; Dental Products of India, Mumbai, India).

2.3. Prosthesis Modification for Facilitation of Insertion/ Removal and Retention. The shape of the palatal obturator was modified to facilitate the easy placement and removal of the prosthesis. The base was made slightly concave along the borders in the region of right canine. This was the area

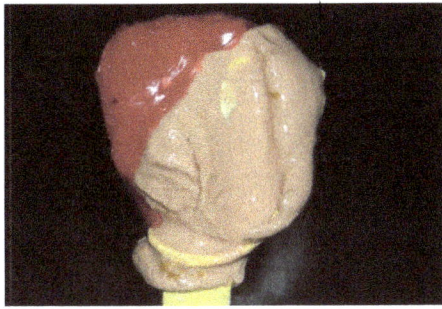

FIGURE 4: Primary impression recorded with irreversible hydrocolloid using modified perforated plastic-stock-tray. Remaining portion of defect area was built up with modelling wax.

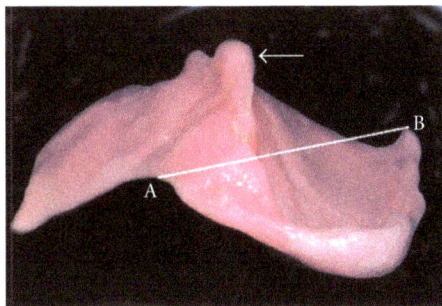

FIGURE 5: Palatal obturator. Note that arrow indicates extension of the resin in undercut areas seen along the defect margins. Line joining A and B indicates maximum stretchable distance of mouth.

around which the prosthesis was planned to turn inside the mouth during insertion and removal (Figure 3). The point A (see Figure 5) indicates concave area of prosthesis at corner of the mouth allowing insertion of the prosthesis in curvilinear path with centre at point A. The point B (Figure 5) indicates the distobuccal end of prosthesis. The concavity provided at this specific area facilitated the reduction of the maximum horizontal length of the prosthesis which was almost similar to that of maximum stretchable distance of the oral aperture during insertion and removal of prosthesis horizontally. The obturator was placed in the mouth as described earlier and tried to evaluate the retention, stability, and the amount of defect closure area. The obturator was selectively trimmed along the edges to sufficiently close the defect margins without displacement during oral functional movements. As the remaining maxillary arch was edentulous, there was hardly anything to depend upon for retention of the prosthesis except the defect margins along the midpalatal area. This area was relined with the permanent resilient liner (Tokuyama Soft-Plus II; Tokuyama Dental Corporation, Tokyo, Japan) to achieve better adaptation and undercut engagement with the available undercut space along the defect margin. The patient was then evaluated for the need of additional retention during speech and deglutition. The undercut engagement was not sufficient to retain the prosthesis during function as the prosthesis tends to fall especially from anterior aspect. The small test was carried out to identify the need of extra retention. The anterior portion of the prosthesis was stabilized with the

one finger and allowed patient to speak and swallow. This time the prosthesis remained in place. So the treatment plan was modified to insert an implant for achieving additional retention with the help of overdenture attachment.

2.4. Implant Placement. The remaining right edentulous maxillary arch was evaluated for the suitability of implant placement. Patient agreed to undergo additional minor surgical procedure of implant placement for the sake of improved retention and stability of the obturator and was convinced for improved eating and swallowing. The site of the implant placement was selected in the anterior most possible area of the right maxilla for implant osteotomy for the implant surgical hand-piece accessibility. The gutta-percha point of 3 mm length was inserted into the same obturator for diagnostic purpose and the periapical radiograph was taken. Bone sounding procedure was carried out in the same region to ensure adequate bone volume. An endosseous self-threading implant of diameter 4.2 mm and length 13 mm (Adin Touareg S; Adin Implant Corporation, Israel) was selected with the help of radiographic evaluation and bone sounding procedure. The flapless surgical procedure was performed by punching out the 3 mm diameter circular attached mucosa to place the implant (Figure 6(a)). The healing abutment was placed to avoid second stage surgery (Figure 6(b)). Four months after surgery, an intraoral periapical radiograph was taken to ensure the osseointegration of the implant (Figure 7). Clinical examination revealed stable implant with healthy peri-implant tissues. The healing abutment was replaced with the overdenture-abutment (ball and socket) (Figure 8). The obturator was then modified from the intaglio surface to accommodate the matrix-components of the attachment relined/fixed with the autopolymerizing acrylic resin (GC Cooliner; GC Corporation, Tokyo, Japan) (Figure 9). The softest available retentive nylon cap along with the metal housing was attached with the direct pick-up technique (Adin overdenture nylon cap with pink colour code). The patient was trained to insert and remove the obturator prosthesis. The possible nasal regurgitation of liquid was evaluated by asking the patient to drink the water. The water regurgitation was found to be reduced and patient could drink with ease compared to previous conditions. The possible leakage areas were identified by evaluating the overextensions and underextensions of the prosthesis margins again and modified accordingly to achieve maximum possible seal during oral functions.

2.5. Obturator Delivery and Recall. The patient was not keen to add anterior teeth to the prosthesis as he was more concerned about the functions rather than the esthetics. Hence the teeth were not added to the prosthesis. Patient learned to masticate by contacting his mandibular remaining natural teeth with the anterior portion of the obturator and could manage to handle the semisolid and soft-solid food. The patient was kept under observation for the implant success by taking the periapical radiograph after initial 6 months and then planned to take the periapical radiographs after every 12 months. The soft nylon cap was replaced regularly after every 6 months. The obturator was relined after

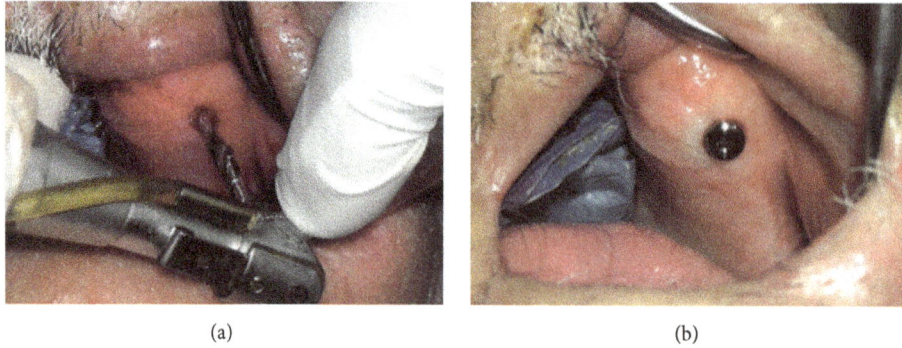

(a)   (b)

FIGURE 6: (a) Flapless implant placement. Note limited access of implant surgical hand-piece. (b) Healing abutment in place.

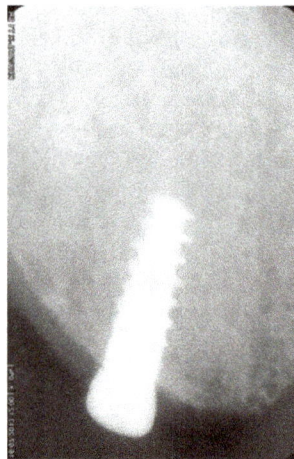

FIGURE 7: Intraoral periapical radiograph of implant after 4 months of osseointegration.

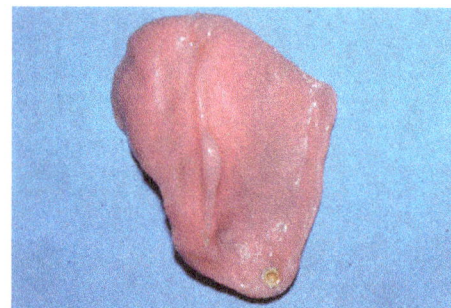

FIGURE 9: Retentive component incorporated in obturator plate.

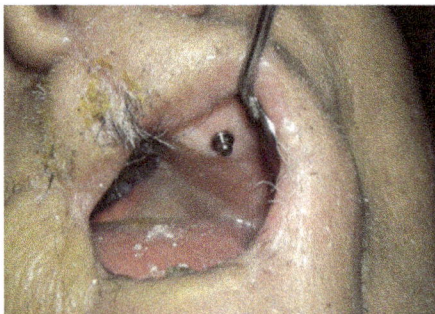

FIGURE 8: Overdenture attachment in place.

every 12 months. Last recall visit was after 18 months of the treatment (Figures 10(a) and 10(b)). The marginal bone loss of 1.5 mm was observed around the implant after 18 months of use. The patient was pleased with the improved functions and eating comfort.

3. Discussion

Management of postsurgical and/or postradiation patients of oral cancer therapy is a clinically challenging situation. The smaller the defect area is, with healthy teeth present in nonresected portion of the arch, the easier the condition to achieve retention, stability, and support for the prosthesis is. The larger the area is, the harder the prosthodontic rehabilitation is. This problem worsens when the remaining arch is having lesser number of teeth, periodontally compromised teeth or completely edentulous ridge. The implants can be used to gain the retention, stability, and support to the prosthesis in such situation. But the prosthesis movement during functions like speech, mastication, and swallowing makes long-term implant success rate questionable. The careful evaluation of such movement must be done before planning the implant treatment for maxillofacial prostheses. In this patient, fortunately, the prosthesis was seated and adapted well on the remaining edentulous arch with little movement of the obturator during functions. The simple obturator prosthesis (without addition of teeth) was used to obdurate the defect. Addition of teeth would have increased the weight of the prosthesis and the chances of lateral forces to dislodge the prosthesis. The patient's desire to have more importance on oral intake of food than the aesthetic appearance made this prosthesis simpler than the prosthesis with teeth. There was no option other than the implant attachment to achieve retention of the prosthesis due to completely edentulous remaining maxillary arch and inadequate tissue undercut on defect side. However implant placement in the irradiated bone was one of the concerns. Nooh [17] performed a systematic review of the literature with 38 articles published between 1990 and 2012. He concluded that overall implant

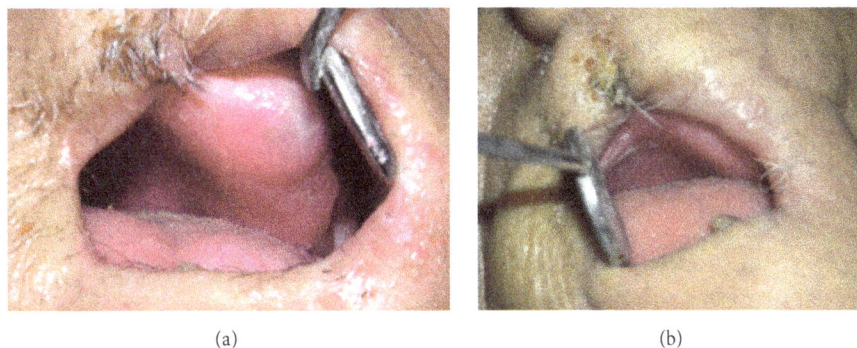

(a)   (b)

FIGURE 10: (a) Left lateral view showing implant-retained obturator in place; (b) midpalatal view indicating closed defect.

survival rates with radiation therapy done before and after implantation were 88.9% and 92.2%, respectively. In this patient the implant was survived till 18 months of the last recall and the marginal bone loss was observed to be 1.5 mm, which is considered to be the success of the implant as well.

There are various types of implant overdenture retentive components available. Any overdenture attachment type (including ball/socket, bar/clip, magnets, and locators) can be used as per the clinical situations and treatment needs. We had used the ball and socket with one single implant to allow 360 degrees of freedom to allow the prosthesis to have micromovements in all spatial directions with the retentive component in place. This would probably reduce the unwanted stress on the implant. The single implant was sufficient in this situation to retain the toothless lightweight obturator. Mastication is not possible with this obturator; however patient can eat semisolid and liquid food. The principal purpose of this obturator was to allow liquid/semisolid food intake orally without masticating, as there are no teeth for mastication purpose in lower arch too.

4. Conclusion

In severe microstomia prosthesis insertion and removal can be achieved with modification of the maximum width of the prosthesis. Dental implant retention is useful treatment option in edentulous patients with maxillary surgical defect provided that sufficient bone volume and accessibility are there for implant placement.

Competing Interests

The authors declare that they have no competing interests.

References

[1] "The glossary of prosthodontic terms," *The Journal of Prosthetic Dentistry*, vol. 94, no. 1, pp. 1–85, 2005.

[2] D. McClure, G. Barker, B. Barker, and P. Feil, "Oral management of the cancer patient, part II: oral complications of radiation therapy," *Compendium*, vol. 8, no. 88, pp. 90–92, 1987.

[3] S. Sakai, T. Kubo, N. Mori et al., "A study of the late effects of radiotherapy and operation on patients with maxillary cancer.

A survey more than 10 years after initial treatment," *Cancer*, vol. 62, no. 10, pp. 2114–2117, 1998.

[4] K. Ichimura and T. Tanaka, "Trismus in patients with malignant tumours in the head and neck," *Journal of Laryngology and Otology*, vol. 107, no. 11, pp. 1017–1020, 1993.

[5] R. L. Engelmeier and G. E. King, "Complications of head and neck radiation therapy and their management," *The Journal of Prosthetic Dentistry*, vol. 49, no. 4, pp. 514–522, 1983.

[6] A. C. Cheng, A. G. Wee, and L. Tat-Keung, "Maxillofacial prosthetic rehabilitation of a midfacial defect complicated by microstomia: a clinical report," *Journal of Prosthetic Dentistry*, vol. 85, no. 5, pp. 432–437, 2001.

[7] R. W. Horst, "Trismus: its causes, effects and treatment," *ORL— Head and Neck Nursing*, vol. 12, no. 2, pp. 11–12, 1994.

[8] S. G. Cohen and P. D. Quinn, "Facial trismus and myofascial pain associated with infections and malignant disease. Report of five cases," *Oral Surgery, Oral Medicine, Oral Pathology*, vol. 65, no. 5, pp. 538–544, 1988.

[9] L. A. al-Hadi, "A simplified technique for prosthetic treatment of microstomia in a patient with scleroderma: a case report," *Quintessence International*, vol. 25, no. 8, pp. 531–533, 1994.

[10] T. Nakajima, H. Sasakura, and N. Kato, "Screw-type mouth gag for prevention and treatment of postoperative jaw limitation by fibrous tissue," *Journal of Oral Surgery*, vol. 38, no. 1, pp. 46–50, 1980.

[11] G. M. Maragakis and M. Garcia-Tempone, "Microstomia following facial burns," *Journal of Clinical Pediatric Dentistry*, vol. 23, no. 1, pp. 69–74, 1998.

[12] P. G. Smith, H. R. Muntz, and S. E. Thawley, "Local myocutaneous advancement flaps. Alternatives to cross-lip and distant flaps in the reconstruction of ablative lip defects," *Archives of Otolaryngology*, vol. 108, no. 11, pp. 714–718, 1982.

[13] P. A. Heasman, J. M. Thomason, and J. G. Robinson, "The provision of prostheses for patients with severe limitation in opening of the mouth," *British Dental Journal*, vol. 176, no. 5, pp. 171–174, 1994.

[14] R. Werner, "Treatment of trismus following radiotherapy in nasopharyngeal cancer (N.P.C.)," *Singapore Medical Journal*, vol. 15, no. 1, pp. 64–68, 1974.

[15] P. U. Dijkstra, T. J. Kropmans, and R. Y. Tamminga, "Modified use of a dynamic bite opener—treatment and prevention of trismus in a child with head and neck cancer: a case report," *Cranio*, vol. 10, no. 4, pp. 327–329, 1992.

[16] Y. Suzuki, M. Abe, T. Hosoi, and K. S. Kurtz, "Sectional col-
     lapsed denture for a partially edentulous patient with micros-
     tomia: a clinical report," *Journal of Prosthetic Dentistry*, vol. 84,
     no. 3, pp. 256–259, 2000.

[17] N. Nooh, "Dental implant survival in irradiated oral cancer
     patients: a systematic review of the literature," *The International
     Journal of Oral & Maxillofacial Implants*, vol. 28, no. 5, pp. 1233–
     1242, 2013.

23

A Rational Approach to Sinus Augmentation: The Low Window Sinus Lift

Terry Zaniol and Alex Zaniol

Studio Dentistico Zaniol, Crocetta del Montello, Italy

Correspondence should be addressed to Terry Zaniol; drterry@studiozaniol.it

Academic Editor: Gilberto Sammartino

Sinus augmentation is a well-known approach to treating alveolar bone ridge atrophy in the posterior maxilla. The preparation of the lateral window is crucial. Its size, design, and position in the vestibular sinus wall may affect the intra- and postsurgical complication rates and affect the intrasurgical activity of both surgeons and assistants. The present paper describes a rational technique that also exploits the guided surgery approach for design and preparation of a lateral window for sinus augmentation, the Low Window Sinus Lift. To illustrate the use of this approach, a case is presented in which the 50-year-old patient had the left maxillary first molar extracted, followed two months later by sinus augmentation and placement of three implants. One year after delivery of the definitive prosthesis, all three implants were successful, and the prosthesis was fully functional. Controlled studies should be undertaken to assess whether this technique provides significant advantages compared to other sinus augmentation approaches.

1. Introduction

Sinus augmentation is one of the most common bone-grafting surgeries, and its execution is within the reach of every oral surgeon with average skills [1]. Since its introduction by Tatum Jr. et al. [2, 3] and Boyne and James [4] in the 1980s, this surgical technique has been extensively studied. Widespread consensus [5, 6] about it has been reached, and it has been further refined [1, 7] to make it less invasive, spare the patient discomfort, and lower the rate of intra- and postsurgical complications. Along with the lateral approach originally proposed by Tatum Jr. et al., and Boyne and James, technique variants involving a crestal approach were later implemented by Summers [8] and other authors [7, 9–11]. The crestal approach, however, is not indicated if the residual bone ridge height is less than 4-5 mm [12]. In such cases, a lateral approach is still preferred.

A key element of lateral sinus lift surgery is designing and carrying out the lateral antrostomy. The design and position of the lateral window define the extent to which the mucoperiosteal flap must be elevated and affect the surgeon's subsequent actions. The window width, height, shape, and distance from the ridge border may have an impact on the angles that the sinus-membrane-elevation instruments must

assume to effectively detach the membrane from the sinus floor. This, in turn, may affect the probability of membrane perforation, one of the most common complications [1, 13, 14]. Additionally, the extent to which the mucoperiosteal flap is elevated can limit easy access to the operatory field because of the need to keep the patient's vestibular tissues retracted for a longer time or to a wider amplitude, causing patient discomfort and operator fatigue.

To the authors' knowledge, no systematic investigation of the effect of the window design, size, and position on complication rates or effort required to carry out sinus lift surgeries has been carried out. Indications concerning the window size vary from author to author [15–21]. Different authors suggest that the lower antrostomy line should be positioned either flush with the sinus floor or up to 2-3 mm above it [1, 12, 22–24]. Analysis of the current clinical literature on lateral sinus lifts reveals great variability in the window shape, design, size, and position. Part of this variability is necessarily due to specific requirements arising from the individual patient anatomy [1], but part seems to depend only on the surgeon's personal habits. In the present paper, the authors propose a specific design for the lateral window based on rational considerations and observations. This design involves positioning the window as low and

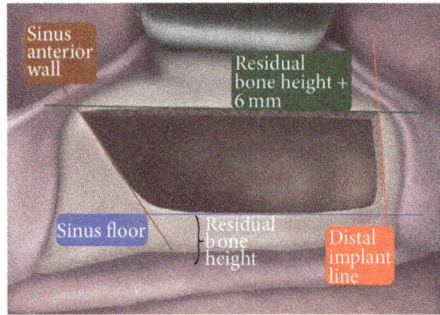

FIGURE 1: The Low Window Sinus Lift antrostomy. The lower osteotomy line (blue) is positioned flush with the sinus floor. The upper one (green) is 6 mm higher; that is, it is placed at a distance from the ridge equal to the residual bone height plus 6 mm. The mesial line (brown) is flush to the sinus anterior wall. The distal one (red) should be placed in correspondence with the position of the most distal implant.

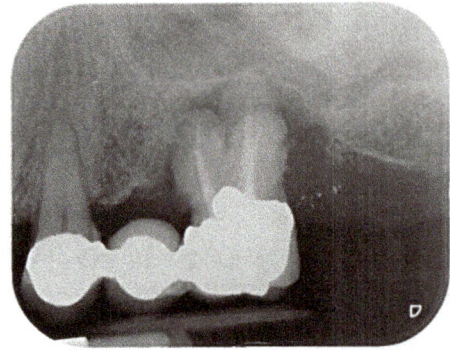

FIGURE 2: Intraoral radiograph at the patient presentation. Tooth 26 is affected by an endoperiodontal lesion and is lost.

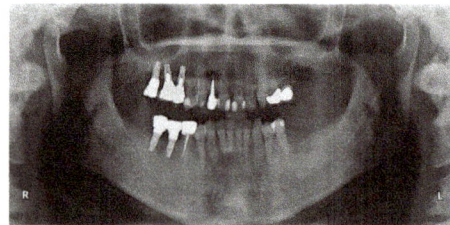

FIGURE 3: OPT recorded after sectioning the prosthesis and extracting the compromised element. The residual ridge presents a significant defect.

mesial as possible and has been named the "Low Window Sinus Lift technique."

The Low Window Sinus Lift technique involves designing the lateral window according to the scheme presented in Figure 1. The lower osteotomy line is always placed flush with the sinus floor. The window optimally should be 6 mm high. Accordingly, the cranial (apical) osteotomy line is positioned 6 mm above the sinus-floor level or, equivalently, at a distance from the ridge border equal to the residual bone height (RBH) plus 6 mm. The distal osteotomy line position varies corresponding to the most distal planned implant. Finally, the mesial osteotomy should be placed flush with the anterior wall of the sinus. Using this approach may allow preparation of the flap to be limited to a linear incision, one that preserves the attached gingiva of the most distal residual element present. Release incisions are not performed, and the mucoperiosteal flap may be elevated by a maximum of 10 mm.

The rationale for creating a low window at the most coronal and mesial possible position is that the more apical and distal the window is, the more difficult the surgical access to the sinus will be. Additionally, the position of the osteotomy lines provides specific surgical advantages. Placement of the lower horizontal osteotomy flush with the sinus floor eliminates any residual bone wall that could hinder detachment of the sinus membrane. The position of the distal osteotomy line is optimized according to the position of the most distal implant; extending it more distally than that provides no advantage and may result in elevation of a wider mucoperiosteal flap. Placing it more mesially forces the surgeon to detach a portion of the membrane in a "blind" condition, with no reference points. The position of the mesial osteotomy line, flush with the anterior sinus wall, allows for easier access to the sinus recess, that is, the zone where detaching the sinus membrane is usually more difficult. A window height of 6 mm is the minimum that allows for easy access of the membrane elevators. A smaller height would be an obstacle to membrane elevation, while a greater one would not provide any significant advantage but would require elevation of a wider mucoperiosteal flap [21].

An additional consideration is that when the maxillary ridge is more atrophic, the upper horizontal osteotomy will be lower (since the distance from the upper osteotomy to the sinus floor must be 6 mm) and less detachment of the mucoperiosteal flap will be required, reducing the overall invasiveness of the surgery.

The following case illustrates the use of the Low Window Sinus Lift technique.

2. Case Presentation

The patient, a 50-year-old male, presented complaining about pain in his upper left maxilla that corresponded to earlier placement of a bridge connecting the first bicuspid to the first molar. The second bicuspid previously had been extracted. The patient underwent clinical examination and radiographic assessment, and the intraoral radiograph (Figure 2) showed an endoperiodontal lesion affecting the first molar. After sectioning the old prosthesis, the affected tooth was atraumatically extracted, and an orthopantomography (OPT) was collected (Figure 3). Two months later, the residual bone height was found to be insufficient to place osseointegrated implants (Figure 4). A CBCT examination was performed to evaluate the health and anatomical status of the left sinus (Figure 5). A rehabilitation plan involving sinus augmentation using the Low Window Sinus Lift approach and concomitant implant placement was developed, and the patient provided informed consent. The implant positioning was preplanned using the CBCT scan in order to have a surgical guide manufactured.

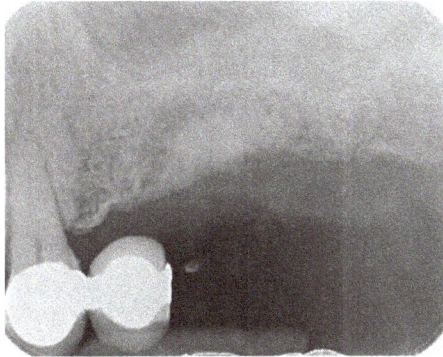

FIGURE 4: Intraoral radiograph collected two months later showing the limited thickness of the residual posterior ridge.

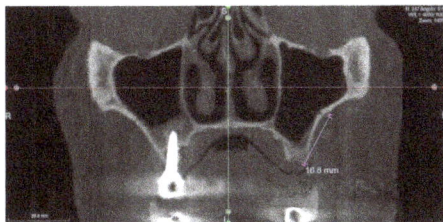

FIGURE 5: CBCT of the sinuses. The maxillary intraosseous anastomosis at the left sinus is 16.8 mm above the ridge coronal bone level.

The design of the surgical guide also included a guide for carrying out the lateral antrostomy according to the low window scheme previously described (Figure 6).

Surgical Procedure. Antibiotic prophylaxis (amoxicillin/ clavulanic acid, Augmentin, Glaxo-SmithKline, Verona, Italy, 1 g 1 hour before surgery and then every 12 hours for 6 days) was initiated. The patient also was instructed to rinse with chlorhexidine 0.2% (Corsodyl, Glaxo-SmithKline) for two weeks after surgery. Ketoprofen 80 mg (Oki, Dompé, L'Aquila, Italy) was prescribed for pain as needed, but not to exceed every eight hours for seven days.

To get easier access to the surgical area, a flexible aid (Optragate, Ivoclar Vivadent AG, Schaan, Liechtenstein) was placed. The surgical area was anesthetized with articaine hydrochloride 40 mg/mL with adrenaline 1 : 100,000. A full-thickness flap that enabled the apical osteotomy line to be drawn 10 mm above the ridge was elevated. Mesially, the incision was paramarginal to the more distal residual element in order to preserve its attached gingiva. No releasing incisions were performed either distally or mesially; that is, the incision had no vertical components (Figures 7 and 8). The access window was then drawn on the vestibular bone using a dermographic pencil and the surgical guide. Using standard piezoelectric tips under sterile saline irrigation, the window in the maxillary sinus lateral wall was then created. The sinus membrane was carefully elevated (Figure 9), and equine-derived cortical-cancellous granules, sized 0.5–1 mm (Osteoxenon, Bioteck, Arcugnano, Italy), were hydrated with sterile saline and inserted into the cavity, applying gentle

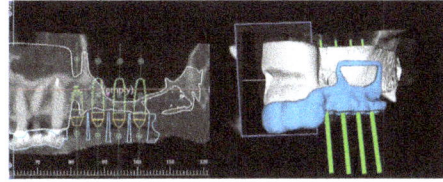

FIGURE 6: The position of the implants is preplanned on the CBCT scan. A surgical guide is designed that includes also the frame of the sinus antrostomy designed according to the low window principles.

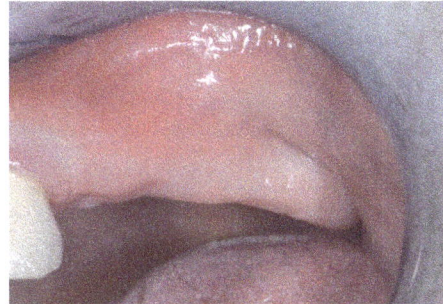

(a)

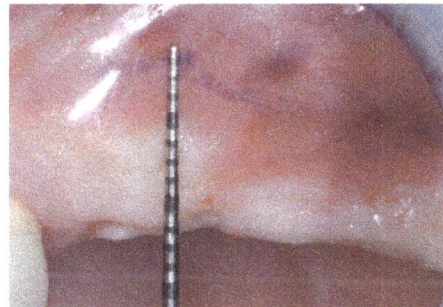

(b)

FIGURE 7: The clinical appearance of the edentulous posterior maxilla (a) and the flap design (b) at no more than 10 mm from the ridge.

pressure to stabilize them. Before the cavity was full, three 4.0 × 13.0 mm osseointegrated implants were placed in the positions indicated by the surgical guide. Filling of the cavity was then completed, and the mucoperiosteal flaps were sutured using nonresorbable 5.0 sutures (Figure 10).

The sutures were removed after 10 days. Six months after placement, the implants were uncovered, and healing screws were attached. Three weeks later, a radiograph was taken, and a dental impression was made using pick-up impression copings in order to manufacture a provisional prosthesis. This was delivered after 10 days, and the patient wore it for approximately three months, at which point the definitive abutments and metal-ceramic crowns were delivered (Figure 11). The maintenance program included professional oral hygiene at six and 12 months after rehabilitation with the definitive prosthesis (Figure 12).

No intraoperative or immediate postoperative complications occurred. The patient healed uneventfully. At the

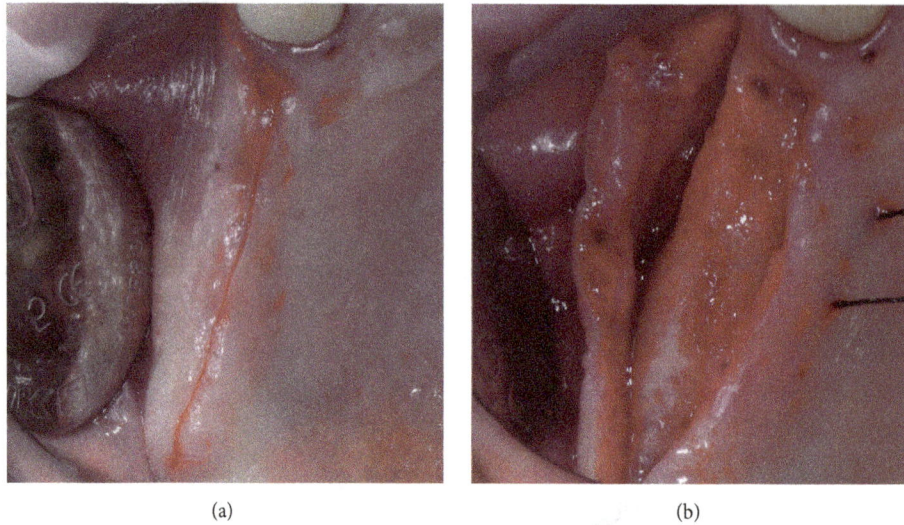

FIGURE 8: A single incision is performed on the medial, occlusal line of the ridge, preserving the papilla of the most distal residual element (a). No release incisions are carried out, and a full-thickness mucoperiosteal flap is elevated (b).

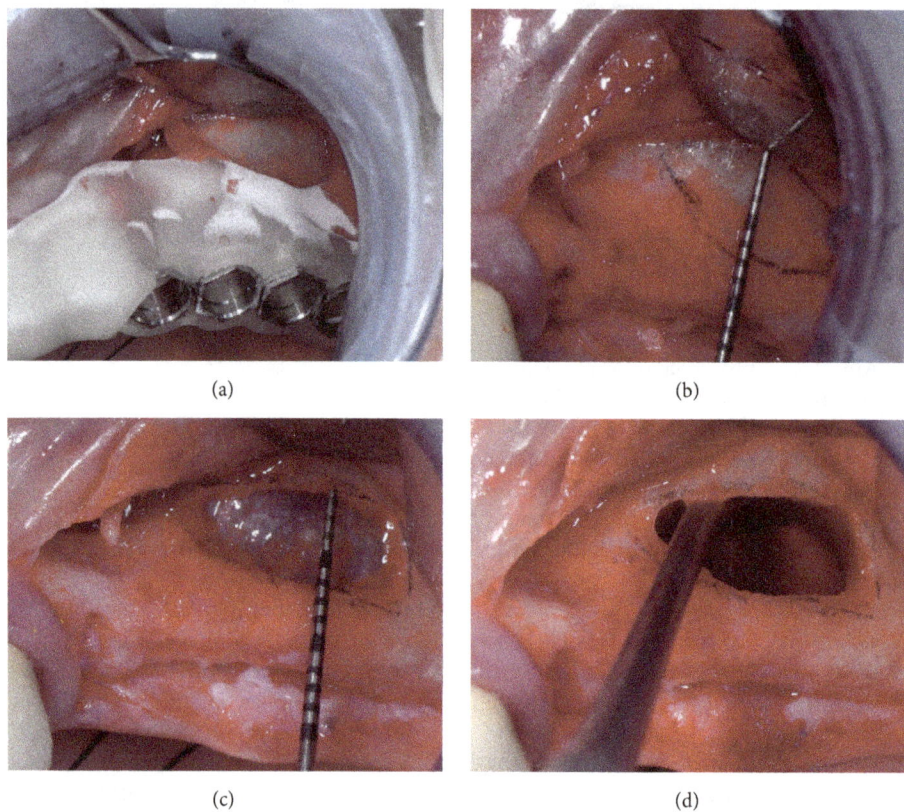

FIGURE 9: The preparation of the antrostomy and the elevation of the sinus membrane. First, the window is drawn on the vestibular bone wall with the aid of the surgical guide (a). The window is no more than 6 mm high (b). After performing the osteotomy (c), the sinus membrane is fully elevated (d).

one-year follow-up, all implants were successful according to the criteria defined by Albrektsson et al. [25] concerning marginal bone levels changes. The prosthesis was fully functional (Figure 12). No significant differences were observed as far as the graft height stability was concerned; that is, the distance between the implant apices and the graft level showed no changes when compared to that at baseline (grafting surgery). The Full Mouth Plaque Score of the patient, which was 10% before surgery, had increased to 20% at the one-year control follow-up. The patient was therefore

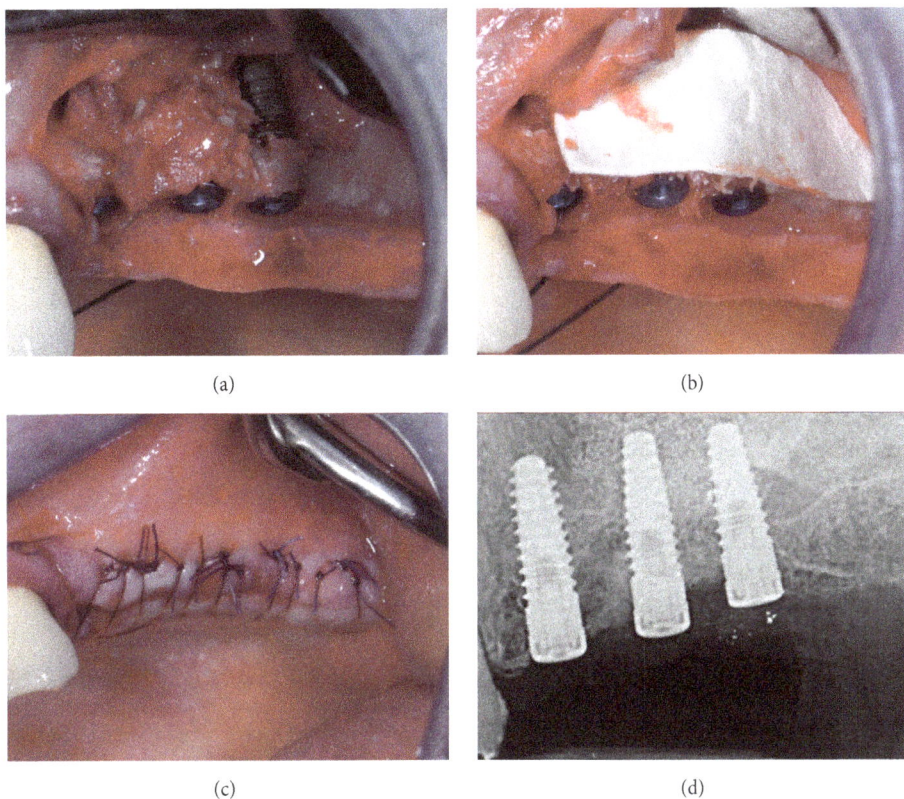

(a)

(b)

(c)

(d)

FIGURE 10: After partially filling the grafting site, implants are being placed with the aid of the surgical guide (a) and filling is complete (b). Implants are left submerged (c), and an intraoral control radiograph is collected (d).

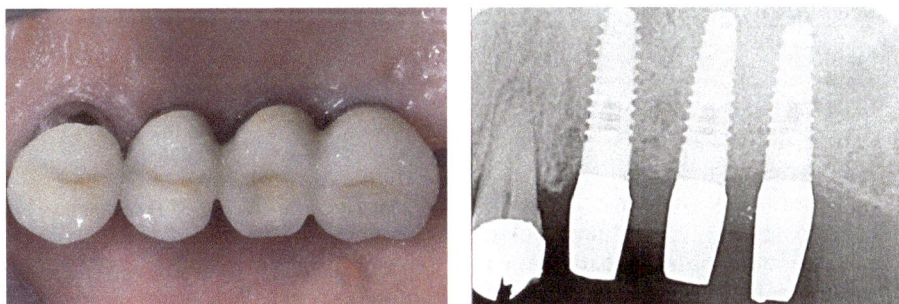

FIGURE 11: The final prosthetic rehabilitation.

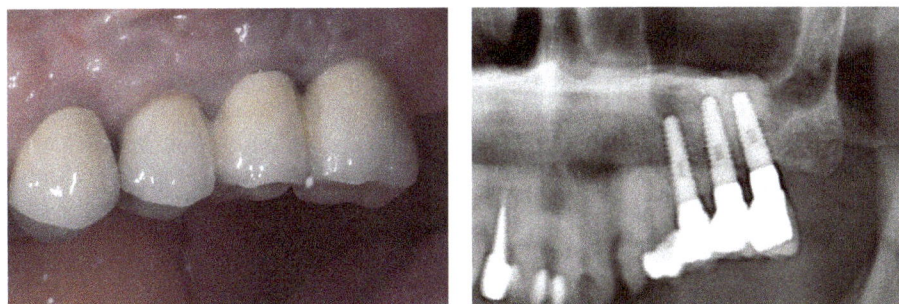

FIGURE 12: At the one-year control after definitive prosthetic rehabilitation, implants are successful and the prosthesis is fully functional.

advised to take greater care of his oral hygiene at home, and more frequent hygiene treatments were planned. The patient was fully satisfied with his rehabilitation.

3. Discussion

The authors have used the Low Window Sinus Lift technique in more than 50 lateral sinus augmentations performed over the past four years. Invasiveness appears to be reduced because a smaller flap is usually necessary than with other lateral antrostomy preparations. Consequently, patients may experience less discomfort and fewer postsurgical complications, such as swelling or pain. The approach has also been surgeon-friendly, with access to the surgical site gained more easily. This in turn often reduces the need for the surgical assistant to provide retraction of lips and cheeks during the surgery. As in the case described, a flexible aid alone may provide sufficient retraction. Because of the low window position, the cortical layer that must be removed tends to be thinner. Osteotomy preparation thus tends to require less time. Moreover, detaching the sinus membrane tends to be accomplished more easily because, given the lower window position, the elevating movement occurs not only laterally but also upward. Together with the greater membrane visibility, these features may also reduce the intraoperative complications (e.g., sinus membrane tearing). Last but not least, positioning the window according to this technique would usually prevent the clinician from encountering the posterior superior alveolar artery [26, 27], thus minimizing the risk of damaging it. The short operative time, reduced invasiveness, and lower risk of membrane tearing and/or superior alveolar artery damage are the possible advantages of this technique over other current approaches.

It should be noted that this technique is effective insofar as it exploits the accuracy that can be achieved by current CAD-CAM manufacturing systems; that is, the surgeon, in order to carry out the technique properly, will need to have a CT or a CBCT scan performed and a surgical guide manufactured. Yet, the surgical guide for implant insertion, modified to incorporate the window frame, can be easily created and used effectively because of the low window position. In contrast, a higher window position tends to hinder correct positioning of such a guide because of the inclination of the vestibular ridge.

The Low Window Sinus Lift technique does not influence other significant sinus augmentation variables, such as the volume of biomaterial required or the length of the implants to be placed, and it does not preclude the possibility of performing a concomitant vertical/horizontal ridge augmentation by guided bone regeneration if necessary. In this case, the flap design will still involve performing release incisions in order to allow suturing without residual tension even if the ridge volume has been augmented.

In the authors' experience, the Low Window Sinus Lift technique has no technique-specific contraindications. The use of the surgical guide also minimizes the risk of creating the lower osteotomy in too low position, that is, one that will cut into the residual crestal bone below the sinus membrane.

Finally, the Low Window Sinus Lift technique requires following specific and replicable operative indications in designing the lateral window. This implies that clinical studies could be designed to investigate its effectiveness at lowering intraoperative complications, postsurgical patient discomfort, or other outcomes of interest, with no bias due to different window designs and positions such as that observed in current studies of lateral sinus augmentation.

The Low Window Sinus Lift technique proposed in the present study appears to be a replicable, rational approach to sinus lift augmentation that may entail significant advantages for both patients and surgeons. Controlled studies should be undertaken to investigate whether this technique provides significant improvements over alternative sinus augmentation approaches.

Competing Interests

The authors declare that they have no competing interests.

References

[1] S. A. Danesh-Sani, P. M. Loomer, and S. S. Wallace, "A comprehensive clinical review of maxillary sinus floor elevation: anatomy, techniques, biomaterials and complications," *British Journal of Oral and Maxillofacial Surgery*, vol. 54, no. 7, pp. 724–730, 2016.

[2] H. Tatum Jr, "Maxillary and sinus implant reconstructions," *Dental clinics of North America*, vol. 30, no. 2, pp. 207–229, 1986.

[3] O. H. Tatum Jr., M. S. Lebowitz, C. A. Tatum, and R. A. Borgner, "Sinus augmentation. Rationale, development, long-term results," *The New York State Dental Journal*, vol. 59, no. 5, pp. 43–48, 1993.

[4] P. J. Boyne and R. A. James, "Grafting of the maxillary sinus floor with autogenous marrow and bone," *Journal of Oral Surgery*, vol. 38, no. 8, pp. 613–616, 1980.

[5] M. Del Fabbro, S. S. Wallace, and T. Testori, "Long-term implant survival in the grafted maxillary sinus: a systematic review," *The International Journal of Periodontics & Restorative Dentistry*, vol. 33, no. 6, pp. 773–783, 2013.

[6] M. Chiapasco, P. Casentini, and M. Zaniboni, "Bone augmentation procedures in implant dentistry," *The International Journal of Oral & Maxillofacial Implants*, vol. 24, pp. 237–259, 2009.

[7] M. Esposito, P. Felice, and H. V. Worthington, "Interventions for replacing missing teeth: augmentation procedures of the maxillary sinus," *The Cochrane database of systematic reviews*, vol. 5, 2014.

[8] R. B. Summers, "A new concept in maxillary implant surgery: the osteotome technique," *Compendium*, vol. 15, no. 2, article 152, pp. 154–156, 1994.

[9] F. Cosci and M. Luccioli, "A new sinus lift technique in conjunction with placement of 265 implants: a 6-year retrospective study," *Implant Dentistry*, vol. 9, no. 4, pp. 363–366, 2000.

[10] P. A. Fugazzotto, "The modified trephine/osteotome sinus augmentation technique: technical considerations and discussion of indications," *Implant Dentistry*, vol. 10, no. 4, pp. 259–264, 2001.

[11] L. Trombelli, G. Franceschetti, C. Stacchi et al., "Minimally invasive transcrestal sinus floor elevation with deproteinized

bovine bone or β-tricalcium phosphate: a multicenter, double-blind, randomized, controlled clinical trial," *Journal of Clinical Periodontology*, vol. 41, no. 3, pp. 311–319, 2014.

[12] T. Testori, M. Del Fabbro, R. Weinstein, and S. Wallace, *Maxillary Sinus Surgery and Alternatives in Treatment*, Quintessence Publishing, 2009.

[13] S. S. Wallace, Z. Mazor, S. J. Froum, S.-O. Cho, and D. P. Tarnow, "Schneiderian membrane perforation rate during sinus elevation using piezosurgery: clinical results of 100 consecutive cases," *International Journal of Periodontics and Restorative Dentistry*, vol. 27, no. 5, pp. 413–419, 2007.

[14] P. Fugazzotto, P. R. Melnick, and M. Al-Sabbagh, "Complications when augmenting the posterior maxilla," *Dental Clinics of North America*, vol. 59, no. 1, pp. 97–130, 2015.

[15] O. T. Jensen, L. B. Shulman, M. S. Block, and V. J. Iacono, "Report of the sinus consensus conference of 1996," *The International Journal of Oral & Maxillofacial Implants*, vol. 13, supplement, pp. 11–45, 1998.

[16] N. U. Zitzmann and P. Schärer, "Sinus elevation procedures in the resorbed posterior maxilla: comparison of the crestal and lateral approaches," *Oral Surgery, Oral Medicine, Oral Pathology, Oral Radiology, and Endodontics*, vol. 85, no. 1, pp. 8–17, 1998.

[17] T. Vercellotti, S. De Paoli, and M. Nevins, "The piezoelectric bony window osteotomy and sinus membrane elevation: introduction of a new technique for simplification of the sinus augmentation procedure," *International Journal of Periodontics and Restorative Dentistry*, vol. 21, no. 6, pp. 561–567, 2001.

[18] A. Barone, S. Santini, S. Marconcini, L. Giacomelli, E. Gherlone, and U. Covani, "Osteotomy and membrane elevation during the maxillary sinus augmentation procedure: a comparative study: piezoelectric device vs. conventional rotative instruments," *Clinical Oral Implants Research*, vol. 19, no. 5, pp. 511–515, 2008.

[19] F. Lambert, G. Lecloux, and E. Rompen, "One-step approach for implant placement and subantral bone regeneration using bovine hydroxyapatite: a 2- to 6-year follow-up study," *International Journal of Oral & Maxillofacial Implants*, vol. 25, no. 3, pp. 598–606, 2010.

[20] A. Simonpieri, J. Choukroun, M. Del Corso, G. Sammartino, and D. M. Dohan Ehrenfest, "Simultaneous sinus-lift and implantation using microthreaded implants and leukocyte- and platelet-rich fibrin as sole grafting material: a six-year experience," *Implant Dentistry*, vol. 20, no. 1, pp. 2–12, 2011.

[21] N. Baldini, C. D'Elia, A. Bianco, C. Goracci, M. de Sanctis, and M. Ferrari, "Lateral approach for sinus floor elevation: large versus small bone window—a split-mouth randomized clinical trial," *Clinical Oral Implants Research*, 2016.

[22] E. Kaufman, "Maxillary sinus elevation surgery: an overview," *Journal of Esthetic and Restorative Dentistry*, vol. 15, no. 5, pp. 272–282, 2003.

[23] A. Stern and J. Green, "Sinus lift procedures: an overview of current techniques," *Dental Clinics of North America*, vol. 56, no. 1, pp. 219–233, 2012.

[24] J. S. Guerrero and B. A. Al-Jandan, "Lateral wall sinus floor elevation for implant placement: revisiting fundamentals and the surgical technique," *Journal of the California Dental Association*, vol. 41, no. 3, pp. 185–195, 2013.

[25] T. Albrektsson, G. Zarb, P. Worthington, and A. R. Eriksson, "The long-term efficacy of currently used dental implants: a review and proposed criteria of success," *The International journal of oral & maxillofacial implants*, vol. 1, no. 1, pp. 11–25, 1986.

[26] M. Velasco-Torres, M. Padial-Molina, J. A. Alarcón, F. Ovalle, A. Catena, and P. Galindo-Moreno, "Maxillary sinus dimensions with respect to the posterior superior alveolar artery decrease with tooth loss," *Implant Dentistry*, vol. 25, no. 4, pp. 464–470, 2016.

[27] G. Rosano, S. Taschieri, J.-F. Gaudy, T. Weinstein, and M. Del Fabbro, "Maxillary sinus vascular anatomy and its relation to sinus lift surgery," *Clinical Oral Implants Research*, vol. 22, no. 7, pp. 711–715, 2011.

24

Peripheral Giant Cell Granuloma in a Child Associated with Ectopic Eruption and Traumatic Habit with Control of Four Years

Luiz Evaristo Ricci Volpato,[1] **Cristhiane Almeida Leite,**[2] **Brunna Haddad Anhesini,**[3] **Jéssica Marques Gomes da Silva Aguilera,**[4] **and Álvaro Henrique Borges**[1]

[1]*Master's Program in Integrated Dental Sciences, University of Cuiabá, Cuiabá, MT, Brazil*
[2]*Department of Oral Pathology, University of Cuiabá, Cuiabá, MT, Brazil*
[3]*Master's Program in Restorative Dentistry, University of São Paulo, São Paulo, SP, Brazil*
[4]*University of Cuiabá, Cuiabá, MT, Brazil*

Correspondence should be addressed to Luiz Evaristo Ricci Volpato; odontologiavolpato@uol.com.br

Academic Editor: Jose López-López

Peripheral giant cell granuloma (PGCG) is a nonneoplastic lesion that may affect any region of the gingiva or alveolar mucosa of edentulous and toothed areas, preferentially in the mandible and rarely occurring in children. This report describes the clinical and histopathological findings of a PGCG diagnosed in the maxilla of a 9-year-old boy associated with a tooth erupting improperly and a traumatic habit. The patient did not present anything noteworthy on extraoral physical examination or medical history, but the habit of picking his teeth and "poking" the gingiva. The oral lesion consisted of an asymptomatic, rounded, pink colored, smooth surface, soft tissue injury with fibrous consistency and approximated size of 1.5 cm located in the attached gingiva between the upper left permanent lateral incisor and the primary canine of the same side. Excisional biopsy was performed through curettage and removal of the periosteum, periodontal ligament, and curettage of the involved teeth with vestibular access. The histopathological analysis led to the diagnosis of PGCG. The prompt diagnosis and treatment of the PGCG resulted in a more conservative surgery and a reduced risk for tooth and bone loss and recurrence of the lesion. After four years of control, patient had no relapse of the lesion and good gingival and osseous health.

1. Introduction

The peripheral giant cell granuloma (PGCG) was first described in 1953 by Jaffe and was originally called reparative giant cell granuloma [1]. PGCG is a nonneoplastic lesion, characterized by reactive hyperplasia in the presence of local irritation, including trauma from extractions, food impaction, calculus, periodontal disease, periodontal surgery, orthodontic appliances, defective restorations with overhanging margins, and ill-fitting removable appliances [2–4]. They affect any region of the gingiva or alveolar mucosa of edentulous and toothed areas [2] and it is believed to be originated from periosteal or periodontal ligament cells [5, 6]. They can occur in different age groups, predominantly between the fourth and sixth decades of life [7, 8].

Clinically, the PGCG presents exophytic growth of sessile or pedicle base, reddish or purplish smooth surface, and consistency ranging from being soft to firm, with the mandible more often involved than the maxilla [2, 8, 9]. The clinical differential diagnosis of a reactive lesion of the gingiva must include pyogenic granuloma, traumatic fibroma, peripheral ossifying fibroma, and other lesions [10]. Early recognition, diagnosis, and treatment of this lesion are important. The treatment consists of local surgical excision below the underlying bone and removal of any irritation agent in the region in order to minimize the risk of relapse [10, 11].

This case report describes the clinical and histopathological findings of a PGCG diagnosed in the maxilla of a pediatric patient associated with a tooth erupting improperly

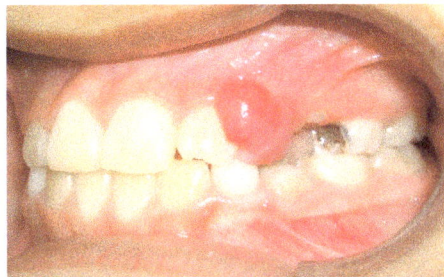

FIGURE 1: Nodular lesion between the upper left permanent lateral incisor and the primary canine.

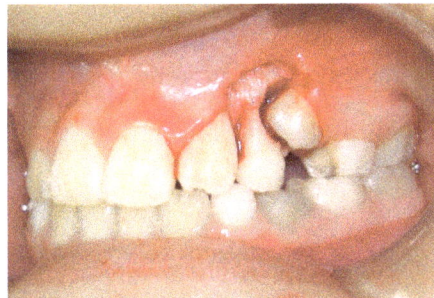

FIGURE 3: Clinical aspect after excisional biopsy of the lesion.

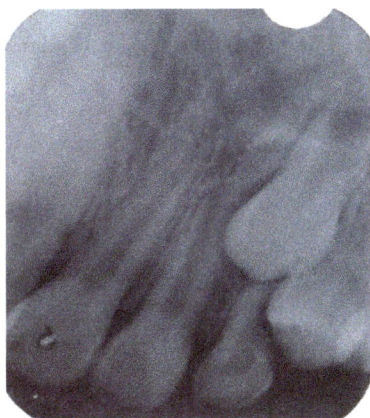

FIGURE 2: Radiographic aspect of the lesion without signs of abnormality.

and a traumatic habit along with four years of clinical and radiographic control.

2. Case Presentation

A 9-year-old boy was referred for treatment in the Pediatric Dentistry Clinic of the Cuiabá Dental School of the University of Cuiabá (UNIC) accompanied by his mother. The main complaint of the patient, reported by his mother, was the presence of a "ball of gingiva" with three months of progressive growth. There was nothing noteworthy at the extraoral physical examination. The medical history revealed no systemic diseases, and he was not in use of any medications at the time. Both the patient and his mother reported that he had the habit of picking his teeth and "poking" the gingiva.

The intraoral examination showed an asymptomatic, rounded, pink colored, smooth surface, soft tissue lesion. It had fibrous consistency, was resilient to the touch, and had the size of approximately 1.5 cm in its largest diameter, located in the attached gingiva between the upper left permanent lateral incisor and the primary canine of the same side (Figure 1). Patient was in mixed dentition with some active carious lesions and poor oral hygiene.

No radiographic change was observed (Figure 2). Faced with clinical and radiographic findings, the presumptive diagnosis was pyogenic granuloma.

The patient was submitted to excisional biopsy of the lesion through curettage and removal of the periosteum, periodontal ligament, and curettage of the involved teeth with vestibular access. Surgical planning of the case included the preservation of the involved teeth which showed vitality and no increased mobility (Figure 3).

Microscopic examination showed noncapsulated nodular proliferation of cellular mesenchymal tissue with abundant multinucleated giant cells dispersed throughout, surfaced by stratified squamous epithelium. Stromal cells consisted of spindle-shaped ovoid plump and mesenchymal cells. Mononuclear inflammatory cells, abundant capillaries, hemorrhage, and hemosiderophages were also observed. The histopathological diagnosis was peripheral giant cell granuloma (Figure 4).

In the postoperative controls of 7 (Figure 5), 14, and 21 days, the area showed a good evolution, with the wound healing.

After four years, the region shows no sign of relapse of the lesion and no clinical or radiographic alteration (Figures 6 and 7).

3. Discussion

The dentist is often faced with conditions involving inflammatory processes related to dental plaque, as gingivitis and periodontitis. However, some patients may have other pathological processes located in periodontium, such as PGCG [12]. The giant cell granuloma (GCG) is not a neoplasm, but a reactive lesion caused by trauma or irritation. Usually it occurs in patients with poor oral hygiene condition [13], as in the presented case. Only 9% of the cases occur in children aged up to 10 years and range from 6.5% to 12.7% in patients of 11–20 years [3, 11].

The origin of giant cells in PGCG is still unclear. Some authors concluded that the multinucleated cells in PGCG are of osteoclastic origin and are derived from differentiated mononuclear cells but the mechanism that activates or recruits osteoclasts in PGCG is still being investigated [14, 15].

In the presented case, the lesion was located in the interdental papilla and the initial clinical hypothesis was pyogenic granuloma (PG). Clinically PGCG, PG, peripheral ossifying fibroma (POF), and gingival fibromatosis (GF) are proliferative gingival lesions that can show very similar characteristics but can present distinct infiltrative features and recurrence

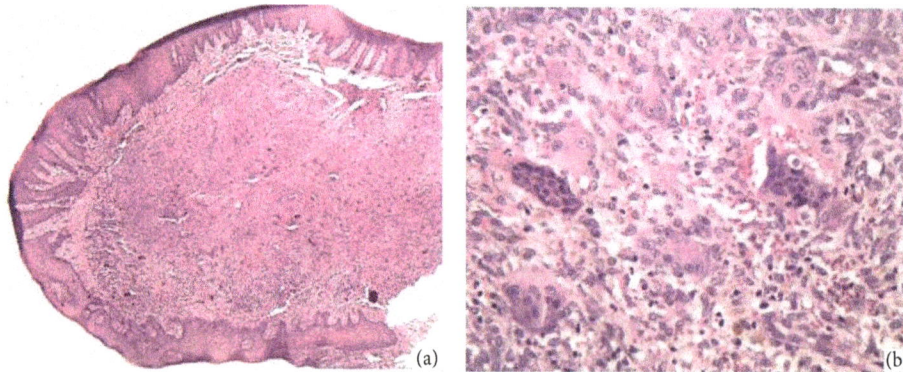

FIGURE 4: (a) Low magnification of PGCG. The stratified squamous epithelium exhibits hyperkeratosis and acanthosis. The subjacent fibrous connective tissue showed noncapsulated nodular proliferation of cellular mesenchymal tissue with abundant multinucleated giant cells dispersed throughout (H&E; original magnification ×20). (b) Higher magnification of PGCG showing giant cells, spindle-shaped ovoid plump stromal cells, inflammatory cells, capillaries, hemorrhage, and hemosiderophages (H&E; original magnification ×400).

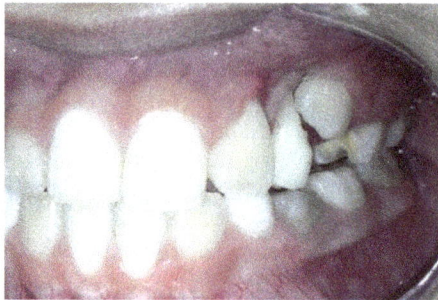

FIGURE 5: Seven-day control.

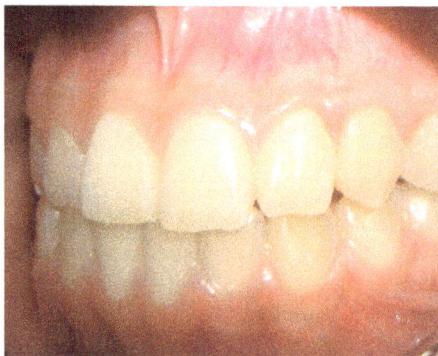

FIGURE 6: Clinical appearance after four years.

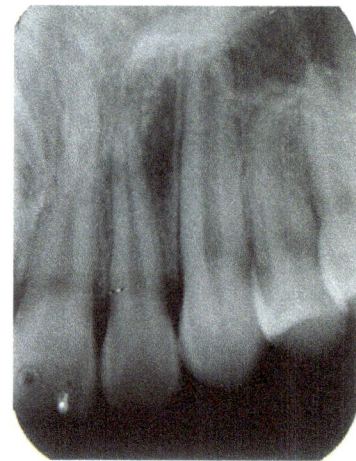

FIGURE 7: Radiographic control after four years without signs of abnormality.

risk [16]. They can be also easily distinguished from parulis, which is frequently associated with a necrotic tooth or with periodontal disorder [17]. PGCG like the peripheral ossifying fibroma is a lesion unique to the oral cavity, occurring only on the gingiva. Unlike peripheral ossifying fibroma, however, it may occur on the alveolar mucosa of edentulous areas. Like pyogenic granuloma and peripheral ossifying fibroma, peripheral giant cell granuloma may represent an unusual response to tissue injury. It is distinguishable from pyogenic granuloma and peripheral ossifying fibroma only on the basis of its unique histomorphology [18, 19].

Peripheral odontogenic fibroma (WHO type) must be considered in the differential diagnosis of dome-shaped or nodular, nonulcerated growths on the gingiva like PGCG. Peripheral odontogenic fibroma is characterized by a fibrous or fibromyxomatous stroma containing varying numbers of islands and strands of odontogenic epithelium that is clearly distinguishable from PGCG histopathology [20].

The diagnosis was confirmed after histopathological analysis of the excised lesion. Histologically the PGCG can be differentiated from other reactive lesions mainly by the abundance of multinucleated giant cells [8, 11, 14], which is the same as central giant cell granuloma [18, 19] and only radiological evaluation can establish the distinction between central and peripheral forms of giant cell granulomas [14]. Radiographs are essential for confirming the oral mucosa origin of the giant cell lesion and refusing a central bony lesion with cortical perforation and soft tissue extension [16].

In the presented case, there was no radiographic evidence of bone involvement and no recurrence was observed.

Other entities need to be considered in differential diagnosis on the basis of histology, namely, brown tumor of hyperparathyroidism, cherubism, and aneurysmal bone cyst. This possibility should be considered, particularly if there are multiple lesions, if the same lesion recurs following appropriate surgical removal, and if there are radiographic alterations. [21, 22] Brown tumor of hyperparathyroidism can perforate the cervical region of the tooth and mimic GCG; alternatively, GCG may be the initial presentation of primary hyperparathyroidism or secondary hyperparathyroidism (generally due to renal insufficiency). Consideration of this disorder is particularly important in cases showing signs of hypercalcemia (renal calculi and neuromuscular, gastrointestinal, or psychiatric disorders), since patients with hyperparathyroidism have been reported to show increased blood levels of calcium, as well as parathormone and alkaline phosphates [23, 24]. However, the medical history of the patient was noncontributory.

Some investigators have suggested that history of trauma might be related to the development of PGCG [11, 15]. Although the patient did not relate any traumatic factor to the occurrence of the lesion, the fact of the left first premolar to be erupting improperly and partially reabsorbing the tooth root of primary canine and the patient's habit of "poking" the gingiva might have contributed to the development of the lesion.

The treatment of the PGCG involves the removal of irritating factors and, mainly, the surgical excision of the lesion, carefully curetting its edges and base, in order to reduce recurrences [10, 11, 25]. In the presented case, the patient was submitted to excisional biopsy of the lesion through its curettage with removal of the periosteum, periodontal ligament, and curettage of the teeth involved with vestibular access and there was no recurrence of the lesion. Surgical planning included the preservation of permanent lateral incisor and primary canine that, although involved, did not show increased mobility.

Early detection of the PGCG results in a more conservative surgery with reduced risk for tooth and bone loss, important issues when treating pediatric patients. After four years of clinical and radiographic control, patient shows no signs of relapse or tissue defects.

Careful medical history followed by complete physical, imaginological, and histopathological examination is critical procedures in the diagnosis process, aiming for a correct treatment plan and thereby reducing the possibility of recurrence and morbidity for patients.

Competing Interests

The authors declare that there is no conflict of interests regarding the publication of this paper.

References

[1] H. L. Jaffe, "Giant-cell reparative granuloma, traumatic bone cyst, and fibrous (fibro-osseous) dysplasia of the jawbones," *Oral Surgery, Oral Medicine, Oral Pathology*, vol. 6, no. 1, pp. 159–175, 1953.

[2] S. R. Lester, K. G. Cordell, M. S. Rosebush, A. A. Palaiologou, and P. Maney, "Peripheral giant cell granulomas: a series of 279 cases," *Oral Surgery, Oral Medicine, Oral Pathology and Oral Radiology*, vol. 118, no. 4, pp. 475–482, 2014.

[3] N. Shadman, S. F. Ebrahimi, S. Jafari, and M. Eslami, "Peripheral giant cell granuloma: a review of 123 cases," *Dental Research Journal*, vol. 6, no. 1, pp. 47–50, 2009.

[4] A. J. Mighell, P. A. Robinson, and W. J. Hume, "Peripheral giant cell granuloma: a clinical study of 77 cases from 62 patients, and literature review," *Oral Diseases*, vol. 1, no. 1, pp. 12–19, 1995.

[5] A. V. Chaparro Avendaño, L. Berini Aytés, and C. Gay Escoda, "Peripheral giant cell granuloma. A report of five cases and review of the literature," *Medicina Oral, Patologia Oral y Cirugia Bucal*, vol. 10, no. 1, pp. 48–57, 2005.

[6] J. M. Gándara, J. L. Pacheco, P. Gándara et al., "Granuloma periférico de células gigantes. Revisión de 13 Casos Clínicos," *Medicina Oral*, vol. 7, pp. 254–259, 2002.

[7] M. H. K. Motamedi, N. Eshghyar, S. M. Jafari et al., "Peripheral and central giant cell granulomas of the jaws: A Demographic Study," *Oral Surgery, Oral Medicine, Oral Pathology, Oral Radiology and Endodontology*, vol. 103, no. 6, pp. e39–e43, 2007.

[8] M. R. Zarei, G. Chamani, and S. Amanpoor, "Reactive hyperplasia of the oral cavity in Kerman province, Iran: a review of 172 cases," *British Journal of Oral and Maxillofacial Surgery*, vol. 45, no. 4, pp. 288–292, 2007.

[9] L. Bodner, M. Peist, A. Gatot, and D. M. Fliss, "Growth potential of peripheral giant cell granuloma," *Oral Surgery, Oral Medicine, Oral Pathology, Oral Radiology*, vol. 83, no. 5, pp. 548–551, 1997.

[10] A. L. Brown, P. C. de Moraes, M. Sperandio, A. B. Soares, V. C. Araújo, and F. Passador-Santos, "Peripheral giant cell granuloma associated with a dental implant: a case report and review of the literature," *Case Reports in Dentistry*, vol. 2015, Article ID 697673, 6 pages, 2015.

[11] N. Katsikeris, E. Kakarantza-Angelopoulou, and A. P. Angelopoulos, "Peripheral giant cell granuloma: clinicopathologic study of 224 new cases and review of 956 reported cases," *International Journal of Oral and Maxillofacial Surgery*, vol. 17, no. 2, pp. 94–99, 1988.

[12] C. M. Flaitz, "Peripheral giant cell granuloma: a potentially aggressive lesion in children," *Pediatric Dentistry*, vol. 22, no. 3, pp. 232–233, 2000.

[13] L. Bodner and J. Bar-Ziv, "Radiographic features of central giant cell granuloma of the jaws in children," *Pediatric Radiology*, vol. 26, no. 2, pp. 148–151, 1996.

[14] A. Z. Abu Gharbyah and M. Assaf, "Management of a peripheral giant cell granuloma in the esthetic area of upper jaw: a case report," *International Journal of Surgery Case Reports*, vol. 5, no. 11, pp. 779–782, 2014.

[15] S. E. Sahingur, R. E. Cohen, and A. Aguirre, "Esthetic management of peripheral giant cell granuloma," *Journal of Periodontology*, vol. 75, no. 3, pp. 487–492, 2004.

[16] F. C. daSilva, C. M. Piazzetta, C. C. Torres-Pereira, J. L. Schussel, and J. M. Amenábar, "Gingival proliferative lesions in children and adolescents in Brazil: a 15-year-period crosssectional study," *Journal of Indian Society of Periodontology*, vol. 20, no. 1, pp. 63–66, 2016.

[17] A. Nekouei, A. Eshghi, P. Jafarnejadi, and Z. Enshaei, "A review and report of peripheral giant cell granuloma in a 4-year-old child," *Case Reports in Dentistry*, vol. 2016, Article ID 7536304, 4 pages, 2016.

[18] L. Andersen, O. Fejerskov, and H. P. Philipsen, "Oral giant cell granulomas. A clinical and histological study of 129 new cases," *Acta Pathologica et Microbiologica Scandinavica A*, vol. 81, no. 5, pp. 606–616, 1973.

[19] J. S. Giansanti and C. A. Waldron, "Peripheral giant cell granuloma: review of 720 cases," *Journal of Oral Surgery*, vol. 27, no. 10, pp. 787–791, 1969.

[20] T. D. Daley and G. P. Wysocki, "Peripheral odontogenic fibroma," *Oral Surgery, Oral Medicine, Oral Pathology*, vol. 78, no. 3, pp. 329–336, 1994.

[21] S. Moghe, M. K. Gupta, A. Pillai, and A. Maheswari, "Peripheral giant cell granuloma: a case report and review of literature," *People's Journal of Scientific Research*, vol. 6, no. 2, pp. 55–59, 2013.

[22] E. J. Burkes Jr. and R. P. White Jr., "A peripheral giant-cell granuloma manifestation of primary hyperparathyroidism: report of case," *The Journal of the American Dental Association*, vol. 118, no. 1, pp. 62–64, 1989.

[23] M. A. Todero, A. Monaco, M. DAmario, M. La Carbonara, and M. Capogreco, "Peripheral gigant cell granuloma (giant cell epulis) associated with metabolic diseases: case report and literature review," *Annali di Stomatologia*, vol. 4, supplement 2, p. 45, 2013.

[24] C. H. Houpis, K. I. Tosios, D. Papavasileiou et al., "Parathyroid hormone-related peptide (PTHrP), parathyroid hormone/parathyroid hormone-related peptide receptor 1 (PTHR1), and MSX1 protein are expressed in central and peripheral giant cell granulomas of the jaws," *Oral Surgery, Oral Medicine, Oral Pathology, Oral Radiology, and Endodontology*, vol. 109, no. 3, pp. 415–424, 2010.

[25] M. T. Vázquez Piñeiro, J. M. González Bereijo, and E. Niembro de Rasche, "Granuloma periférico de células gigantes: caso clínico y revisión de la literatura," *RCOE*, vol. 7, no. 2, pp. 201–206, 2002.

25

Management of the Amniotic Band Syndrome with Cleft Palate

Carolina Cortez-Ortega, José Arturo Garrocho-Rangel, Joselín Flores-Velázquez, Socorro Ruiz-Rodríguez, Miguel Ángel Noyola-Frías, Miguel Ángel Santos-Díaz, and Amaury Pozos-Guillén

Pediatric Dentistry Postgraduate Program, Faculty of Dentistry, San Luis Potosi University, 78290 San Luis Potosí, SLP, Mexico

Correspondence should be addressed to José Arturo Garrocho-Rangel; agarrocho@hotmail.com

Academic Editor: Daniel Torrés-Lagares

Amniotic Band Syndrome (ABS) is a group of congenital malformations that includes the majority of typical constriction rings and limb and digital amputations, together with major craniofacial, thoracic, and abdominal malformations. The syndrome is caused by early rupture of the amniotic sac. Some of the main oral manifestations include micrognathia, hyperdontia, and cleft lip with or without cleft palate, which is present in 14.6% of patients with this syndrome. The purpose of this report was to describe the clinical characteristics and the oral treatment provided to a 6-month-old male patient affected with ABS with cleft lip and palate.

1. Introduction

Amniotic Band Syndrome (ABS), also known as ADAM (acronym for *Amniotic Deformity, Adhesions,* and *Mutilations*), is a rare condition consisting of a broad group of congenital malformations caused mainly by the rupture of the amniotic sac, which produces a series of alterations due to the appearance of fibrous mesodermal amniotic tissue bands [1]. The syndrome exhibits different clinical manifestations at birth, such as constriction rings and limb and digital amputations, together with diverse craniofacial malformations and thoracic-abdominal wall anomalies [1, 2]. These defects represent disruptions not occurring along the known lines of embryologic development [2, 3].

According to recent epidemiologic data, the occurrence of ABS is around 1 in 1,200–15,000 live births and it exhibits no special preference for a specific gender or race [4]; however, some studies report a slight preference for Afro-Caribbean individuals [2]. The pathogenesis of the ABS has not been totally elucidated, but it probably has a genetic origin. Two theories have been proposed to explain the multiple causal factors associated with this syndrome. First, the *intrinsic model*, described by Streeter in 1930 [5], which suggests the existence of an early embryolesion with alterations of the germinal disc that would produce an inflammatory response of the adjacent amnions and that would then develop a fibrous band. Second, the *extrinsic model*, the more widely accepted theory, developed by Torpin in 1968 [6], in which the authors proposed that the rupture of the amnions during early pregnancy allows the embryo or fetus to enter into the chorionic cavity and to contact the chorionic side of the amnions. Thus, fetal structures may be trapped by the fibrous septum that protrudes into the chorionic cavity. Compression and adhesion of these amniotic bands, which float freely, may cause disruption of the fetal structures [7]. The fetus' arms and legs, tangled around the amniotic bands, may be amputated during intrauterine development due to loss of blood flow [4, 8, 9]. The variability in the type and severity of the anomalies caused by this syndrome can be attributed to the moment at which the amniotic membranes rupture. Other related manifestations comprising congenital heart defects, renal anomalies, polydactyly, supernumerary nipples, and skin tags [2].

In their reviews, Muraskas et al. [10] and Bouguila et al. [11] mention that the most common craniofacial anomalies characteristic of the syndrome include corneal and orbital defects, anencephaly, meningocele or encephalocele, palpebral colobomas, nose malformations, and facial nerve paralysis; in the oral cavity, there may be micrognathism, hyperdontia, and cleft lip with or without cleft palate, representing 14.6% of patients who are afflicted with this condition [12, 13]. Multiple anomalies are present in 77% of cases [10].

Prenatal diagnosis of ABS, as early as 12 weeks of gestation, is performed in 29–50% of cases, depending on the severity of the disorder and the time when the lesions appear [10, 14]. Diagnosis of the syndrome consists of the identification of a fibrous band that deforms the distal part of a body limb, which renders it difficult for the limb to move [15]. Fetal compromise may be suspected with the use of Doppler studies, which exhibit reversal of end-diastolic flow in the umbilical artery [10]. When the child is born, it is possible to confirm the diagnosis of ABS by performing a histopathological analysis of the placenta, which can inform about persistence of the amniotic chorionic rupture [16].

The purpose of this report was to provide a review of the literature related to the syndrome and to describe the case of a 6-month-old male patient with ABS, his systematic, craniofacial, and oral clinical characteristics and reconstructive/oral management provided.

2. Literature Search Strategy and Results

An exhaustive Web literature search of relevant references was conducted in March/June 2016 in the following five Internet databases, without language or publication-date restrictions: MEDLINE (via PubMed); EMBASE (Elsevier Science); Google Scholar; Latin Index; and Scielo. The study selection criteria were methodological designs comprised of clinical trials, cohort and case-control studies, and clinical case reports, carried out on infants, children, and adolescents. Articles had to include any type of relevant oral management process or intervention, such as diagnosis tests, craneofacial surgical/rehabilitation procedures, or dental restorative treatments; in vitro studies were excluded. The main search algorithm was the following: (("Amniotic Band Syndrome" [Mesh]) OR ("Amniotic Deformity" [Mesh]) AND ("Pediatric Dentistry") OR ("Maxillofacial Surgery" [Mesh])). Other search terms employed were as follows: "Craniofacial Anomalies"; "Orofacial Cleft"; "Lip Cleft", and "Palate Cleft", or "Pediatric Patients", "Pediatrics"; "Children"; "Childhood"; "Child Dentistry", and "Dentistry for Children", all of these alone or with their different combinations. The filter "Age" was set at "Child: birth–18 years." Subsequently, titles, abstracts, and keywords were objectively and independently reviewed. The papers selected were retrieved in full-text and read in detail. In addition, the authors hand-searched the content pages of the reference lists of these papers.

The literature search identified a total of 145 potential citation references; after reviewing titles and abstracts, 107 of these clearly did not meet the desired criteria and were discarded. The full-text of the remaining 38 citations was retrieved and screened in greater detail; finally, 28 relevant papers were identified for inclusion in the literature review, including 7 dental and 3 medical case reports.

3. Case Report

The patient was a 6-month-old boy who was born at 37 weeks of pregnancy who was referred from the Department of Maxillofacial Surgery of Hospital Central "Dr. Ignacio Morones Prieto" to the Pediatric Dentistry Postgraduate Clinic (San Luis Potosi University, Mexico) for a dental examination and the possible placement of a palatal obturator.

In relation to the perinatal medical history, the child's parents were healthy, nonconsanguineous at 39 and 38 years of age; the mother reported vaginal bleeding during the first month of pregnancy and a urinary tract infection in month 2 of pregnancy. At that time, the mother began prenatal care, including the intake of folic acid. As part of the medical history, no hereditary anomalies were reported, nor smoking, alcoholic-beverage consumption, or drug abuse during pregnancy. The baby-in-question was the mother's fourth pregnancy and he was born within the normal time period (body weight: 2,800 g, size: 51 cm).

Clinically, the patient exhibited multiple craniofacial anomalies, including a fissure on the upper part of the face, encephalocele, corneal opacity of the right eye, hypertelorism, severe hearing loss on the left side, and evident asymmetry (Figure 1). The remainder of his body manifested constriction rings and anomalies in hands and feet (amputation and lymphedema) (Figure 2). The intraoral clinical examination demonstrated a "Y"-shaped lip-palatal fissure from the soft palate terminating with a bifurcation in the upper lip and nose (Figure 3). A karyotype study was performed, whose result revealed the absence of chromosomal alterations. The final ABS diagnosis was determined based on the clinical findings. The patient underwent a reconstructive surgical procedure at 5 months of age.

Based on the intraoral clinical findings compiled, we decided to provide instruction to the parents with oral-hygiene indications, particularly on the cleaning of the infant's alveolar ridge with wet gauze at least once a day, preferably at night after the patient's finishing drinking his bottle. A condensation silicone impression was obtained of the upper dental arch for the fabrication of a palatal obturator; the device was fabricated using autopolymerizable acrylic. After placement of the obturator, its use was recommended for 24 hours a day, with a thoroughly washing each night. Then, control and review appointments were scheduled every 3 months in order to observe how well the palatal obturator adapted and to monitor the patient's craniofacial/oral development and the dental eruption process.

The most recent oral/general examination appointment was 10 months after the first examination. According to the patient's mother, the child was in good general health. He showed a brachyfacial pattern and midface/maxillary arch hypoplasia (Figure 4) but a poor oral-hygiene level; the obturator had been properly used, and marked improvement in swallowing and feeding during the previous 3 months was manifested. However, the device was not well adapted because the upper primary central incisors and first molars were in the eruption process; therefore, the corresponding acrylic trimmings were performed (Figure 5). At the same time, we reinforced the hygiene instructions and began

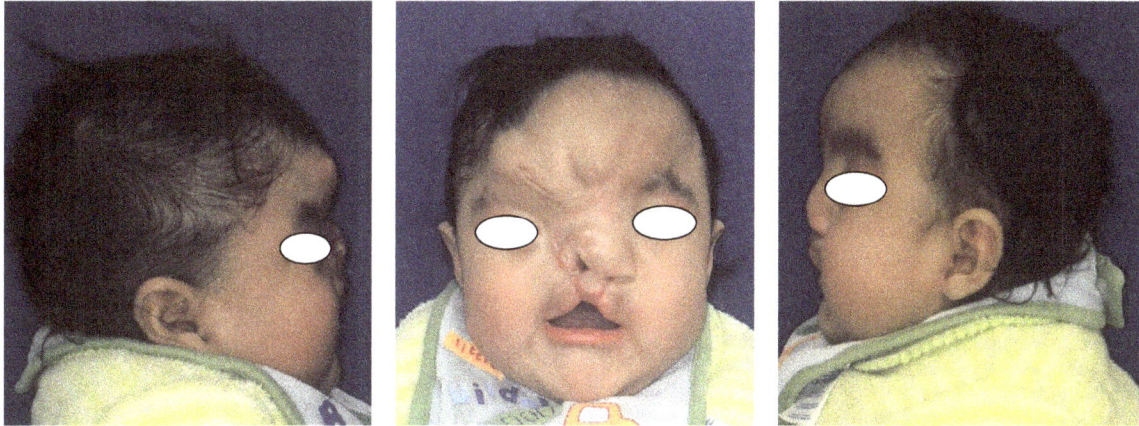

FIGURE 1: Extraoral views.

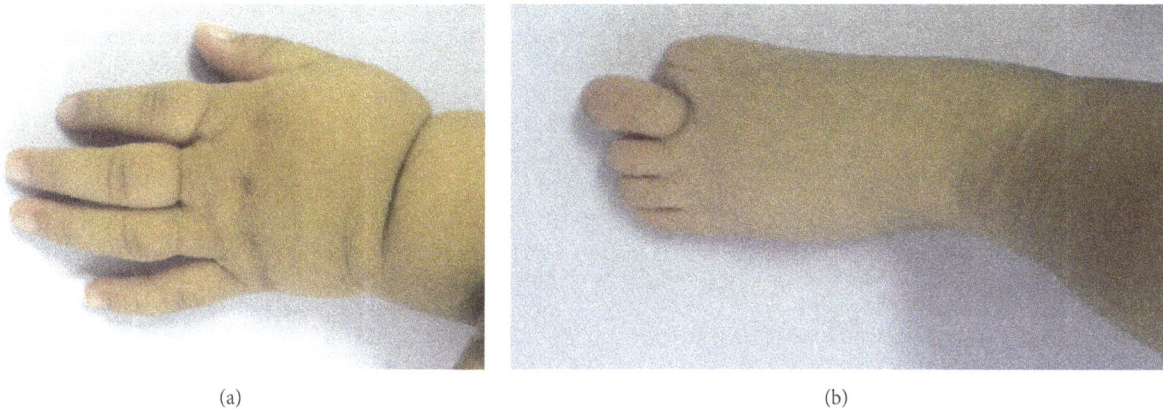

(a)   (b)

FIGURE 2: (a) Right hand. (b) Right foot.

to apply topical high-concentration fluoride varnish on the enamel of these erupting teeth. The manufacture of a new palatal obturator was programmed in the following 4 weeks. Additionally, control and review appointments were scheduled in order to monitor the patient's craniofacial/oral development and his dental eruption progression. Thus, in the short/medium term, we will be able to plan the next reconstructive surgical procedure.

4. Discussion

The occurrence of the ABS with facial/lip/palate is a sporadic event; around 50 medical and dental cases have been reported in the literature over the past 25 years [4, 17]. Although this disorder includes diverse anomalies of the craniofacial and body structures, it is very difficult to specify exclusive clinical features [9, 18]. The observed variability in the type and severity of the anomalies depends on the time of rupture of the amniotic membranes; if this occurs during the first 45 days of pregnancy, the defects are more severe, mainly in the craniofacial structures, along with other anomalies of the central nervous system, visceral defects, and limb anomalies (such as syndactyly or polydactyly). However, if

the fibrous bands appeared after week 12 of pregnancy, the characteristic adherences and constriction rings would only be evident at birth [12, 13, 19]. In the present case, the amniotic membranes' rupture probably took place during the first 45 days of pregnancy, according to the anomalies observed in the patient, such as encephalocele, facial fissure, constriction rings, and toe amputation [18, 20, 21].

Management of patients with ABS requires a multidisciplinary approach with a collaborative medical/dental team. Depending on its severity and the malformations present, the team is integrated by diverse specialists, such as Orthodontists, Pediatric Surgeons, Plastic and Maxillofacial Surgeons, Ophthalmologists, Neurologists, Geneticists, and Psychologists [22, 23]. In addition to being familiar with ABS, Pediatric Dentists must also collaborate actively, both in the prevention and the rehabilitation of oral-dental anomalies, bearing in mind the importance of active early intervention [1, 10]. Considering these issues, some authors have recommended a relatively novel procedure, the fetoscopy or in uterosurgery [10], with the intent of preventing limb amputation and repairing other small or complex ABS malformations. Basically, the procedure consists of releasing the constriction membranes of the limbs at risk; this therapeutic

(a)   (b)   (c)

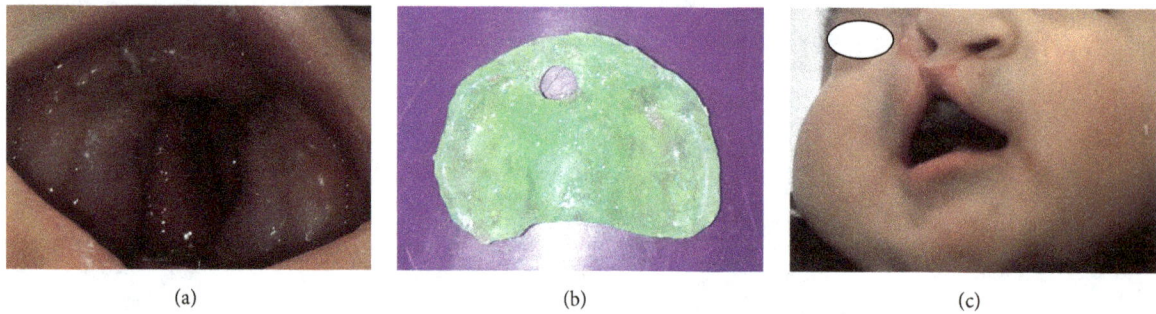

FIGURE 3: (a) Palate cleft view. (b) The obturator device (the hole was created to permit the recent eruption of the right central incisor). (c) Intraoral placement of the obturator.

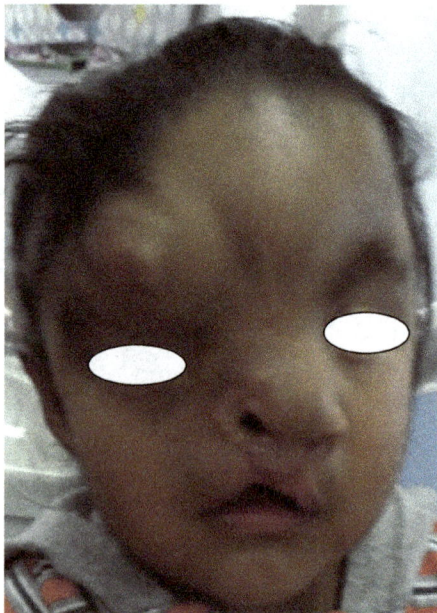

FIGURE 4: The patient's facial view, 10 months after the first examination.

option is slightly invasive and is performed during the early stages of pregnancy [3], and its prognosis depends on the severity of the disorder [8, 23].

For the patient reported in the present work, the pediatric dental treatment provided consisted mainly of the placing of a palatal obturator and the suggestion of some oral-hygiene habits [24, 25]. A palatal obturator is a device that possesses the following several therapeutic effects: (1) it enhances the esthetic result of nasolabial structures and reduces the need for additional surgical procedures by bringing the soft and bone structures surrounding the palatal cleft closer together [25–27]; (2) it creates a seal between the oral and nasal cavities to control the flow of liquids and solid foods [28]; and (3) it restores some basic oral functions such as chewing, swallowing, and speech [25, 28]. Additionally, the obturator creates a rigid surface that allows the child to press her/his mother's nipple and create sufficient negative pressure to achieve proper suction of breast milk, facilitating

the feeding process [24, 28]. The device also reduces nasal regurgitation and the possibility of asphyxiation and aids in achieving correct positioning of the tongue, thus enhancing the functional development of the maxillaries and speech [26]. Because of the horizontal position of the Eustachian tube, abnormal insertion of elevators and soft palate tensor, and the child's muscle hypoplasia, all characteristic findings of patients with ABS, a permanent significant risk is present of food passing through the nasopharynx [25]. The palatal obturator reduces such a risk, thus the incidence of otitis media and nasopharynx infections [24]. These orthopedic devices are considered essential during the presurgical phase, a technique initially developed by McNeil and Burston [24, 26]. Due to all of these preventive and therapeutic reasons, we placed the palatal obturator in our patient prior to the reconstructive procedures.

It is also noteworthy that the oral cavity of an edentate child, such as the patient mentioned herein, should be cleaned at least once a day, preferably at night, using wet gauze with saline solution or filtered water on the alveolar ridges [20]. If the mouth is cleaned each day, the child will grow up with the sensation of having a healthy mouth and will become accustomed to the manipulation of the oral cavity's soft and hard structures [22]. Once the primary teeth have erupted, a special toothbrush with soft bristles for infants should be used, and later, an electrical toothbrush may be implemented; this recommendation would be especially useful in cases of children with motor or neuronal alterations [12].

5. Conclusions

Pediatric Dentists have the obligation of possessing the essential knowledge of the ABS, not only to advise the patient's parents, but also to refer the child to other health professionals. Additionally, active participation by the practitioner is necessary in the management process of ABS patients, for instance, timely diagnosis, prevention, and treatment of the different craniofacial/oral anomalies, control of the growth and development of teeth and maxillary area, and collaboration during the correction of the diverse structural anomalies. In order to achieve these objectives, it is essential to obtain an exhaustive medical history, which allows the

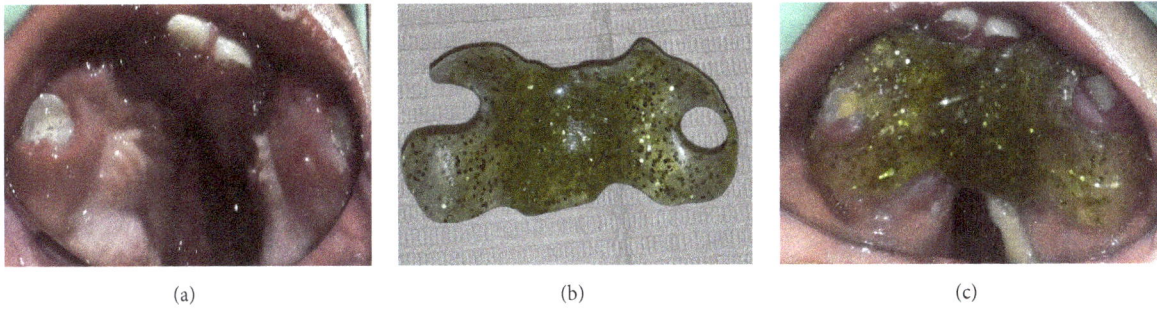

FIGURE 5: (a) Most recent view of the maxillary arch. (b) Adjustments made to the palatal obturator, according to the eruption process of primary teeth. (c) Palatal obturator well adapted in mouth.

specialist to evaluate thoroughly all craniofacial anomalies, design a proper dental treatment plan, and prevent possible complications during the management of these vulnerable patients.

Competing Interests

The authors declare that they have no conflict of interests.

References

[1] K. Hotwani and K. Sharma, "Oral rehabilitation for amniotic band syndrome: an unusual presentation," *International Journal of Clinical Pediatric Dentistry*, vol. 8, no. 1, pp. 55–57, 2015.

[2] E. Koskimies, J. Syvänen, Y. Nietosvaara, O. Mäkitie, and N. Pakkasjärvi, "Congenital constriction band syndrome with limb defects," *Journal of Pediatric Orthopaedics*, vol. 35, no. 1, pp. 100–103, 2015.

[3] B. L. Eppley, L. David, M. Li, C. A. Moore, and A. M. Sadove, "Amniotic band facies," *The Journal of Craniofacial Surgery*, vol. 9, no. 4, pp. 360–365, 1998.

[4] Y. Doi, H. Kawamata, K. Asano, and Y. Imai, "A case of amniotic band syndrome with cleft lip and palate," *Journal of Maxillofacial and Oral Surgery*, vol. 10, no. 4, pp. 354–356, 2011.

[5] G. L. Streeter, *Carnegie Institution Focal deficiencies in fetal tissues and their relation to intra-uterine amputation of Washington*, 1930.

[6] R. Torpin, *Fetal Malformations caused by Amnion Rupture during Gestation*, Charles Thomas, Springfield, Ill, USA, 1968.

[7] Y. Kino, "Clinical and experimental studies of the congenital constriction band syndrome, with an emphasis on its etiology," *Journal of Bone and Joint Surgery*, vol. 57, no. 5, pp. 636–643, 1975.

[8] M. S. E. Coady, M. H. Moore, and K. Wallis, "Amniotic band syndrome: the association between rare facial clefts and limb ring constrictions," *Plastic and Reconstructive Surgery*, vol. 101, no. 3, pp. 640–649, 1998.

[9] S. M. Purandare, L. Ernst, L. Medne, D. Huff, and E. H. Zackai, "Developmental anomalies with features of disorganization (Ds) and amniotic band sequence (ABS): a report of four cases," *American Journal of Medical Genetics, Part A*, vol. 149, no. 8, pp. 1740–1748, 2009.

[10] J. K. Muraskas, J. F. McDonnell, R. J. Chudik, K. E. Salyer, and L. Glynn, "Amniotic band syndrome with significant orofacial clefts and disruptions and distortions of craniofacial structures," *Journal of Pediatric Surgery*, vol. 38, no. 4, pp. 635–638, 2003.

[11] J. Bouguila, N. Ben Khoud, A. Ghrissi et al., "Amniotic band syndrome and facial malformations," *Revue de Stomatologie et de Chirurgie Maxillo-Faciale*, vol. 108, no. 6, pp. 526–529, 2007.

[12] S. Coyle, J. M. Karp, and A. Shirakura, "Oral rehabilitation of a child with amniotic band syndrome," *Journal of Dentistry for Children*, vol. 75, no. 1, pp. 74–79, 2008.

[13] D. Das, G. Das, S. Gayen, and A. Konar, "Median facial cleft in amniotic band syndrome," *Middle East African Journal of Ophthalmology*, vol. 18, no. 2, pp. 192–194, 2011.

[14] J. Hukki, P. Balan, R. Ceponiene, E. Kantola-Sorsa, P. Saarinen, and H. Wikstrom, "A case study of amnion rupture sequence with acalvaria, blindness, and clefting: clinical and psychological profiles," *The Journal of Craniofacial Surgery*, vol. 15, no. 2, pp. 185–191, 2004.

[15] T. K. Pedersen and S. G. Thomsen, "Spontaneous resolution of amniotic bands," *Ultrasound in Obstetrics and Gynecology*, vol. 18, no. 6, pp. 673–674, 2001.

[16] C. G. Morovic, F. Berwart, and J. Varas, "Craniofacial anomalies of the amniotic band syndrome in serial clinical cases," *Plastic and Reconstructive Surgery*, vol. 113, no. 6, pp. 1556–1562, 2004.

[17] A. M. Buccoliero, F. Castiglione, F. Garbini et al., "Amniotic band syndrome: a case report," *Pathologica*, vol. 103, no. 1, pp. 11–13, 2011.

[18] P. Cignini, C. Giorlandino, F. Padula, N. Dugo, E. V. Cafà, and A. Spata, "Epidemiology and risk factors of amniotic band syndrome, or ADAM sequence," *Journal of Prenatal Medicine*, vol. 6, no. 4, pp. 59–63, 2012.

[19] M. C. Obdeijn, P. J. Offringa, R. R. M. Bos, A. A. E. Verhagen, F. B. Niessen, and N. A. Roche, "Facial clefts and associated limb anomalies: description of three cases and a review of the literature," *Cleft Palate-Craniofacial Journal*, vol. 47, no. 6, pp. 661–667, 2010.

[20] P. J. Taub, J. P. Bradley, Y. Setoguchi, L. Schimmenti, and H. K. Kawamoto Jr., "Typical facial clefting and constriction band anomalies: an unusual association in three unrelated patients," *American Journal of Medical Genetics*, vol. 120, no. 2, pp. 256–260, 2003.

[21] C. A. Perlyn, R. Schmelzer, D. Govier, and J. L. Marsh, "Congenital scalp and calvarial deficiencies: principles for classification and surgical management," *Plastic and Reconstructive Surgery*, vol. 115, no. 4, pp. 1129–1141, 2005.

[22] M. A. Jabor and E. D. Cronin, "Bilateral cleft lip and palate and limb deformities: a presentation of amniotic band sequence?" *Journal of Craniofacial Surgery*, vol. 11, no. 4, pp. 388–393, 2000.

[23] O. O. Adeosun, D. James, V. I. Akinmoladun, and T. Owobu, "Amniotic band syndrome associated with orofacial clefts: a report of two cases," *Oral Surgery*, vol. 5, no. 4, pp. 185–189, 2012.

[24] R. Narendra, C. R. Sashi Purna, S. D. Reddy, N. Simhachalam Reddy, P. Sesha Reddy, and B. Rajendra Prasad, "Feeding obturator-a presurgical prosthetic aid for infants with cleft lip and palate-clinical report," *Annals and Essences of Dentistry*, vol. 5, no. 2, pp. 1–5, 2013.

[25] M. Goyal, R. Chopra, K. Bansal, and M. Marwaha, "Role of obturators and other feeding interventions in patients with cleft lip and palate: a review," *European Archives of Paediatric Dentistry*, vol. 15, no. 1, pp. 1–9, 2014.

[26] K. S. Ravichandra, K. E. Vijayaprasad, A. A. K. Vasa, and S. Suzan, "A new technique of impression making for an obturator in cleft lip and palate patient," *Journal of Indian Society of Pedodontics and Preventive Dentistry*, vol. 28, no. 4, pp. 311–314, 2010.

[27] M. A. Papadopoulos, E. N. Koumpridou, M. L. Vakalis, and S. N. Papageorgiou, "Effectiveness of pre-surgical infant orthopedic treatment for cleft lip and palate patients: a systematic review and meta-analysis," *Orthodontics & Craniofacial Research*, vol. 15, no. 4, pp. 207–236, 2012.

[28] K. F. M. Britton, S. H. McDonald, and R. R. Welbury, "An investigation into infant feeding in children born with a cleft lip and/or palate in the West of Scotland," *European Archives of Paediatric Dentistry*, vol. 12, no. 5, pp. 250–255, 2011.

26

New Approach to Managing Onychophagia

O. Marouane,[1] M. Ghorbel,[2] M. Nahdi,[3] A. Necibi,[3] and N. Douki[1]

[1]*Restorative Dentistry, Dental Surgery Department, University Hospital Sahloul, Sousse, Tunisia*
[2]*Department of Removable Prosthodontics, Faculty of Dental Medicine of Monastir, Monastir, Tunisia*
[3]*Orthodontic Department, Faculty of Dental Medicine of Monastir, Monastir, Tunisia*

Correspondence should be addressed to O. Marouane; marouane.omar@yahoo.com

Academic Editor: Daniel Torrés-Lagares

Onychophagia is defined as a chronic habit of biting nails, commonly observed in both children and young adults. This oral habit may lead to various medical and dental problems. To date, onychophagia is considered an unsolved problem in medicine and dentistry. In this paper we describe an exclusive nonpunitive fixed appliance utilizing a stainless steel twisted round wire bonded from canine to canine, in the mandibular arch, as a treatment of onychophagia. It was used successfully in young adult patients and maintained for a month. With 9-month follow-up the treatment has satisfied the patients' expectations which may eventually yield promising implications of this new treatment to similar situations.

1. Introduction

Onychophagia is defined as a chronic habit of biting nails, commonly observed in both children and young adults, and it is classified among nail diseases caused by repeated injuries [1–3].

Only few epidemiological studies provide the frequency or the prevalence of this habit and most data are limited to children and adolescents [3]. Onychophagia is usually not observed before the age of 3 or 4 years. The prevalence of nail biting increases from childhood to adolescence and decreases in adulthood [2].

It ranges from 20 to 33% during childhood and approximately 45% of teenagers are nail biters [4–7]. By the age of 18 years the frequency of nail biting decreases; however it may persist in some adults [8].

To date, the exact etiology of onychophagia remains as yet unclear. Although it has been observed that nail biters have more anxiety than those who do not have the habit, no relevant relationship was found between nail biting and anxiety [9]. Others support that onychophagia is a learned behavior from family members, which most likely seems consistent with a process of imitation [10].

Nail biting is associated with a variety of medical and dental problems. Besides the persistently embarrassing and socially undesirable cosmetic problem, onychophagia is responsible for recurrent chronic paronychia, subungual infection, onychomycosis, or severe damage to the nail bed causing onycholysis [3, 11].

On the other hand, just like any other oral parafunction, onychophagia may cause temporomandibular dysfunction [12]. Moreover, biting pressure can be transferred down from the crown to the root leading to small fractures at the edges of incisors, apical root resorption, alveolar destruction, or gingivitis [2, 7].

Continuous nonphysiological mechanical forces induced by this habit may also lead to clinical dental crowding, rotations, or malocclusion [2].

To date, several treatments have been proposed to manage nail biting. Some of them focus on the psychological aspect of this oral habit aiming to obtain a behavioral change such as psychotherapy or pharmacotherapy [2, 13]. Others focus on target areas as they fetch solutions to keep the hands away from the mouth among which the application of a bitter-tasting nail polish or the use of an occlusive dressing on fingertips is mainly cited [2].

Unfortunately, even nowadays there has not been a strong deterrent to onychophagia which therefore remains an unsolved problem in medicine and dentistry [2].

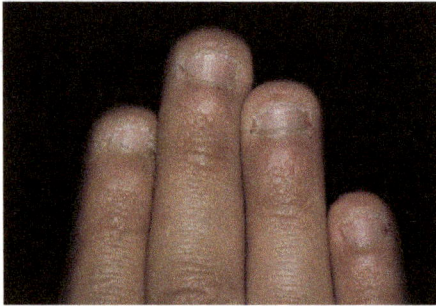

FIGURE 1: Fingertip mutilation associated with generalized parony-chia and onycholysis.

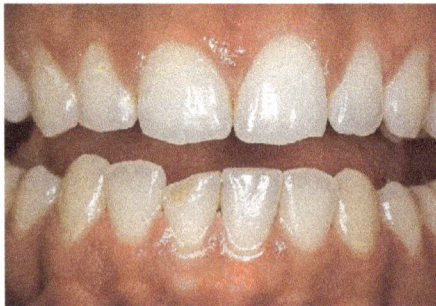

FIGURE 3: Patient simulating the occlusal position of nail biting. Note the coinciding outlines of the incisal notch and the antagonist incisal-edge surfaces.

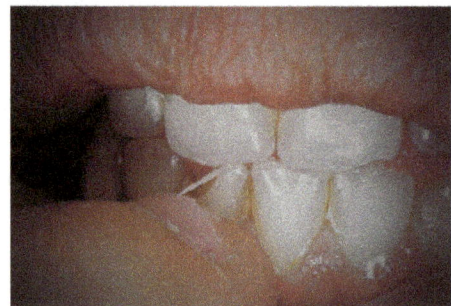

FIGURE 2: A V-shaped notching of the incisal edges of both right maxillary central and lateral incisors is associated with occlusal position of nail biting (scroll-up).

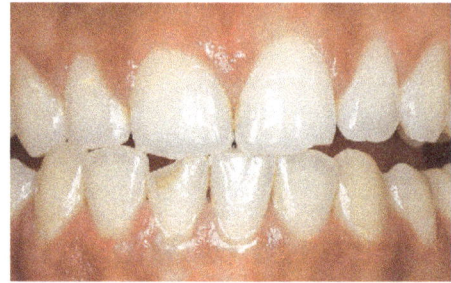

FIGURE 4: Patient simulating nail biting.

The aim of this paper is to describe a nonpunitive fixed appliance utilizing a stainless steel twisted round wire bonded from canine to canine, on the mandibular arch, as a treatment of onychophagia.

2. Case Description

A 26-year-old male patient was referred to our Department of Dental Medicine to treat his onychophagia with the chief complaint of the hideous aspect of his fingers. The medical history of the patient revealed regular nail biting associated with recurrent infections of fingernails; otherwise it was grossly unremarkable.

The anamnesis also showed first symptoms of nail biting since early childhood. The patient stated several failed attempts to quit biting his nails which left him powerless against breaking this habit. Clinical examination showed fingertip mutilation associated with generalized paronychia and onycholysis (Figure 1). After a thorough intraoral examination, we noticed the presence of an enamel fracture on the left maxillary central incisor with an enamel-dentin fracture of the right mandibular central incisor following a trauma during the patient's adolescence. Aside from these fractures, V-shaped notches of the incisal edges of both right maxillary central and lateral incisors were present. Misshapen incisal edge occurs as a result of the patient-specific-mandibular posture sustained when he bites his nails (Figures 2 and 3). Furthermore, the meticulous exploration of the oral habit

in this particular case revealed a tendency towards tapping the fingers preferentially against the right maxillary and the right mandibular central incisors (Figure 4). So, based on this habitual specific nail biting incision position, an appliance utilizing stainless steel twisted round wire was made to help the patient break this habit. In fact, this appliance is designed to adapt to engaging the lingual surfaces of the mandibular incisors towards the incisal edges with a horizontal segment, from which are strung out three vertical extensions lying on the incisal surfaces each. The appliance is retained with buccal extensions occupying a very small interincisal space aiming to prevent anterior incision and, thus, all dental interincisal contacts are prohibited whenever nail biting is then attempted (Figures 5 and 6).

By this method, we stop mechanically the action of nail biting. Thus, the aim of this nonremovable appliance is to constantly remind the patient to quit his unwanted behavior. Also, by punishing all attempts of nail biting, this appliance works as an aversion-based behavioral modification technique.

After obtaining an informed consent from the patient, the appliance was bonded (Figure 7). The patient was further called for follow-up every two weeks, and except for his first-week evaluation during which the patient reported an unusual sensation in his mouth, a significant decrease in nail biting was noted.

However, during his regular clinical examination, plaque accumulation was observed requiring further motivation of the patient to improve oral hygiene compliance (Figure 8). One month later, the patient eventually stopped his nail

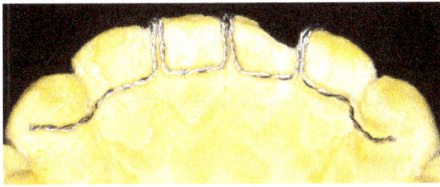

FIGURE 5: Lingual view of the appliance.

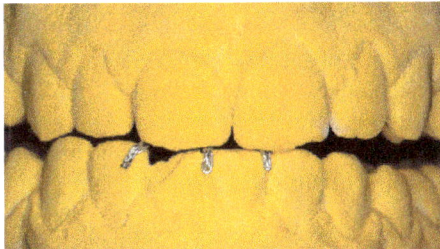

FIGURE 6: Buccal view of the appliance showing the eventual deliberate interference with the nail biting contact position of the patient.

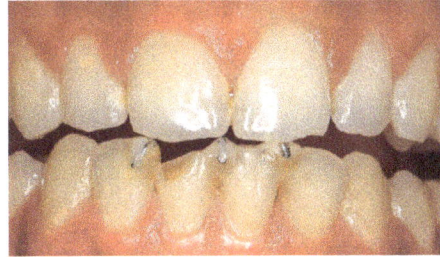

FIGURE 7: Intraoral view of the bonded appliance interfering and shifting out the nail biting contact position assumed by the patient.

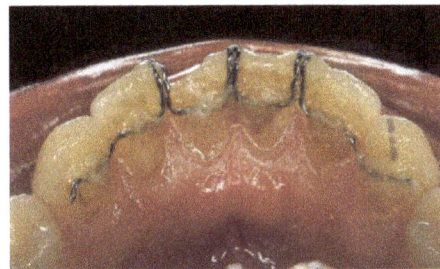

FIGURE 8: Intraoral lingual view of the bonded appliance showing plaque accumulation.

biting addiction and during all this period of time, excellent results were observed as every attempt to start this behavior again was mechanically unsuccessful. Clinically, from a dermatological point of view, the nails started to grow out smoothly and most of the mutilated parts of the patients' nails were cicatrized along with a progressive resolution of paronychia (Figure 9). With regard to the favorable treatment outcome, the appliance was removed. Furthermore, a constant assessment of the behavioral symptoms followed a monthly clinical evaluation which was planned to control and prevent the recurrence of the patient's desire to bite his nails whenever he feels the urge to. The clinical examination after 9 months shows a normal appearance of his fingernails which continued to grow out as the patient has stopped biting them (Figure 10).

3. Discussion

To date, several treatments have been developed in order to treat onychophagia. However nail biting remains an unsolved problem in medicine and dentistry [2].

Among the treatment options available today, the psychological aspect and the dermatological side effects of such an oral habit both remain the major therapeutic focus [2, 13]. The idea behind using appliances was developed to make the habit physically and mechanically difficult to maintain and eventually remind the patient to keep his fingertips away from his mouth. Basically this dental nail biting deterrent appliance can be considered analogous to purpose compared to bluegrass appliance that works as an aid to stop thumb sucking [14].

Psychologically, the nonremovable appliance constantly reminds the patient to quit his behavior.

Also, by punishing all attempts of nail biting, this appliance works as an aversion-based behavioral modification technique [15]. The aversion technique essentially involves reinforcement learning, but it also constitutes a reminder, which is self-terminating and requires reactivation [15].

Specifically, although the mechanical presence serves as a discriminative stimulus, it also serves as a reminder of one's goal of avoiding nail biting. Indeed, as suggested by Koritzky and Yechiam, the use of constantly present reminders broadens the target population that can benefit from reminders in the course of behavior modification [15].

Nail biting is genuinely a sequence of 4 distinct phases. Once the finger has been inspected visually or felt by palpation by another finger, the hands are then placed close to the mouth. Subsequently, the mandible is placed in a laterotrusive (or just lateral) edge-to-edge contact position; then, the fingers are quickly tapped against the front teeth followed by a series of quick spasmodic biting actions. In this case the patient will have his fingernails pressed tightly against the biting edges of the teeth. And finally the fingers are withdrawn from the mouth [2].

The aim of this exclusive appliance is to prevent the biting phase of this oral habit. Mechanically, it renders the chisel-shaped teeth that meet in an edge-to-edge bite to become inoperative. As was illustrated in the clinical case, this appliance disabled efficiently the front teeth from making any damage to the nails and the surrounding cuticles. After about one month from the day of bonding, it led to the patient cut-out of his habit addiction and, overtime, a full oppression of the nail biting urge has been noted.

By the end of a nine-month posttreatment follow-up, the patient completely stopped his nail biting habit after the removal of the appliance showing a total disappearance of unaesthetic fingertips with no relapse periods observed.

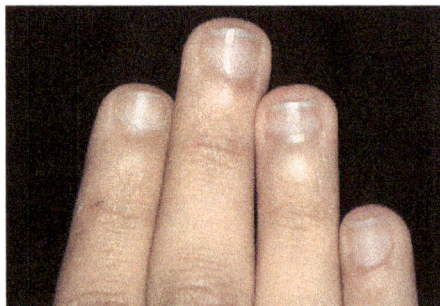

FIGURE 9: Retrieval of a normal appearance of the fingertips after one month of treatment.

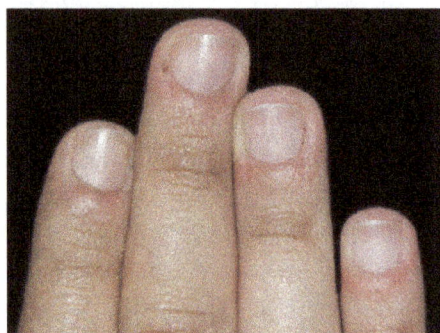

FIGURE 10: 9 months after the removal of the appliance, the patient has quit the oral habit with persistence of normal appearance of his fingertips (scroll-up).

Concerning the acceptance of the bonded appliance, it significantly subsides later on in spite of a few disadvantages as in eating and speech difficulties experienced by the patient few days after placement. Moreover, the duration, frequency of the habit, the cooperation, and motivation of the patient are all important factors to be considered in ensuring treatment success. Ample time should be given to educate the patients, stimulate good habits, and develop conscious awareness [16].

Accordingly, in addition to the bonded appliance role, effective results may be expected. From a dentistry point of view, since onychophagia is a common behavior, usually with no or minimal sequelae, clinician should be aware of the potential complications of this habit. Moreover, dentists need to be cognizant to establish a correct diagnosis of this oral habit, inform patients of potential ramifications of fingernail biting, and suggest the appropriate solutions to quit this behavior.

4. Conclusion

Onychophagia is a common oral habit that may lead to dermatological, esthetic, dental, or psychological complications. Since numerous treatments have been suggested to treat several other different oral habits, there always remains a lack of a tangible dental treatment for nail biting nowadays. This paper describes a fixed oral appliance placed by the dentist, aiming to make nail biting rather unpleasant and difficult for the affected patient. The case report discussed in

this paper shows an innovative successful treatment for nail biters providing efficient results within a 9-month follow-up. Further studies and clinical follow-ups are still required in order to confirm the effectiveness of this appliance.

Competing Interests

The authors declare that they have no conflict of interests.

Acknowledgments

The authors acknowledge Research Laboratory of Oral Health and Orofacial Rehabilitation LR12 ES11, Faculty of Dental Medicine, Monastir University, Tunisia. And also they want to acknowledge Fadwa Chtiou for her contribution with the proofreading and English revision.

References

[1] A. W. Pelc and A. K. Jaworek, "Interdisciplinary approach to onychophagia," *Przeglad Lekarski*, vol. 60, no. 11, pp. 737–739, 2003.

[2] O. M. Tanaka, R. W. F. Vitral, G. Y. Tanaka, A. P. Guerrero, and E. S. Camargo, "Nailbiting, or onychophagia: a special habit," *American Journal of Orthodontics and Dentofacial Orthopedics*, vol. 134, no. 2, pp. 305–308, 2008.

[3] P. Pacan, M. Grzesiak, A. Reich, and J. C. Szepietowski, "Onychophagia as a spectrum of obsessive-compulsive disorder," *Acta Dermato-Venereologica*, vol. 89, no. 3, pp. 278–280, 2009.

[4] D. Wechsler, "The incidences and significance of fingernail biting in children," *The Psychoanalytic Review (1913–1957)*, vol. 18, p. 201, 1931.

[5] L. B. Birch, "The incidence of nail biting among school children," *British Journal of Educational Psychology*, vol. 25, no. 2, pp. 123–128, 1955.

[6] M. Nilner, "Relationships between oral parafunctions and functional disturbances and diseases of the stomatognathic system among children aged 7–14 years," *Acta Odontologica Scandinavica*, vol. 41, no. 3, pp. 167–172, 1983.

[7] A. K. C. Leung and W. L. M. Robson, "Nailbiting," *Clinical Pediatrics*, vol. 29, no. 12, pp. 690–692, 1990.

[8] L. Gregory, "Stereotypic movement disorder and disorder of infancy, childhood, or adolescence NOS," in *Comprehensive Textbook of Psychiatry*, pp. 2360–2362, Williams & Wilkins, Baltimore, Md, USA, 6th edition, 1995.

[9] P. A. Deardoff, A. J. Finch Jr., and L. R. Royall, "Manifest anxiety and nail-biting," *Journal of Clinical Psychology*, vol. 30, no. 3, p. 378, 1974.

[10] M. Massler and A. J. Malone, "Nail biting-a review," *American Journal of Orthodontics*, vol. 36, no. 5, pp. 351–367, 1950.

[11] D.-Y. Lee, "Chronic nail biting and irreversible shortening of the fingernails," *Journal of the European Academy of Dermatology and Venereology*, vol. 23, no. 2, p. 185, 2009.

[12] E. Winocur, D. Littner, I. Adams, and A. Gavish, "Oral habits and their association with signs and symptoms of temporomandibular disorders in adolescents: a gender comparison," *Oral Surgery, Oral Medicine, Oral Pathology, Oral Radiology, and Endodontology*, vol. 102, no. 4, pp. 482–487, 2006.

[13] A. Ghanizadeh, "Nail biting; etiology, consequences and management," *Iranian Journal of Medical Sciences*, vol. 36, no. 2, pp. 73–79, 2011.

[14] B. S. Haskell and J. R. Mink, "An aid to stop thumb sucking: the 'Bluegrass' appliance," *Pediatric dentistry*, vol. 13, no. 2, pp. 83–85, 1991.

[15] G. Koritzky and E. Yechiam, "On the value of nonremovable reminders for behavior modification: an application to nail-biting (onychophagia)," *Behavior Modification*, vol. 35, no. 6, pp. 511–530, 2011.

[16] A. Sachan and T. P. Chaturvedi, "Onychophagia (Nail biting), anxiety, and malocclusion," *Indian Journal of Dental Research*, vol. 23, no. 5, pp. 680–682, 2012.

27

Absorbable Suture as an Apical Matrix in Single Visit Apexification with Mineral Trioxide Aggregate

Ayush Goyal, Vineeta Nikhil, and Padmanabh Jha

Department of Conservative Dentistry & Endodontics, Subharti Dental College, Meerut, Uttar Pradesh, India

Correspondence should be addressed to Ayush Goyal; ayush2106.goyal@gmail.com

Academic Editor: Jiiang H. Jeng

Several procedures have been recommended to induce the root end barrier formation in teeth with open apices. Conventional treatment for such cases will require many appointments with an average duration of 12.9 months. During this period, the root canal is susceptible to reinfection from around the provisional restoration, which may promote apical periodontitis and arrest of apical repair. Mineral trioxide aggregate (MTA) has been successfully used for one visit apexification wherein the root canal can be obturated within 24 hours after placement of MTA. Using a matrix prior to the placement of MTA avoids its extrusion, reduces leakage in the sealing material, and allows favorable response of the periapical tissues. This report presents a case of apexification where an absorbable suture was used as an apical matrix. Use of an absorbable suture circumvents all the problems associated with other conventional materials. *Conclusion.* Placement of the matrix made from the suture material is predictable and is easily positioned at the apex and the length can be adjusted as required. 10-month follow-up of the case shows resorbed matrix and bone healing in the periapical region. The patient was asymptomatic during the whole follow-up period and tooth exhibited mobility within physiologic limits and was functioning normally.

1. Introduction

When teeth with incomplete root formation suffer trauma, the root development ceases and the apical closure cannot be achieved. Luxation injuries appear to be associated with greatest risk of incomplete root development and according to J. O. Andreasen and F. M. Andreasen, about 15 to 59% teeth lose their vitality [1]. The maxillary central incisor is the most common tooth affected in both dentitions [1].

Root canal treatment of a tooth with immature apex is an arduous task because of large size of the canal, thin and fragile roots, and absence of an apical barrier against which to condense the obturating material. Apexification is a treatment modality which induces a calcified barrier in teeth with immature apices. The purpose of this barrier is twofold [2], (a) to prevent the passage of toxins and bacteria from the root canal into the periapical tissues and (b) to allow the compaction of the root filling material.

Calcium hydroxide has been a widely reported and probably the most studied material for apexification. Granath was the first to report the use of the material for apical closure [3]. Though its efficiency has been reported by many authors, it has certain disadvantages, like unpredictability in the duration of treatment (average duration is 12.9 months) [4], patient compliance due to multiple recalls, and increased risk of root fracture following several calcium hydroxide dressings.

It is possible to circumvent all the above problems with MTA which has achieved widespread acceptance in this field. The main advantages of MTA are (a) reduction in the treatment time leading to better patient compliance, (b) decreased risk of fracture of root as the tooth can be permanently restored with minimal delay, and (c) minimal alteration of mechanical properties of dentin.

Although MTA is reported to be biocompatible, overfilling of root canals with MTA yielded significantly inferior results compared to obturation performed at the limit of the cemental canal [5]. Using a matrix prior to the placement of MTA avoids its extrusion, reduces leakage in the sealing material, and allows favorable response of the periapical tissues [6]. Several materials have been recommended to create a matrix, like hydroxyapatite-based materials, resorbable

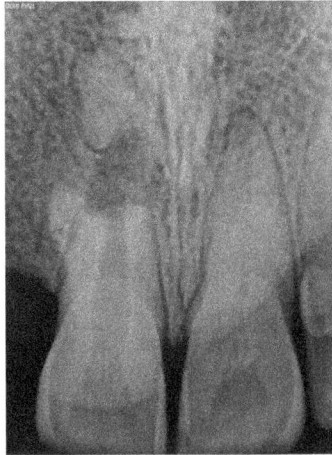

FIGURE 1: Preoperative intraoral periapical (IOPA) radiograph showing open apex in relation to 11.

collagen, platelet-rich fibrin, and calcium sulphate [7–9]. All these materials share a common disadvantage that once placed, their position cannot be adjusted.

The present case demonstrates the use of an absorbable suture that was modified to form an apical matrix in a single visit apexification procedure with MTA with a 10-month follow-up.

2. Case Report

A 19-year-old male patient reported to the Department of Conservative Dentistry and Endodontics, Subharti Dental College, Meerut, with a chief complaint of pain in relation to his upper front teeth region since few weeks. On examination, it was found that the tooth in question was maxillary right central incisor (11). Pain was moderate in intensity, nonradiating, and aggravated on biting. Clinical examination revealed an Ellis class I fracture in relation to 11. The patient reported a history of trauma around 5 years back. Tooth was moderately tender on percussion. Radiograph in relation to 11 showed a wide-open apex along with an area of periapical rarefaction (Figure 1). Pulp sensibility tests in relation to 11 did not elicit any response. Cold test was performed using Endo Ice® (Coltène/Whaledent Inc., Cuyahoga Falls, USA). The tooth did not respond to electric pulp testing also. Based on clinical and radiographic findings, a diagnosis of pulpal necrosis with symptomatic apical periodontitis was made.

The crown-root ratio of the subject tooth was 1:1 (approx.). Though the crown-root ratio may be considered inadequate by some clinicians, the tooth exhibited no abnormal mobility and the patient and his parents were not willing for extraction (at any cost!). It was decided to carry out single visit apexification using MTA.

After administration of local anaesthesia, Lignocaine HCl with adrenaline 1:80000 (Lignox 2% A, Indoco Remedies Ltd., Mumbai, India) and rubber dam isolation, access was opened. The canal was debrided using Hedström files followed by copious irrigation with 3% sodium hypochlorite

(Novodent Equipments & Materials Ltd., Mumbai, India). Working length was determined radiographically with a file placed in the canal (Figure 2(d)). The canal was dried using sterile paper points (Meta® BioMed, Korea). Braided coated polyglactin-based, 3-0 absorbable suture material VICRYL™ (Johnson and Johnson Ltd., Aurangabad, India) was used for the formation of apical matrix. The suture was tied to form a knot and was tied 2 more times to form a thicker knot (Figure 2(a)). The thickness of the knot can be approximately determined by gauging the apex with a large size file. This knot would serve as an apical matrix and the free end of the suture material can be used to adjust its length. The suture material was placed in an iopamidol solution (61%) (ISOVUE®-300, Bracco Diagnostics, Italy) for 15 minutes to make it radiopaque (Figures 2(b) and 2(c)). The "matrix" was then placed in the canal and was pushed to position it at the apex using a set of preselected hand pluggers. The position of the matrix was confirmed radiographically (Figure 2(e)). Once the matrix was in position, MTA (White Pro-Root MTA®, Dentsply Maillefer, Ballaigues, Switzerland) was mixed according to the manufacturer's instructions to a thick creamy consistency and placed in the canal using an MTA carrier (Messing Gun®, Produits Dentaires, Vevey, Switzerland). MTA was condensed with the butt end of sterile damp paper points to form a 3 mm MTA plug. After this, free end of the suture was cut with a thin scissor as close as possible to the MTA plug and another 1 mm MTA plug was packed. This was done to avoid any suture material remaining inside the canal which may result in a longitudinal filling defect at the tooth-restoration interface. A moist cotton pellet was placed in the canal and the access cavity was temporized with Cavit™ G (3M ESPE, Neuss, Germany). The patient was recalled next day and the root canal was obturated using lateral condensation technique with gutta percha (Meta® BioMed, Korea) and AH Plus sealer (Dentsply Detrey GmbH, Germany). Finally, the access cavity was restored with resin composite (Figure 2(f)). The patient was recalled 2 weeks later and demonstrated no clinical signs and symptoms. At 3-month recall, the tooth exhibited mobility within physiologic limits and no evidence of periodontal pockets and was functioning normally. Radiographic examination revealed ongoing resorption of the apical matrix (Figure 2(g)). 10-month follow-up of the case shows resorbed matrix and bone healing in the periapical region (Figure 5).

3. Discussion

Apexification is defined as "a method to induce a calcified barrier in a root with an open apex or the continued apical development of an incomplete root in teeth with necrotic pulp" [10]. Traditionally, calcium hydroxide has been used extensively for apexification. Dominguez Reyes et al. [4] reported 100% success rate with calcium hydroxide. However, there are a number of factors which might lead to failure of the apexification procedure in this technique [2]; for example, high pH (12.7) of calcium hydroxide can induce a necrotic zone in the periapical area, risk of contamination of the root canal space since a permanent restoration cannot be placed until the treatment is complete, and resultant decrease in

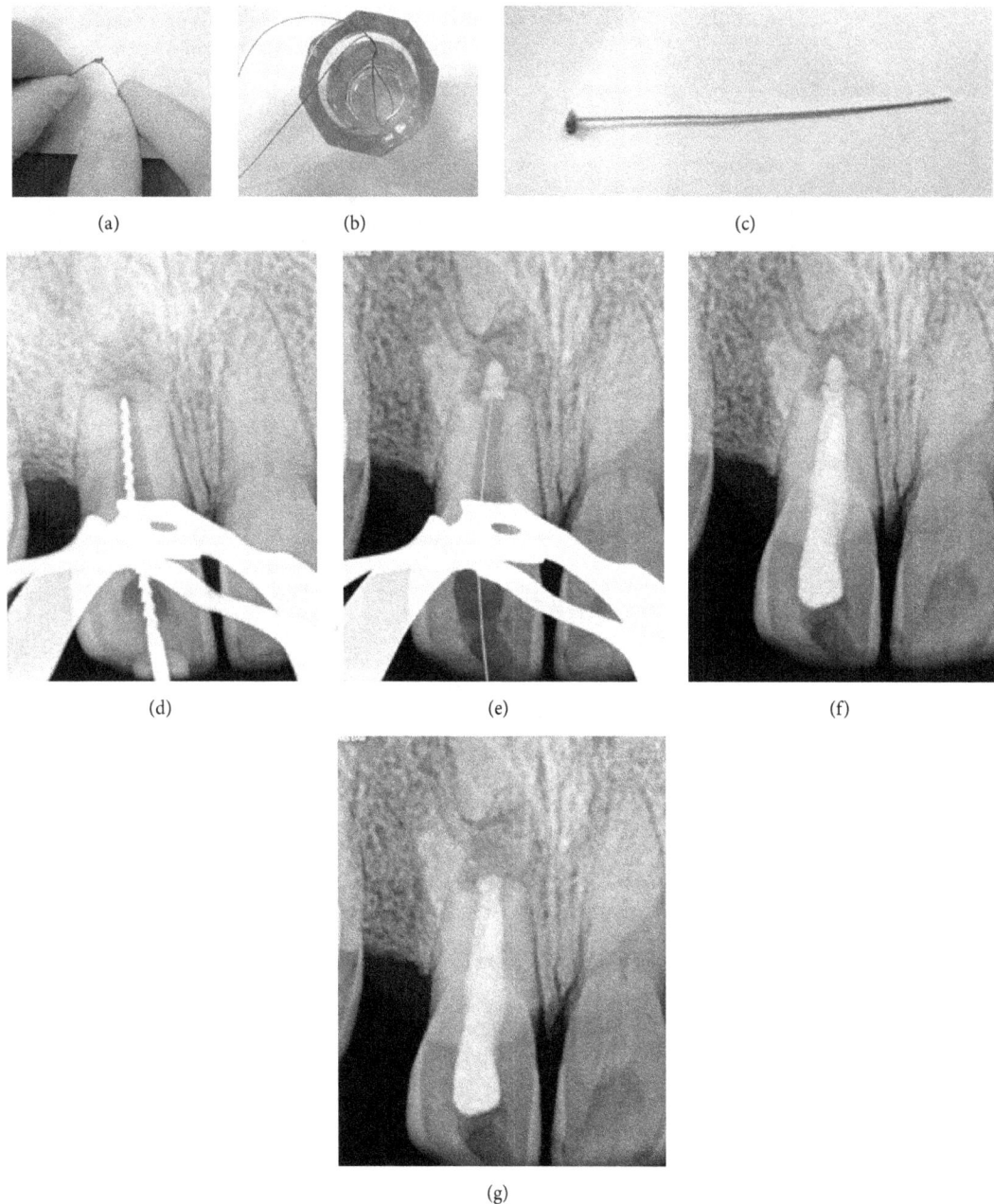

FIGURE 2: (a)–(c) Fabrication of the matrix. (a) Formation of the "apical matrix" by tying a knot with the suture material. (b) The suture material was kept in the radio-opaque dye for 15 minutes. (c) "Modified suture apical matrix" ready for placement in the root canal. (d)–(g) Intracanal procedures. (d) Working length radiograph. (e) Apical matrix was placed at the apex and the free end was left outside for adjustment. (f) Radiograph taken after placement of MTA, obturation, and coronal restoration with composite. (g) 3-month recall shows absorption of the "apical matrix."

the strength of roots which ultimately may lead to fracture even before the treatment is complete. On the other hand, in a single visit apexification procedure with MTA, obturation and coronal restoration can be done within 24 hours after the placement of MTA. This is a definite advantage when compared to the traditional technique of apexification.

In a prospective study by Simon et al. [2], forty-three cases were followed up for one year after one-visit apexification procedure with MTA. The authors reported a high success rate (81%) with this technique and concluded that apexification with MTA is a predictable and reproducible procedure. As mentioned above, use of an internal matrix makes the compaction of MTA easier and placement predictable.

Various materials, like platelet-rich fibrin, calcium sulphate, hydroxyapatite, and resorbable collagen, have been used as internal matrix. However, all these materials possess certain disadvantages. Calcium sulphate has a short setting time of 1-2 minutes [7]. This is a major drawback of this material. If not placed correctly inside the canal, there is hardly any time to readjust it. Secondly, it requires placement using specialized devices like Messing gun or Dovgan carriers. Thirdly, care has to be taken while placement so that calcium sulphate does not contact the root canal walls as it interferes with the close adaptation of MTA. Lastly, the tip of the carrier has to be cleaned immediately after placement, otherwise calcium sulphate sets and is difficult to remove. Placement of collagen membranes is technique sensitive and requires high level of accuracy in positioning [6]. Hydroxyapatite is difficult to manipulate, is granular in consistency, has poor adaptability to the walls, and does not set [11]. Moreover, it is an expensive material. Platelet-rich fibrin, though it has shown promising results in various case reports, has an inherent disadvantage of being radiolucent. Radiographic confirmation can only be done after the apical plug has been placed with a barrier material.

Coated VICRYL (polyglactin 910) suture is a synthetic absorbable sterile surgical suture composed of a copolymer made from 90% glycolide and 10% L-lactide [12]. It is commonly used in subcutaneous, intracutaneous, abdominal, and thoracic surgeries. Coated VICRYL suture is prepared by coating the suture material with a mixture composed of equal parts of copolymer of glycolide and lactide (polyglactin 370) and calcium stearate [13]. Calcium stearate is a salt of calcium and stearic acid, both of which are present in the body and constantly metabolized and excreted [13]. Coated VICRYL has been found to be nonantigenic and nonpyrogenic and elicit only a mild tissue reaction during absorption [14, 15]. Absorption of coated VICRYL suture is complete between 56 and 70 days by hydrolysis [13]. Lactide and glycolide acids are readily eliminated from the body, primarily in urine [13]. Manufacturers of VICRYL suture material state that the absorption of the suture material may be accelerated if the suture is contaminated with blood or water prior to suturing procedure. Since the suture material was placed in a radio-opaque dye for 15 minutes, it is possible that the absorption process would have initiated earlier. However, since the patient was recalled only after 3 months, it is difficult to quote the exact time of absorption.

The certain advantages of this technique over conventional techniques and materials mentioned previously are as follows: (a) easy "fabrication" of the matrix, (b) length being adjusted as required using the free end of the suture, (c) simple placement technique using pluggers, (d) easy availability of absorbable sutures, (e) being inexpensive, and (f) VICRYL being not a newly introduced suture material; it has been in use for surgeries for more than three decades. Since a suture material was modified to form a knot which in turn serves as a matrix, the authors would like to term this technique "modified suture apical matrix" technique.

The dye iopamidol was used to impart radiopacity to the matrix. Iopamidol has been used as diagnostic agent for clinical CT protocols since 1981 [16]. High water solubility coupled with very low toxicity makes it an ideal contrast agent for various diagnostic purposes [16]. It has been used

for angiography throughout cardiovascular system, pediatric angiocardiography, selective visceral arteriography and aortography, phlebography, adult and pediatric intravenous excretory urography, and intravenous adult and pediatric Contrast Enhancement of Computed Tomographic (CECT) Head and Body Imaging [17]. It is available in various concentrations, from 200 to 370 mg/mL. ISOVUE®-300 used in the present case contains 300 mg organically bound iodine per mL. Presence of iodine atoms endows iopamidol molecule with high X-ray radiopacity [16].

Iodine and iodinated contrast agents have been shown to cross the placenta [18] and have been reported to pass into breast milk [19]. Hence, when used as a contrast media, it is contraindicated for pregnant patients and lactating mothers. However, when used as an apical matrix for endodontic purpose, it is unclear whether it should be used in such patients or not. It is best to avoid iopamidol until further data is available on the same. Also, iopamidol is advised against use in cases of active infection. However, most data available on iopamidol is based on its indications as a contrast media. Further studies could probably throw some light on this subject. Iopamidol is eliminated by the body, primarily in urine [17]. McKinstry et al. [17] have reported a urinary recovery of 90% or more of the dose within 72 to 96 hours after intravenous injection of iopamidol. Figure 3 shows a schematic representation of the whole procedure.

An unusual finding in the present case was the wide-open apex even though the tooth was traumatized at 14 years of age, that is, after the root formation was complete for central incisors. A careful look at the preoperative radiograph will reveal a "root-tip" shaped radiopacity about 5 mm from the apex of the tooth. It is the opinion of the authors that the trauma must have caused the tooth to suffer a horizontal root fracture in addition to intrusion. With time, the intruded tooth may have erupted until it reached its original position in the arch while leaving the root tip behind. The radiopacity is surrounded by a thin radiolucency very similar to periodontal ligament. This supports the fact that radiopacity may in fact be the root tip. One might feel that the data provided by the patient regarding the time of trauma may be incorrect. But careful history was taken before arriving at any conclusion and the patient and his parents were most certain of the time of trauma. Another finding that the authors would like to share is a silhouette of the resorbed suture material when the image is zoomed in to 140% (Figure 4). It is possible that scattered radio-opaque filaments may have imparted this appearance. It may be speculated that there is some effect on the absorption rate of dye when combined with suture material. It remains unclear whether this finding is of any clinical significance.

The technique mentioned in this report is easy to carry out and very importantly allows for adjustment of the position during the placement. The authors encourage further research on this subject using different suture materials like, for example, Coated VICRYL® Plus Antibacterial (polyglactin 910) Suture which has an antibacterial coating on it. Research investigating the reaction of periapical tissues to the suture material and the radio-opaque dye is further encouraged.

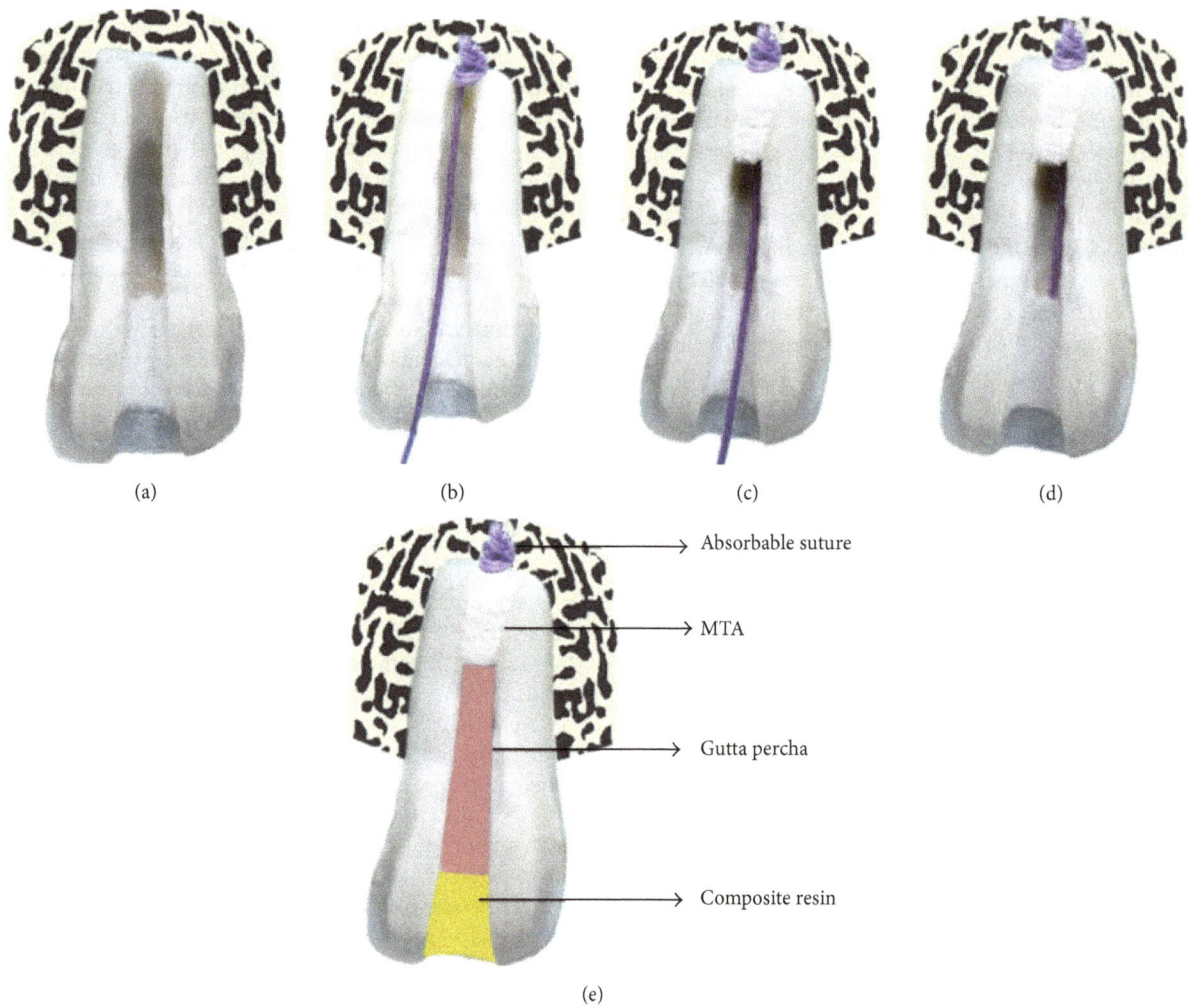

(a)   (b)   (c)   (d)

→ Absorbable suture

→ MTA

→ Gutta percha

→ Composite resin

(e)

FIGURE 3: Modified suture apical matrix concept. (a) Tooth with immature apex. (b) Suture matrix placed at the apex. (c) MTA is condensed against the matrix. (d) The free end of the suture is cut. (e) Obturation is done followed by a permanent coronal restoration.

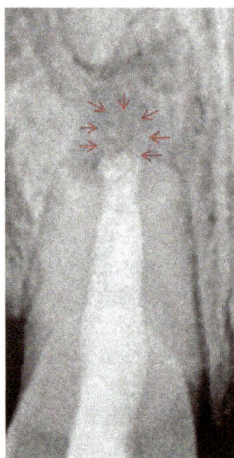

FIGURE 4: Silhouette of the resorbed suture material when the image is zoomed in to 140%.

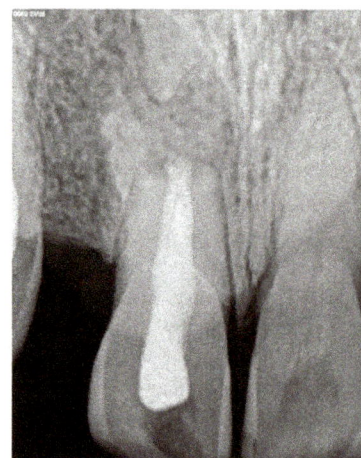

FIGURE 5: 10-month follow-up of the case shows completely resorbed matrix and bone healing in the periapical area.

4. Conclusion

The technique mentioned in this report is new. However, the materials used for it are not. The suture material and the radio-opaque die have been approved by the Food and Drug Administration (FDA) and have been in use for several years. The technique makes it possible for the clinicians to bypass certain disadvantages encountered with other techniques mentioned in the literature. More case reports and long-term follow-up periods with this technique are required for it to establish a firm foot in the field of endodontics.

Competing Interests

The authors of this manuscript declare that there are no competing interests regarding the publication of this manuscript.

References

[1] J. O. Andreasen, "Luxation injuries," in *Textbook and the Color Atlas of Traumatic Dental Injuries to the Teeth*, J. O. Andreasen and F. M. Andreasen, Eds., chapter 9, pp. 315–378, Munksgaard, Copenhagen, Denmark, 3rd edition, 1993.

[2] S. Simon, F. Rilliard, A. Berdal, and P. Machtou, "The use of mineral trioxide aggregate in one-visit apexification treatment: a prospective study," *International Endodontic Journal*, vol. 40, no. 3, pp. 186–197, 2007.

[3] L.-E. Granath, "Nagra synpunkter pa behandlingen av traumatiserade incisiver parbn," *Odontologisk Revy Journal*, vol. 10, article 272, 1959.

[4] A. Dominguez Reyes, L. Muñoz Muñoz, and T. Aznar Martín, "Study of calcium hydroxide apexification in 26 young permanent incisors," *Dental Traumatology*, vol. 21, no. 3, pp. 141–145, 2005.

[5] R. Holland, L. Mazuqueli, V. de Souza, S. S. Murata, E. Dezan Júnior, and P. Suzuki, "Influence of the type of vehicle and limit of obturation on apical and periapical tissue response in dogs' teeth after root canal filling with mineral trioxide aggregate," *Journal of Endodontics*, vol. 33, no. 6, pp. 693–697, 2007.

[6] R. Khatavkar and V. Hegde, "Use of a matrix for apexification procedure with mineral trioxide aggregate," *Journal of Conservative Dentistry*, vol. 13, no. 1, pp. 54–57, 2010.

[7] H. A. Alhadainy, V. T. Himel, W. B. Lee, and Y. M. Elbaghdady, "Use of a hydroxylapatite-based material and calcium sulfate as artificial floors to repair furcal perforations," *Oral Surgery, Oral Medicine, Oral Pathology, Oral Radiology, and Endodontics*, vol. 86, no. 6, pp. 723–729, 1998.

[8] C. Bargholz, "Perforation repair with mineral trioxide aggregate: a modified matrix concept," *International Endodontic Journal*, vol. 38, no. 1, pp. 59–69, 2005.

[9] P. Yadav, P. J. Pruthi, R. R. Naval, S. Talwar, and M. Verma, "Novel use of platelet-rich fibrin matrix and MTA as an apical barrier in the management of a failed revascularization case," *Dental Traumatology*, vol. 31, no. 4, pp. 328–331, 2015.

[10] AAE, *Glossary of Endodontic Terms*, American Association of Endodontists, Chicago, Ill, USA, 2003.

[11] S. Taneja and M. Kumari, "Effect of internal matrices of hydroxyapatite and calcium sulfate on the sealing ability of mineral trioxide aggregate and light cured glass ionomer cement," *Journal of Conservative Dentistry*, vol. 14, no. 1, pp. 6–9, 2011.

[12] S. J. Aston and T. D. Rees, "Vicryl sutures," *Aesthetic Plastic Surgery*, vol. 1, no. 1, pp. 289–293, 1976.

[13] *Ethicon Wound Closure Manual*, Ethicon, Inc, 2007.

[14] G. J. Reul Jr., "Use of vicryl (polyglactin 910) sutures in general surgical and cardiothoracic procedures," *The American Journal of Surgery*, vol. 134, no. 2, pp. 297–299, 1977.

[15] P. H. Craig, J. A. Williams, K. W. Davis et al., "A biologic comparison of polyglactin 910 and polyglycolic acid synthetic absorbable sutures," *Surgery Gynecology and Obstetrics*, vol. 141, no. 1, pp. 1–10, 1975.

[16] S. Aime, L. Calabi, L. Biondi et al., "Iopamidol: exploring the potential use of a well-established x-ray contrast agent for MRI," *Magnetic Resonance in Medicine*, vol. 53, no. 4, pp. 830–834, 2005.

[17] D. N. McKinstry, A. J. Rommel, and A. A. Sugerman, "Pharmacokinetics, metabolism and excretion of iopamidol in healthy subjects," *Investigative Radiology*, vol. 19, no. 5, pp. S171–S174, 1984.

[18] J. Kelleher, P. J. Feczko, M. Radkowski, and N. T. Griscom, "Neonatal intestinal opacification secondary to transplacental passage of urographic contrast medium," *American Journal of Roentgenology*, vol. 132, no. 1, pp. 63–65, 1979.

[19] C. Schaefer, P. Peters, and R. K. Miller, *Drugs During Pregnancy and Lactation: Treatment Options and Risk Assessment*, chapter 4, Elsevier, 3rd edition, 2015.

28

Radiographic Enlargement of Mandibular Canal as an Extranodal Primary Non-Hodgkin's Lymphoma Early Sign in an Asymptomatic Patient

Luciana Munhoz,[1] **Felipe Pereira Marcos Marsan,**[1] **and Emiko Saito Arita**[2]

[1]*Department of Stomatology, School of Dentistry, University of São Paulo, 2227 Lineu Prestes Avenue, 05508-000 São Paulo, SP, Brazil*
[2]*Department of Odontology, University of São Paulo, 448-475 Cesário Galeno Street, 03071-000 São Paulo, SP, Brazil*

Correspondence should be addressed to Luciana Munhoz; dra.lucimunhoz@gmail.com

Academic Editor: Luis M. J. Gutierrez

Non-Hodgkin's lymphoma (NHL) is a lymphoproliferative disorder, from a subgroup of heterogeneous hematologic malignancies; the term "extranodal" refers to malignant involvement of tissues other than lymph nodes, tonsils, spleen, pharyngeal lymphatic ring, or thymus. Only 0.6% of all NHL are at mandible alone, and it may involve the inferior alveolar canal. We describe a case of bilateral enlargement of the mandibular canal without symptomatology, which was shown in a panoramic radiograph and cone beam computed tomography in a rehabilitation routine exam, as an early sign of primary extranodal NHL.

1. Introduction

Non-Hodgkin's lymphoma (NHL) is a lymphoproliferative disorder, from a subgroup of heterogeneous hematologic malignancies that also includes other three different lymphoproliferative disorders: Hodgkin disease, lymphocytic leukemia, and multiple myeloma [1]. The term "extranodal" refers to malignant involvement of tissues other than lymph nodes, tonsils, spleen, pharyngeal lymphatic ring, or thymus [1].

Approximately 20% to 30% of NHL occur at extranodal sites [2]; at head and neck the most common involvement of extranodal NHL is at sinonasal site [3]. When NHL affects oral cavity, around only 15% to 45% arise in maxilla or mandible [4]. The most usual sites are maxilla, mandible, palatal soft tissue, and gum, respectively [5]. Only 0.6% of all NHL are at mandible alone [5], and it may involve the inferior alveolar canal, frequently without any radiographic sign of bony changes [6].

In oral cavity, extranodal sites of NHL may be found as solid masses of spongy consistency [7, 8]. Bone marrow infiltration by malignant lymphomas is influenced by the characteristic pattern according to the lymphoma subtyping [9], and these malignant patters may provide diagnostic hints for NHL subtyping [10].

Considering head and neck sites, primary NHL occurs more often in male patients than female [11, 12], in the fifth to seventh decades of life [11, 12]. Male Caucasians patients are more often affected than other genders [11–13].

In radiographic findings, enlargement of inferior alveolar canal is extremely unusual, and it is often related to malformations or benign lesions [14, 15]. The presence of mandibular canal widening in extranodal NHL patients is even rarer; primary extranodal NHL frequently arises in the medullar cavity of single long bones [13]. A review of English language medical literature using Pubmed database from 1990 to 2016 reveled only four previous reports of NHL associated with mandibular canal enlargement [13, 14, 16, 17]. In the present report, we describe a case of bilateral enlargement of the mandibular canal without symptomatology, which was shown in a panoramic radiograph and cone beam computed tomography in a rehabilitation routine exam.

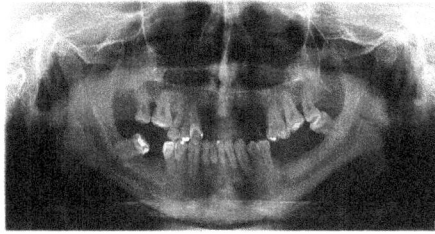

FIGURE 1: Panoramic Radiograph of the case. Enlargement of mandibular canal in both sides.

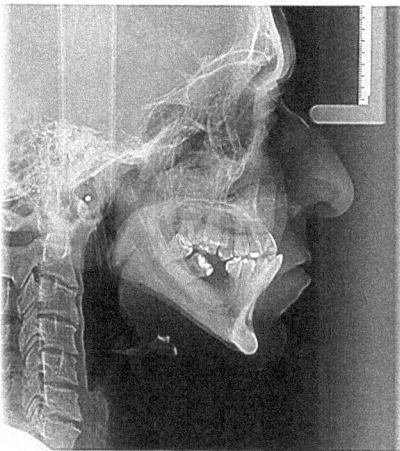

FIGURE 2: Teleradiograph; the enlargement is also observed.

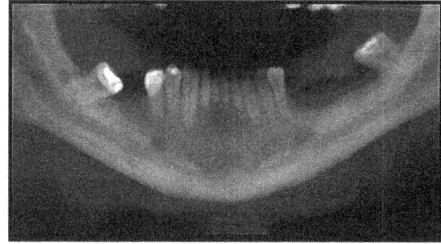

FIGURE 3: CBCT panoramic slice.

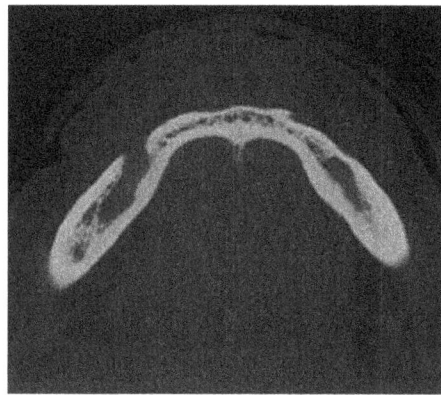

FIGURE 4: CBCT axial slice demonstrating rupture of the mandibular cortex.

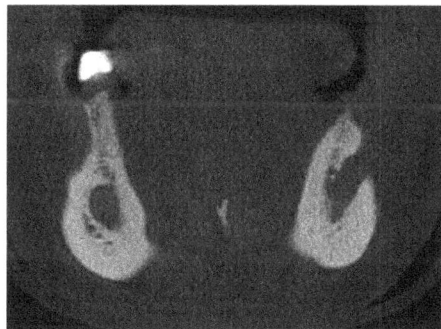

FIGURE 5: Frontal slice; enlargement of mental foramen.

2. Case Report

2.1. Case History and Clinical Findings. Male Caucasian patient, 39-year-old, was referred to a private Radiologic Clinic in São Paulo, Brazil, for radiographic exams with the purpose of planning oral rehabilitation. At the moment of evaluation, the patient did not report any clinical symptoms or showed clinical signs of intraoral or extraoral alterations. The systemic health history did not provide relevant information, and the patient denied carrying any syndrome or having knowledge of any carrier relative.

2.2. Imaging Evaluations. The panoramic radiograph showed the absence of 11 teeth (4 at mandible), alveolar bone loss, trabecular bone with increased thickening as well as mandibular cortical erosion (indicating reduction of bone mineral density), and elongated styloid process. The mandibular canal and mental foramen presented inferior-superior enlargement, bilaterally (Figure 1). The lateral teleradiography also demonstrated the mandibular canal enlargement, beginning in the retromolar trigone and affecting the mandibular ramus (Figure 2).

In the cone beam computed tomography (CBCT), multiplanar reconstruction demonstrated marked increase in the diameter of the mandibular canal throughout their length, on both sides, as well as the enlargement of mental foramens. Right and left side mandibular canal's bone cortices were preserved but they were thinning. At the right side, in

axial and coronal sections, foramen's bone cortex exhibited discontinuity at medial wall. The radiolucent unilocular fusiform areas apparently were unconnected with the teeth or root tips (Figures 3, 4, and 5).

The initial diagnostic hypotheses were bilateral hemangioma, malignant lymphangiona [18], any related syndrome that would affect neural sheath Schwann cells, like neurofibromatosis [19, 20]; multiple endocrine neoplasia type 2b with bilateral involvement and bifurcated inferior alveolar canals [21], arteriovenous malformation [22], vascular leiomyoma associated with mandibular canal [23], and extranodal NHL [14].

The final diagnosis was provided by the histopathological examination and hematologic examinations.

3. Discussion

A better understanding of the clinical and imaging features of this type of lesion is necessary to avoid diagnostic confusion, especially with benign alterations or vascular malformations with involvement of multiple sites. Previous reports on lymphoma demonstrated a single expansion of the bone, with no bone destruction [24, 25]. A classical but not frequent [17, 26] radiologic finding in head and neck lymphoma is ill defined or lytic destruction, suggestive of malignant neoplasms or osteomyelitis [11]; however, the imaging features of the present case resemble a benign lesion more than a malignancy. Probably, as described by the two latest mandibular canal extranodal NHL report [13, 14], the lymphoma encroached so slowly into mandibular canal such that surrounding bone did not lose its characteristic of subtle sclerosis that marks the canal wall; and the limits seen were well defined.

The patient of the present case reported was asymptomatic, with primary complaint of teeth absence. In spite of this finding, clinical presentation of NHL extranodal bone lesions usually includes history of swelling, pain, paresthesia, or hyperesthesia along alveolar nerve extension and distribution, as well as lymphadenopathy [11]. Hyperesthesia may be related to compression or infiltration of the inferior alveolar nerve [24]. Other unspecific symptoms, such as tooth mobility, may refer to dental abscess or osteomyelitis [27, 28], especially to lymphomas at alveolar process, which are confounders to the NHL diagnostic [13].

Establishing the diagnostic hypothesis based on routine X-rays techniques, such as panoramic and lateral teleradiography, is quite difficult, especially in the absence of local and systemic clinical alterations or further accurate patient's clinical history information. However, panoramic images are considered an important tool of investigation at early stage of malignancies like NHL, due to the fact that it allows the professionals to detect and visualize the first signs of the disease. CT may confirm these findings [5].

In the present case, panoramic radiograph was crucial to initiating deep imaging investigations due to the evident radiolucent fusiform lesion with notch-like margins and with no bony septae at inferior alveolar canal especially because of the asymptomatic characteristic presented by the patient. Notwithstanding, compared with standard x-ray techniques, MRI and CTC scans provide much more valuable information for diagnostic hypothesis postulation and preoperative planning [15].

On computed tomography (CT) scans, beyond the expansion of the mandibular canal path walls, erosion of the cortex of mandibular canal should be studied, as well as other radiographic signs, such as thinning or disruption of bone cortices associated with the neoplasms. Magnetic resonance imaging (MRI) findings, unfortunately, have not been reported to our knowledge. MRI findings would help to differentiate NHL from solid purely cystic lesions, before the histopathological exam.

The bilateral presence of the neoplasm has raised questions as to whether the patient is carrying syndromes, genetic disorders, or even vascular malformations. The differential diagnostic hypothesis first included neurofibromatosis, due to the particular aspect of widening of the mandibular canal [19, 20]. Other hypotheses were multiple endocrine neoplasia type 2b [21] with bilateral mandibular canal involvement and arteriovenous malformation [22]. Unilateral or localized intramandibular canal lesions such as solitary neurofibromas [29, 30], traumatic neuroma of the inferior alveolar nerve [31], localized hypertrophic neuropathy (intraneural perineurioma) [32], vascular leiomyoma [23], and schwannomas were excluded [15] after CT examination. Extranodal NHL was not considered at first, due to its frequency at mandible, or even malignant pathologies, because of the radiographic features.

Although rich information was provided by radiological examination, the definitive diagnosis was reached through histopathological exam followed by hematological studies. Immunohistochemical phenotyping is also applied for NHL [13]. The prognosis is determined by clinical staging and histological grade; primary extranodal NHL progression may also lead to a fatal outcome [13].

The recommended treatment for intraosseous lymphomas of the jaws may include nonconservative surgery, although surgical eradication is not the first choice of treatment; frequently chemotherapy or radiation or both are used [12].

Thus, regarding the features of intraosseous NHL of inferior alveolar nerve on plain radiographs and CBCT, it is important to consider this NHL as a diagnostic hypothesis to benign tumors, especially when it is at a bilateral site, despite its rarity. Due the severity of the disease and the possibility of a fatal outcome, it is important to avoid delaying to definitive diagnosis.

Competing Interests

The authors declare no conflict of interests.

References

[1] N. P. Leite, N. Kased, R. F. Hanna et al., "Cross-sectional imaging of extranodal involvement in abdominopelvic lymphoproliferative malignancies," *Radiographics*, vol. 27, no. 6, pp. 1613–1634, 2007.

[2] Q. Cai, J. Westin, K. Fu et al., "Accelerated therapeutic progress in diffuse large B cell lymphoma," *Annals of Hematology*, vol. 93, no. 4, pp. 541–556, 2014.

[3] O. Zagolski, R. Dwivedi, S. Subramanian, and R. Kazi, "Non-Hodgkin's lymphoma of the sino-nasal tract in children," *Journal of Cancer Research and Therapeutics*, vol. 6, no. 1, pp. 5–10, 2010.

[4] A. L. Weber, A. Rahemtullah, and J. A. Ferry, "Hodgkin and non-Hodgkin lymphoma of the head and neck: clinical, pathologic, and imaging evaluation," *Neuroimaging Clinics of North America*, vol. 13, no. 3, pp. 371–392, 2003.

[5] A. Cortese, G. Pantaleo, I. Ferrara et al., "Bone and soft tissue non-Hodgkin lymphoma of the maxillofacial area: report of two cases, literature review and new therapeutic strategies," *International Journal of Surgery*, vol. 12, supplement 2, pp. S23–S28, 2014.

[6] C. C. Wang and D. J. Fleischli, "Primary reticulum cell sarcoma of bone. With emphasis on radiation therapy," *Cancer*, vol. 22, no. 5, pp. 994–998, 1968.

[7] R. I. F. van der Waal, P. C. Huijgens, P. van der Valk, and I. van der Waal, "Characteristics of 40 primary extranodal non-Hodgkin lymphomas of the oral cavity in perspective of the new WHO classification and the International Prognostic Index," *International Journal of Oral and Maxillofacial Surgery*, vol. 34, no. 4, pp. 391–395, 2005.

[8] S. Kemp, G. Gallagher, S. Kabani, V. Noonan, and C. O'Hara, "Oral non-Hodgkin's lymphoma: review of the literature and World Health Organization classification with reference to 40 cases," *Oral Surgery, Oral Medicine, Oral Pathology, Oral Radiology and Endodontology*, vol. 105, no. 2, pp. 194–201, 2008.

[9] M. Kremer, L. Quintanilla-Martínez, J. Nährig, C. Von Schilling, and F. Fend, "Immunohistochemistry in bone marrow pathology: a useful adjunct for morphologic diagnosis," *Virchows Archiv*, vol. 447, no. 6, pp. 920–937, 2005.

[10] F. Fend and M. Kremer, "Diagnosis and classification of malignant lymphoma and related entities in the bone marrow trephine biopsy," *Pathobiology*, vol. 74, no. 2, pp. 133–143, 2007.

[11] A. W. Gusenbauer, N. F. Katsikeris, and A. Brown, "Primary lymphoma of the mandible: report of a case," *Journal of Oral and Maxillofacial Surgery*, vol. 48, no. 4, pp. 409–415, 1990.

[12] J. B. Bavitz, D. W. Patterson, and S. Sorensen, "Non-Hodgkin's lymphoma disguised as odontogenic pain," *The Journal of the American Dental Association*, vol. 123, no. 3, pp. 99–100, 1992.

[13] N. Burić, G. Jovanović, Z. Radovanović, M. Burić, and M. Tijanić, "Radiographic enlargement of mandibular canal as first feature of non-Hodgkin's lymphoma," *Dentomaxillofacial Radiology*, vol. 39, no. 6, pp. 383–388, 2010.

[14] T. Yamada, Y. Kitagawa, T. Ogasawara, S. Yamamoto, Y. Ishii, and Y. Urasaki, "Enlargement of mandibular canal without hypesthesia caused by extranodal non-Hodgkin's lymphoma," *Oral Surgery, Oral Medicine, Oral Pathology, Oral Radiology, and Endodontics*, vol. 89, no. 3, pp. 388–392, 2000.

[15] V. M. Vartiainen, M. Siponen, T. Salo, J. Rosberg, and M. Apaja-Sarkkinen, "Widening of the inferior alveolar canal: a case report with atypical lymphocytic infiltration of the nerve," *Oral Surgery, Oral Medicine, Oral Pathology, Oral Radiology and Endodontology*, vol. 106, no. 4, pp. e35–e39, 2008.

[16] H. Dexter Barber, J. C. B. Stewart, and W. D. Baxter, "Non-Hodgkin's lymphoma involving the inferior alveolar canal and mental foramen: report of a case," *Journal of Oral and Maxillofacial Surgery*, vol. 50, no. 12, pp. 1334–1336, 1992.

[17] M. Bertolotto, G. Cecchini, C. Martinoli, R. Perrone, and G. Garlaschi, "Primary lymphoma of the mandible with diffuse widening of the mandibular canal: report of a case," *European Radiology*, vol. 6, no. 5, pp. 637–639, 1996.

[18] H. Zainab, A. D. Kale, and S. Hallikerimath, "Intraosseous schwannoma of the mandible," *Journal of Oral and Maxillofacial Pathology*, vol. 16, no. 2, pp. 294–296, 2012.

[19] V. Visnapuu, S. Peltonen, T. Ellilä et al., "Periapical cemental dysplasia is common in women with NF1," *European Journal of Medical Genetics*, vol. 50, no. 4, pp. 274–280, 2007.

[20] S. D. Shapiro, K. Abramovitch, M. L. Van Dis et al., "Neurofibromatosis: oral and radiographic manifestations," *Oral Surgery, Oral Medicine, Oral Pathology*, vol. 58, no. 4, pp. 493–498, 1984.

[21] M. E. Schenberg, J. D. Zajac, S. Lim-Tio, N. A. Collier, A. M. V. Brooks, and P. C. Reade, "Multiple endocrine neoplasia syndrome—type 2b: case report and review," *International Journal of Oral and Maxillofacial Surgery*, vol. 21, no. 2, pp. 110–114, 1992.

[22] B. B. Horswell and A. D. Holmes, "Arteriovenous malformation in the mandible of a young child," *Australian and New Zealand Journal of Surgery*, vol. 58, no. 1, pp. 73–76, 1988.

[23] E. J. Burkes Jr., "Vascular leiomyoma of the mandible. Report of a case," *Journal of Oral and Maxillofacial Surgery*, vol. 53, no. 1, pp. 65–66, 1995.

[24] K. T. Robbins, L. M. Fuller, J. Manning et al., "Primary lymphoma of the mandible," *Head & Neck Surgery*, vol. 8, no. 3, pp. 192–199, 1986.

[25] E. S. Delpassand and J. B. Kirkpatrick, "Cavernous sinus syndrome as the presentation of malignant lymphoma: case report and review of the literature," *Neurosurgery*, vol. 23, no. 4, pp. 501–504, 1988.

[26] R. Yagan, M. Radivoyevitch, and E. M. Bellon, "Involvement of the mandibular canal: early sign of osteogenic sarcoma of the mandible," *Oral Surgery, Oral Medicine, Oral Pathology*, vol. 60, no. 1, pp. 56–60, 1985.

[27] S. J. Parrington and A. Punnia-Moorthy, "Primary non-Hodgkin's lymphoma of the mandible presenting following tooth extraction," *British Dental Journal*, vol. 187, no. 9, pp. 468–470, 1999.

[28] E. F. Mendonça, T. O. Sousa, and C. Estrela, "Non-hodgkin lymphoma in the periapical region of a mandibular canine," *Journal of Endodontics*, vol. 39, no. 6, pp. 839–842, 2013.

[29] M. Polak, G. Polak, C. Brocheriou, and J. Vigneul, "Solitary neurofibroma of the mandible: case report and review of the literature," *Journal of Oral and Maxillofacial Surgery*, vol. 47, no. 1, pp. 65–68, 1989.

[30] C. Apostolidis, D. Anterriotis, A. D. Rapidis, and A. P. Angelopoulos, "Solitary intraosseous neurofibroma of the inferior alveolar nerve: report of a case," *Journal of Oral and Maxillofacial Surgery*, vol. 59, no. 2, pp. 232–235, 2001.

[31] R. H. Kallal, F. G. Ritto, L. E. Almeida, D. J. Crofton, and G. P. Thomas, "Traumatic neuroma following sagittal split osteotomy of the mandible," *International Journal of Oral and Maxillofacial Surgery*, vol. 36, no. 5, pp. 453–454, 2007.

[32] M. Ethunandan, R. O. Weller, I. H. McVicar, and S. E. Fisher, "Localized hypertrophic neuropathy involving the inferior alveolar nerve," *Journal of Oral and Maxillofacial Surgery*, vol. 57, no. 1, pp. 84–89, 1999.

29

Morquio's Syndrome: A Case Report of Two Siblings

Sathish Muthukumar Ramalingam,[1] Daya Srinivasan,[2] Sandhya ArunKumar,[1] Joe Louis ChiriyanKandath,[2] and Sriram Kaliamoorthy[1]

[1]*Department of Oral and Maxillofacial Pathology, Chettinad Dental College & Research Institute, Tamil Nadu, India*
[2]*Department of Pedodontia and Preventive Dentistry, Chettinad Dental College & Research Institute, Tamil Nadu, India*

Correspondence should be addressed to Daya Srinivasan; dayaswathi@gmail.com

Academic Editor: Michael W. Roberts

Morquio syndrome or MPS IVA is a rare type of lysosomal storage disease associated with highly specific dental abnormalities. We present two siblings with enamel hypoplasia and skeletal abnormalities. A diagnosis of mucopolysaccharidosis type IVA was reached based on the clinical, radiographic, and dental findings of the patients. The dental findings are useful diagnostic aid for the early diagnosis of this debilitating disorder.

1. Introduction

Glycosaminoglycans (GAGs), formerly known as mucopolysaccharides, are long-chained carbohydrates that are vital for the formation of bone, cartilage, tendons, corneas, skin, and connective tissue. The deficiency of lysosomal enzymes required for the metabolism of the various mucopolysaccharides results in the accumulation of the respective substrate in the cells, leading to progressive cellular damage and clinic pathological changes. Mucopolysaccharidosis (MPS) is comprised of at least seven recognized phenotypes that are assigned by numbers and eponyms.

2. Case Report

Two siblings, a 13-year-old girl (case 1, Figures 1(a)–1(d)) and a 10-year-old boy (case 2, Figures 2(a)–2(d)) of normal intelligence had come to Chettinad Dental College and Research Institute, Chennai, with a complaint of decayed teeth. The physical appearances were similar, characterized by short stature, short neck, protuberant chest, scoliosis, and a waddling gait. Their facial feature presented frontal bossing and flat nasal bridge. The history revealed that the patients had pain in the hip region on walking that subsides at rest. The

parents did not belong to different ethnicity. They had a nonconsanguineous marriage and a family history free from any skeletal disorder. On oral examination, exposed teeth with sharp cusps and rough enamel texture were found (Figures 1(a), 1(b), 2(a), and 2(b)). The orthopantomograph showed thin hypoplastic enamel of normal radiodensity (Figures 1(c) and 2(c)).

A multispecialty approach was adopted and medical examination of all major systems revealed no dysfunctional changes. However, the orthopedic and radiographic evaluation indicated gross skeletal deformity. The hand-wrist radiograph showed proximally narrow metacarpals. The anteroposterior view of the spine expressed curvature of the thoracolumbar vertebral segment. The lateral spinal view revealed anterior beaking of the vertebral body (Figure 1(d)). The pelvic view radiograph revealed an irregularly outlined square-shaped head of the femur and coxa valga defect (Figure 2(d)).

A diagnosis of mucopolysaccharidosis type IVA was reached based on the clinical, dental, and radiographic findings of the patients. The diagnosis would need to be confirmed by analysis of GALNS enzyme activity and molecular genetic testing of GALNS gene. Unfortunately, parents' consent could not be obtained for this analysis.

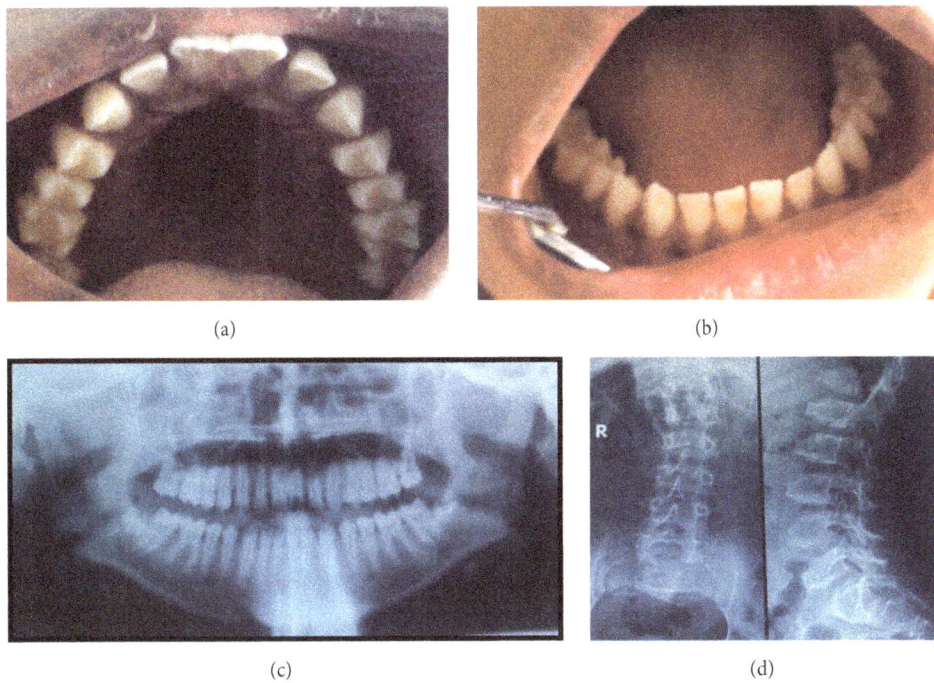

FIGURE 1: (a), (b) Spade-shaped incisors, pointed cusps, and spacing between teeth in case 1. (c) Orthopantomograph showing thin enamel with normal radio density. (d) Spinal radiographs revealing kyphoscoliosis and tongue-like projections from anterior surface of vertebral bodies in case 1.

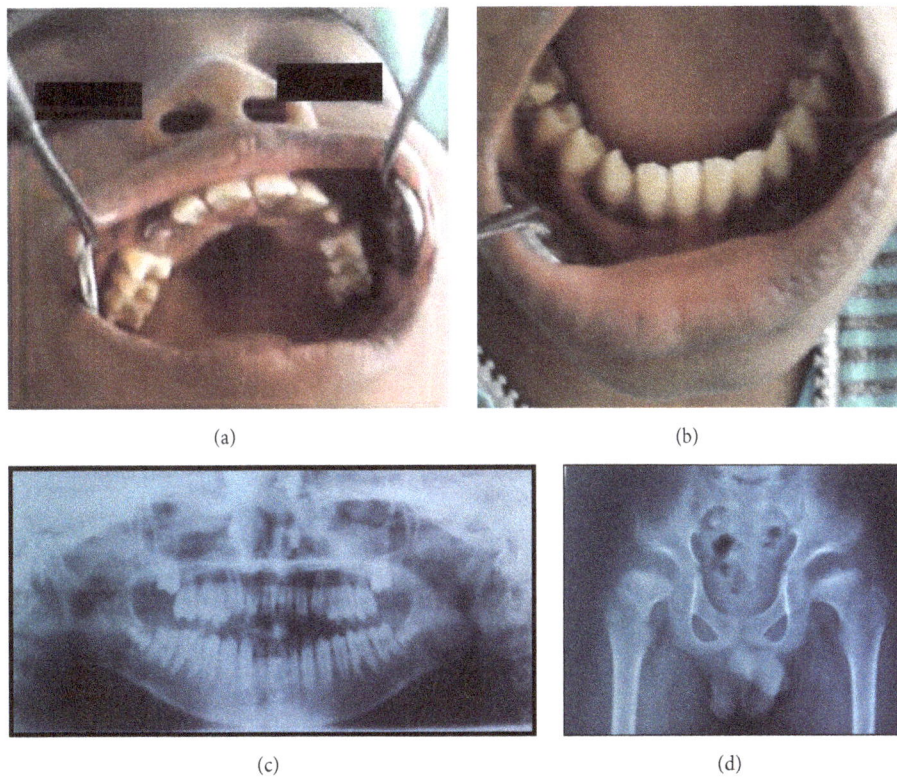

FIGURE 2: (a), (b) Spade-shaped incisors, pointed cusps, and spacing between teeth in both maxillary and mandibular teeth in case 2. (c) Orthopantomograph showing thin enamel with normal radio density. (d) Pelvic radiograph showing shallow acetabula and square-shaped femoral head in case 2.

3. Discussion

Mucopolysaccharidosis type IV (MPS type IV) is a rare disorder which presents with a number of musculoskeletal defects. The clinical condition was first described independently in 1929 by Morquio and Brailsford. Matalon et al. in 1974 identified the deficiency of enzyme N-acetyl-galactosamine-6-sulfatase causing intracellular accumulation of keratan sulfate responsible for Morquio's syndrome type IVA [1]. MPS type IVB is due to deficiency of beta-galactosidase [2]. A non keratan sulfate excretion variety is labeled as MPS type IV C [3].

The parents did not belong to different ethnicity, yet they were not consanguineously related (first cousins, double first cousins, second cousins, double second cousin, or uncle niece relationship) [4]. Morquio patients usually do not present with any clinical signs or symptoms until the end of first year of life, but, as the age advances, they show signs of muscular atrophy, pectus carinatum, and knock knee deformity [5]. Obvious symptoms such as waddling gait and dwarfism due to dorsilumbar kyphoscoliosis can be observed at an earlier age [1]. Atlantoaxial subluxation and spinal cord compression especially in the upper cervical region are frequently noted. This is a sequela of odontoid dysplasia which is a major complication of MPS type IV [5, 6]. The later manifestations include corneal opacity, deafness, hypermobility of joints, cardiac abnormalities, quadriplegia and respiratory paralysis [7].

GAGs and proteoglycans provide the extracellular polyanionic macromolecules for the biomineralization process of several biologic systems. GAGs regulate the enamel maturation during the transitional and maturation stage of amelogenesis. Typical dental changes are characterized by surface pitting and thin hypoplastic enamel resulting in altered shape and discoloration [8]. The maxillary anterior teeth are widely spaced and the posteriors are occlusally tapered with pointed cusps [9, 10]. Enamel hypoplasia is a prominent feature in all forms of MPS type IVA. It is absent in MPS type IVB and MPSIVC. Thus, dental findings can be an important diagnostic aid for MPS type IVA [9–12]. GAGs serve as a matrix for anchoring amelogenin at the enamel dentinal junction so that a close bond is established between enamel and dentine [13]. Lack of sulfatase enzyme would remove the GAGS from dentinal tubule site which can cause lack of integration at enamel dentinal junction. Mineralization of enamel starts in the secretory stage of formation of enamel. Thickening of enamel crystallites to a preferred degree of orientation occurs in the maturation stage. Thus, texture of enamel is determined at both secretory and maturation stages. This could be the possible reason for rough enamel surface being noted [13, 14].

Inclination of the distal ends of the radius and ulna towards each other, hand bones being short, and squat help in radiological diagnosis. Convergence of proximal surfaces of metacarpals gives a "bullet-"shaped appearance [5–7]. Other findings which are observed in the present cases include coxa valga defect, odontoid hypoplasia, platyspondyly, and anterior beaking of the vertebral bodies. The pelvic deformity is characterized by short and square iliac wings associated with flat acetabula roof [5]. The anteroposterior spinal radiograph features thoracolumbar kyphoscoliosis as seen in the present case.

Diagnostic methods available are blood and urine analysis to quantify the keratan sulfate level, direct enzyme assay in leukocytes or fibroblasts, and the wide range of radiographic views to demonstrate the skeletal abnormalities. Although the elevated urinary keratan sulfate is diagnostic of MPS, mucopolysaccharide excretion reduces with age and cases of Morquio with absence of excessive keratan sulfate in the urine have also been reported [6, 7]. Odontoid hypoplasia or dysplasia and spinal cord compression are the most consistent features in Morquio's syndrome. A prenatal diagnosis for the disorder is possible by performing amniocentesis or chorionic villi sampling when there is a family history of Morquio's syndrome. The diagnosis has to be confirmed with GALNS enzyme activity and molecular genetic testing of GALNS gene [15]. In the present case, the children are born out of a nonconsanguineous marriage and no family members are affected. The final diagnosis is based on clinical, radiographic, and dental findings.

In conclusion, MPS IVA is a rare type of mucopolysaccharidosis associated with highly specific dental abnormalities. As there is no cure for Morquio's syndrome, periodic monitoring and intervention are mandatory. Bone marrow transplant and enzyme replacement therapy (ERT) have been used with some success. This case illustrates the importance of systemic evaluation and inclusion of MPS type IVA in the differential diagnosis of enamel hypoplasia. As both the primary and permanent dentitions are affected, an early diagnosis is possible even in the clinically atypical cases. Early systemic evaluation and follow-up will help in improving the quality of life of the patients.

Competing Interests

There are no competing interests.

References

[1] R. Matalon, B. Arbogast, and A. Dorfman, "Deficiency of chondroitin sulfate N-acetylgalactosamine 4-sulfate sulfatase in Maroteaux-Lamy syndrome," *Biochemical and Biophysical Research Communications*, vol. 61, no. 4, pp. 1450–1457, 1974.

[2] J. S. O'Brien, E. Gugler, A. Giedion et al., "Spondyloepiphyseal dysplasia, corneal clouding, normal intelligence and acid β galactosidase deficiency," *Clinical Genetics*, vol. 9, no. 5, pp. 495–504, 1976.

[3] V. A. McKusick, *Heritable Disorders of Connective Tissue*, C. V. Mosby, St. Louis, Mo, USA, 4th edition, 1972.

[4] H. Hamamy, "Consanguineous marriages: preconception consultation in primary health care settings," *Journal of Community Genetics*, vol. 3, no. 3, pp. 185–192, 2012.

[5] J. Nelson and M. Kinirons, "Clinical findings in 12 patients with MPS IV A (Morquio's disease). Further evidence for heterogeneity. Part II: dental findings," *Clinical Genetics*, vol. 33, no. 2, pp. 121–125, 1988.

[6] L. E. Swischuk, *Imaging of New Born, Infant and Young Child*, Lippincott Williams & Wilkins, 5th edition, 2004.

[7] P. Jenkins, G. R. Davies, and P. S. Harper, "Morquio Brailsford disease: a report of four affected sisters with absence of excessive keratan sulphate in the urine," *British Journal of Radiology*, vol. 46, no. 549, pp. 668–675, 1973.

[8] I. Rølling, N. Clausen, B. Nyvad, and S. Sindet-Pedersen, "Dental findings in three siblings with Morquio's syndrome," *International Journal of Paediatric Dentistry*, vol. 9, no. 3, pp. 219–224, 1999.

[9] L. S. Levin, R. J. Jorgenson, and C. F. Salinas, "Oral findings in the Morquio syndrome (mucopolysaccharidosis IV)," *Oral Surgery, Oral Medicine, Oral Pathology*, vol. 39, no. 3, pp. 390–395, 1975.

[10] J. Fitzgerald and S. J. Verveniotis, "Morquio's syndrome. A case report and review of clinical findings," *The New York State Dental Journal*, vol. 64, no. 8, pp. 48–50, 1998.

[11] A. Oyarzún, "Immunohistochemical localization of glycosaminoglycans and proteoglycans involved in enamel formation," *European Cells and Materials*, vol. 14, no. 2, p. 117, 2007.

[12] M. J. Kinirons and J. Nelson, "Dental findings in mucopolysaccharidosis type IV A (Morquio's disease type A)," *Oral Surgery, Oral Medicine, Oral Pathology*, vol. 70, no. 2, pp. 176–179, 1990.

[13] R. M. H. Ravindranath and S. R. M. Basilrose, "Localization of sulfated sialic acids in the dentinal tubules during tooth formation in mice," *Acta Histochemica*, vol. 107, no. 1, pp. 43–56, 2005.

[14] M. Al-Jawad, O. Addison, M. A. Khan, A. James, and C. J. Hendriksz, "Disruption of enamel crystal formation quantified by synchrotron microdiffraction," *Journal of Dentistry*, vol. 40, no. 12, pp. 1074–1080, 2012.

[15] C. J. Hendriksz, K. I. Berger, R. Giugliani et al., "International guidelines for the management and treatment of Morquio a syndrome," *American Journal of Medical Genetics A*, vol. 167, no. 1, pp. 11–25, 2015.

30

Mandibular Symmetrical Bilateral Canine-Lateral Incisors Transposition: Its Early Diagnosis and Treatment Considerations

Yehoshua Shapira, Tamar Finkelstein, Rana Kadry, Shirley Schonberger, and Nir Shpack

Department of Orthodontics, The Maurice and Gabriela Goldschleger School of Dental Medicine, Tel Aviv University, Tel Aviv, Israel

Correspondence should be addressed to Yehoshua Shapira; yehoshua.shapira@gmail.com

Academic Editor: Asja Celebić

Bilateral mandibular tooth transposition is a relatively rare dental anomaly caused by distal migration of the mandibular lateral incisors and can be detected in the early mixed dentition by radiographic examination. Early diagnosis and interceptive intervention may reduce the risk of possible transposition between the mandibular canine and lateral incisor. This report illustrates the orthodontic management of bilateral mandibular canine-lateral incisor transposition. Correct positioning of the affected teeth was achieved on the left side while teeth on the right side were aligned in their transposed position. It demonstrates the outcome of good alignment of the teeth in the dental arch.

1. Introduction

A tooth may deviate from its normal path of eruption usually as a result of severe crowding or presence of an obstacle such as a supernumerary tooth or an odontoma. Such eruption deviation can occur with no apparent local or systemic cause, resulting in ectopic eruption of the tooth in a place normally occupied by another permanent tooth. The most frequently ectopically erupted tooth is the mandibular permanent lateral incisor which may occur unilaterally and bilaterally [1–4]. A study on the occurrence of ectopic erupting permanent teeth has shown that 30% involved the mandibular permanent lateral incisors unilaterally and bilaterally [5].

Early diagnosis of a disturbed eruption of a mandibular permanent lateral incisor can be made in young children during the early mixed dentition at the age of 6–8 years, though some variation in timing of eruption of that tooth has been reported [6]. The permanent lateral incisor during this period is in its preeruptive migration and the deciduous lateral incisor root is resorbing. The lateral incisor may, for unknown reasons, deviate from its normal eruption path and become distally displaced, resulting in overretention of the deciduous lateral incisor, and could ectopically erupt in a transposed position with the permanent canine [7].

Tooth transposition is defined as an interchange in position of two adjacent permanent teeth in the same quadrant of the dental arch or eruption of a tooth in a place normally occupied by another tooth [8]. It is a type of ectopic eruption that results in an abnormal sequence of the permanent teeth in the dental arch. Transposition occurs most frequently between the maxillary canine and first premolar and occasionally between the maxillary canine and lateral incisor [9, 10]. Rare cases of transposition between a canine and a second premolar or an incisor have been reported [11]. Transposition of a tooth may be complete, where both the crowns and roots of the involved teeth are in transposed position. It may be incomplete when only the crown is transposed but the root is within its normal place. Unilateral transpositions are more often than bilateral ones, with left side predominance, and are found more often in females than in males [11, 12].

Transposition in the mandible is relatively rare and occurs between the canine and lateral incisor and is usually unilateral. Only few cases of bilateral transposition of a canine and lateral incisor in the mandible have been reported [13, 14]. The prevalence of tooth transposition varies according to different studies and was found to be 0.43% of patients in India [15], 0.38% in Turkish population [16], and 0.14% of patients in Nigeria [17, 18], whereas the prevalence of mandibular canine-lateral incisor transposition is only 0.03% [19].

The etiology of transposition is unknown and the reason why a tooth deviates from its normal path of eruption is still obscure. Several theories have been suggested such as genetic factors [20, 21], interchange in the position of the developing tooth buds, early loss or prolonged retention of deciduous teeth, and trauma and mechanical interference to the erupting permanent teeth [11, 21].

Tooth transposition has been reported to be associated with other dental anomalies such as missing teeth, small or peg-shaped maxillary lateral incisors, retained deciduous mandibular lateral incisors and canines, rotations and malposition of adjacent teeth, and root dilacerations and impactions [22].

The literature on early detection and treatment procedures for this abnormality is relatively sparse. The purpose of this article is primarily to emphasize early diagnosis and detection of bilateral mandibular tooth transposition and describe its orthodontic management and outcome.

2. Clinical Diagnosis and Evaluation

The early mixed dentition period, between 6 and 8 years, is the best time for assessing the development and path of eruption of the mandibular permanent lateral incisors. These age group children are usually first examined by a pediatric or general dentist who should evaluate both the dental health condition and the dental development. Using a panoramic radiograph is very useful for early diagnosis of the position and path of eruption of the unerupted teeth.

3. Clinical and Radiographic Examination

A routine panoramic radiograph of a 6-year-old boy, taken at the Pedodontic Department of Tel Aviv University School of Dental Medicine, demonstrated normal dental position and development of the mandibular permanent lateral incisors, which are expected to erupt into their proper position in the arch uneventfully (Figure 1). Surprisingly enough and for unknown reason, a follow-up panoramic radiograph taken two years later, at the age of 8 years, demonstrated bilateral distal deflection of the mandibular permanent lateral incisors bypassing the deciduous lateral incisors and canines and ectopically erupted rotated in the place of the deciduous first molars causing their early exfoliation (Figure 2). His intraoral examination revealed Class I interarch relationship with normal overbite and overjet in the early mixed dentition. The mandibular permanent lateral incisors have ectopically erupted bilaterally distal to the deciduous canines with 90 degrees of rotation, causing early exfoliation of the deciduous first molars (Figure 3).

4. Treatment Objectives

The primary objectives were to derotate the mandibular permanent lateral incisors and upright and reposition them to their normal position next to the central incisors. This

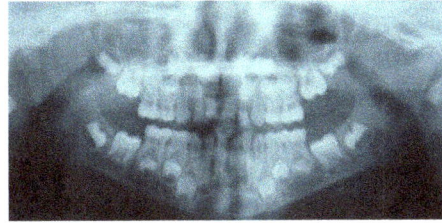

FIGURE 1: Panoramic radiograph of a 6-year-old boy with normal dental position and development of the mandibular permanent lateral incisors.

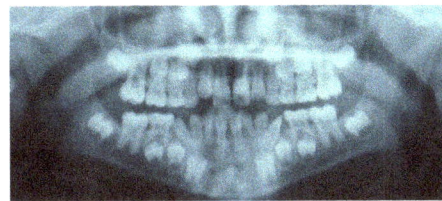

FIGURE 2: Panoramic radiograph at the age of 8 years, showing the mandibular permanent lateral incisors ectopically erupted and rotated in the place of the first deciduous molars causing their early exfoliation.

will allow the canines and first premolars to erupt into their normal place and avoid the possible development of transposition between the canines and lateral incisors.

5. Treatment Plan, Procedure, and Outcome

The early diagnosis is of crucial importance for establishing a correct treatment planning. The retained deciduous lateral incisors and canines were immediately removed at the age of 8 years (Figure 4). Edgewise fixed appliances were used, first to correct the severely rotated lateral incisors and upright them and then to move them mesially to their normal place next to the central incisors (Figure 5).

Periodic radiographs taken during treatment showed that the right permanent canine was already erupting between the central and lateral incisors, while the left canine and lateral incisor were almost overlapping each other (Figure 6). It would have been dangerous to continue the movement of the right lateral incisor to its normal position as it could cause interference between their roots and possible root resorption. Therefore, it was decided at that point that it would be safer to align them in their transposed position. The left lateral incisor was uprighted and moved to its normal place next to the central incisor allowing the left canine to erupt into its normal position in the arch, while the right permanent canine was erupting in transposition with the lateral incisor (Figure 7). The right canine's cusp tip was slightly reshaped to resemble an incisor. Following completion of the orthodontic treatment at the age of 12 years permanent retainers were bonded on the upper and lower anterior teeth. The very nice outcome of the treatment is presented in the final intraoral photographs (Figure 8) and panoramic radiograph (Figure 9).

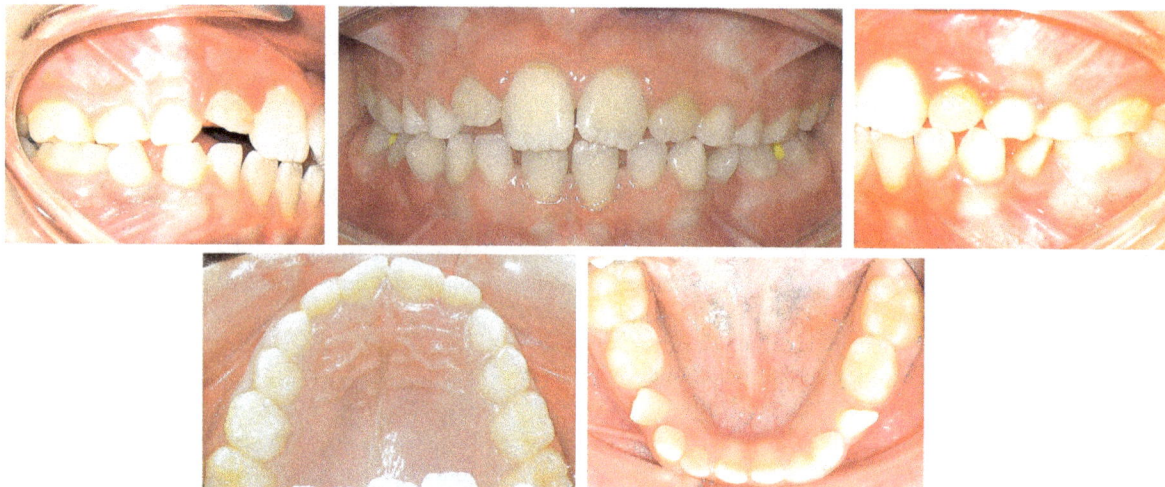

FIGURE 3: Pretreatment intraoral photographs showing the mandibular right and left lateral incisors ectopically erupted rotated in the place of the early exfoliated first deciduous molars.

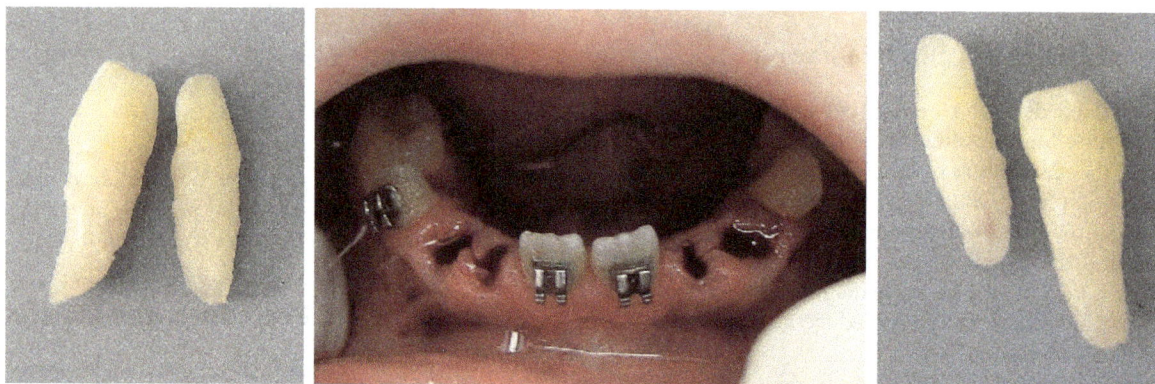

FIGURE 4: Extraction of the deciduous lateral incisors and canines.

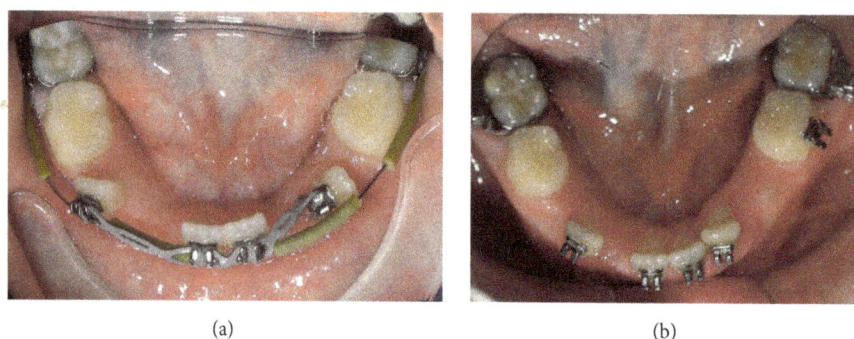

(a)   (b)

FIGURE 5: Derotation (a) and mesial movement of the permanent lateral incisors (b).

6. Discussion

The developing mandibular permanent lateral incisor normally resorbs the root of the deciduous tooth during the process of eruption into the oral cavity. It is still unclear what causes a tooth to deviate from its normal path of eruption and erupt ectopically. The presence of an obstacle such as a supernumerary tooth or an odontoma could be a factor causing the deflection and migration of a tooth. Several theories have been suggested as etiological factors to explain why a tooth deviates from its normal path of eruption to become transposed: interchange in position of the anlage at the very early stage of tooth development [23], genetic control within the dental follicle [20, 21, 24], prolonged retention of the deciduous lateral incisor [25, 26], crowding and inadequate arch length [2]. Crowding did not

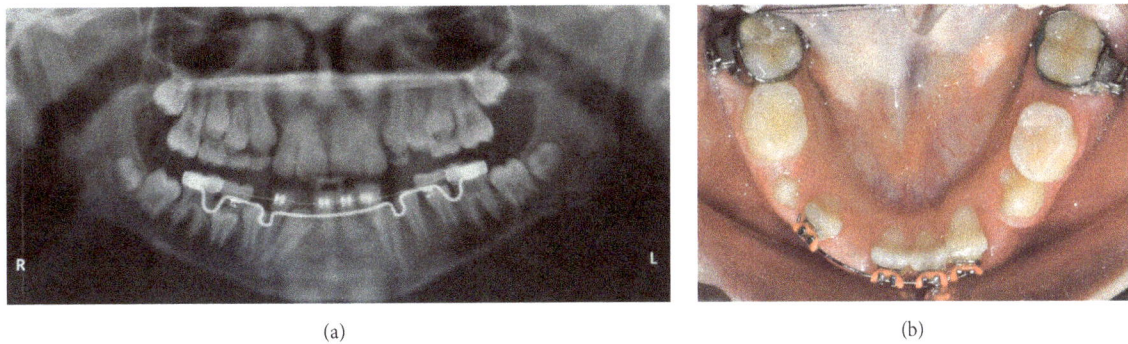

(a)   (b)

FIGURE 6: Panoramic radiograph (a) and intraoral photograph (b) showing the right permanent canine in position to erupt between the lateral and central incisors.

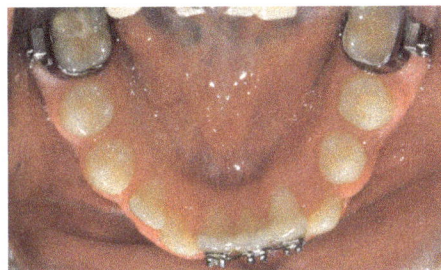

FIGURE 7: The right permanent canine is erupting in transposition with the lateral incisor. The left permanent canine is erupting into its normal position in the arch.

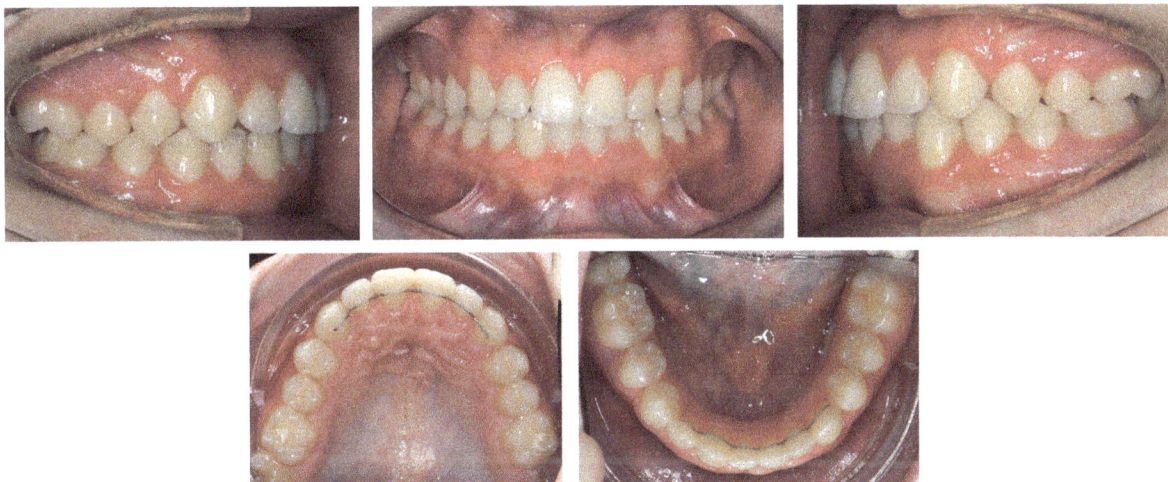

FIGURE 8: Posttreatment intraoral photographs showing mandibular right canine in complete transposition with the lateral incisor, while the left canine is in its normal position in the arch.

seem to be a primary cause of the anomaly as sufficient space to accommodate all the permanent teeth was found in the presented case, which is in agreement with previous reported cases [11]. Another possible explanation suggested that the retained mandibular deciduous lateral incisor could be the cause of the displacement of the permanent lateral incisor resulting in transposition [27].

It is not yet clear whether the retained deciduous tooth is the cause or the result of the displacement and ectopic eruption of its successor.

Treatment considerations for transposed teeth include repositioning them in their normal place in the dental arch, maintaining them in their transposed position, or extracting one of the transposed teeth.

In managing treatment for mandibular tooth transposition several factors should be considered such as the amount of distally displaced lateral incisor and the intrabony position of the permanent canine. Early detection of the abnormal eruption path of the lateral incisor allows for early intervention by uprighting and moving the lateral incisor

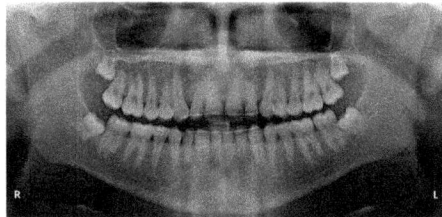

FIGURE 9: Posttreatment panoramic radiograph showing complete transposition between the mandibular right canine and lateral incisor. The left canine erupted in its normal position.

to its normal place in the arch prior to the eruption of the canine into transposition with the lateral incisor. This was successfully achieved in our presented case only on the left side. On the contralateral side, however, the position of the canine was already between the central and lateral incisors and to avoid a possible risk of root resorption it was allowed to erupt into complete transposition with the lateral incisor. The canine's cusp tip was reshaped to resemble a lateral incisor.

7. Conclusions

Early detection of a distally displaced mandibular permanent lateral incisor at the early mixed dentition, at the age of 6–8 years, and timely interceptive intervention may reduce the risk of tooth transposition in the mandible and avoid complex orthodontic therapy. The early orthodontic management and treatment outcome of mandibular bilateral canine-lateral incisor transposition have been described.

Ethical Approval

This work has been approved by the Ethics Committee of the university.

Competing Interests

The authors of the manuscript state that sources of support and institutional affiliations are proper and do not imply any conflict of interests.

Authors' Contributions

All authors have made substantive contribution to this study and/or manuscript, and all have reviewed the final paper prior to its submission.

Acknowledgments

The authors wish to thank Mr. Amir Shapira for his valuable help in the preparation of this article.

References

[1] G. S. Taylor and M. C. Hamilton, "Ectopic eruption of lower lateral incisors," *Journal of Dentistry for Children*, vol. 38, no. 4, pp. 282–284, 1971.

[2] T. D. Schaad and H. E. Thompson, "Extreme ectopic eruption of the lower permanent lateral incisor," *American Journal of Orthodontics*, vol. 66, no. 3, pp. 280–286, 1974.

[3] E. J. Bradley and R. A. Bell, "Eruptive malpositioning of the mandibular permanent lateral incisors: three case reports," *Pediatric dentistry*, vol. 12, no. 6, pp. 380–387, 1990.

[4] Y. Shapira and M. M. Kuftinec, "The ectopically erupted mandibular lateral incisor," *American Journal of Orthodontics*, vol. 82, no. 5, pp. 426–429, 1982.

[5] W. F. O'Meara, "Ectopic Eruption Pattern in Selected Permanent Teeth," *Journal of Dental Research*, vol. 41, no. 3, pp. 607–616, 1962.

[6] V. O. Hurme, "Ranges in normalcy in the eruption of permanent teeth," *Journal of Dentistry for Children*, vol. 16, no. 2, pp. 11–15, 1949.

[7] Y. Shapira and M. M. Kuftinec, "Early detection and prevention of mandibular tooth transposition," *Journal of Dentistry for Children*, vol. 70, no. 3, pp. 204–207, 2003.

[8] Y. Shapira and M. M. Kuftinec, "Tooth transposition: a review of the literature and treatment considerations," *The Angle Orthodontist*, vol. 59, no. 4, pp. 271–276, 1989.

[9] Y. Shapira, "Transposition of canines," *The Journal of the American Dental Association*, vol. 100, no. 5, pp. 710–712, 1980.

[10] Y. Shapira and M. M. Kuftinec, "Maxillary canine-lateral incisor transposition: orthodontic management," *American Journal of Orthodontics & Dentofacial Orthopedics*, vol. 95, no. 5, pp. 439–444, 1989.

[11] M. R. Joshi and N. A. Bhatt, "Canine transposition," *Oral Surgery, Oral Medicine, Oral Pathology*, vol. 31, no. 1, pp. 49–54, 1971.

[12] S. Peck and L. Peck, "Classification of maxillary tooth transpositions," *American Journal of Orthodontics and Dentofacial Orthopedics*, vol. 107, no. 5, pp. 505–517, 1995.

[13] R. G. Pifer, "Bilateral transposed mandibular teeth," *Oral Surgery Oral Medicine and Oral Pathology*, vol. 36, no. 1, p. 145, 1973.

[14] Y. Shapira, "Bilateral transposition of mandibular canines and lateral incisors: orthodontic management of a case," *British Journal of Orthodontics*, vol. 5, no. 4, pp. 207–209, 1978.

[15] A. Ruprecht, S. Batniji, and E. El-Neweihi, "The incidence of transposition of teeth in the dental patients," *Journal of Pedodontics*, vol. 9, no. 3, pp. 244–249, 1985.

[16] H. H. Yilmaz, H. Türkkahraman, and M. Ö. Sayin, "Prevalence of tooth transpositions and associated dental anomalies in a Turkish population," *Dentomaxillofacial Radiology*, vol. 34, no. 1, pp. 32–35, 2005.

[17] S. E. Burbett, "Prevalence of maxillary canine-first premolar transposition in a composite African sample," *Angle Orthodontics*, vol. 69, no. 2, pp. 187–189, 1999.

[18] A. A. Umweni and M. A. Ojo, "The frequency of tooth transposition in Nigerians, its possible aetiologic factors and clinical implications," *The Journal of the Dental Association of South Africa*, vol. 52, no. 9, pp. 551–554, 1997.

[19] S. Järvinen, "Mandibular incisor-cuspid transposition: a survey," *The Journal of pedodontics*, vol. 6, no. 2, pp. 159–163, 1982.

[20] A. Chattopadhyay and K. Srinivas, "Transposition of teeth and genetic etiology," *The Angle Orthodontist*, vol. 66, no. 2, pp. 147–152, 1996.

[21] S. Peck, L. Peck, and M. Kataja, "Mandibular lateral incisor-canine transposition, concomitant dental anomalies, and

genetic control," *Angle Orthodontist*, vol. 68, no. 5, pp. 455–466, 1998.

[22] Y. Shapira and M. M. Kuftinec, "Maxillary tooth transpositions: characteristic features and accompanying dental anomalies," *American Journal of Orthodontics and Dentofacial Orthopedics*, vol. 119, no. 2, pp. 127–134, 2001.

[23] E. C. Stafne, *Stafne's Oral Radiographic Diagnosis*, W.B. Saunders, Philadelphia, Pa, USA, 1958.

[24] N. J. Ely, M. Sherriff, and M. T. Cobourne, "Dental transposition as a disorder of genetic origin," *European Journal of Orthodontics*, vol. 28, no. 2, pp. 145–151, 2006.

[25] J. S. Rose, "Atypical path of eruption: some causes and effects," *Dental Practitioner*, vol. 9, pp. 69–76, 1958.

[26] M. E. Gellin and J. V. Haley, "Managing cases of overretention of mandibular primary incisors where their permanent successors erupt lingually," *ASDC journal of dentistry for children*, vol. 49, no. 2, pp. 118–122, 1982.

[27] K. M. Platzer, "Mandibular incisor-canine transposition," *The Journal of the American Dental Association*, vol. 76, no. 4, pp. 778–784, 1968.

31

Giant Cell Fibroma in a Two-Year-Old Child

Anna Carolina Volpi Mello-Moura,[1,2] **Ana Maria Antunes Santos,**[3]
Gabriela Azevedo Vasconcelos Cunha Bonini,[1,4] **Cristina Giovannetti Del Conte Zardetto,**[5,6]
Cacio Moura-Netto,[7] **and Marcia Turolla Wanderley**[1]

[1]*Research and Clinical Center of Dental Trauma in Primary Teeth, Department of Orthodontics and Pediatric Dentistry,
School of Dentistry, University of São Paulo-FOUSP, São Paulo, SP, Brazil*
[2]*Ibirapuera University (UNIB) Master Program, São Paulo, SP, Brazil*
[3]*Santa Cecília University (UNISANTA), Santos, SP, Brazil*
[4]*Graduate Program in Dentistry, School of Dentistry, São Leopoldo Mandic, Campinas, SP, Brazil*
[5]*Department of Orthodontics and Pediatric Dentistry, School of Dentistry, University of São Paulo-FOUSP, São Paulo, SP, Brazil*
[6]*Clinical Oncology Service, Hospital Santa Catarina, São Paulo, SP, Brazil*
[7]*Graduate Program in Dentistry, Cruzeiro do Sul University, São Paulo, SP, Brazil*

Correspondence should be addressed to Ana Maria Antunes Santos; amas.odonto@gmail.com

Academic Editor: Pablo I. Varela-Centelles

The giant cell fibroma is a benign nonneoplastic fibrous tumor of the oral mucosa. It occurs in the first three decades of life in the mandibular gingiva, predominantly, showing predilection for females. This article reports a case of giant cell fibroma in a 2-year-old girl, which is an uncommon age for this lesion. The patient was brought for treatment at the Research and Clinical Center of Dental Trauma in Primary Teeth, where practice for the Discipline of Pediatric Dentistry (Faculty of Dentistry, University of São Paulo, Brazil) takes place. During clinical examination, a tissue growth was detected on the lingual gingival mucosa of the lower right primary incisors teeth. The lesion was excised under local anesthesia and submitted to histological examination at the Oral Pathology Department of the Faculty of Dentistry, University of São Paulo, which confirmed the diagnosis of giant cell fibroma. There was no recurrence after 20 months of monitoring. This instance reinforces the importance of oral care from the very first months of life in order to enable doctors to make precocious diagnosis and offer more appropriate treatments for oral diseases, as well as to promote more efficient oral health in the community.

1. Introduction

The giant cell fibroma is a nonneoplastic lesion with distinctive clinic-pathologic features [1]. The name "giant cell fibroma" has been assigned due to the presence of large stellate and multinucleated fibroblasts which are mainly in the lamina propria near the epithelium [1–4].

The giant cell fibroma usually occurs at young age, and it is more common in the second and third decades of life [5–7]. The prevalence is reported to be high in Caucasians with a slight female predilection [4, 8]. Lesions diagnosed in older people are likely to have already existed for many years [2]. Most cases predominantly occur on the mandibular gingiva [4, 8, 9]. However, the apex and lateral border of the tongue,

buccal mucosa, palate, lip, and floor of the mouth are also common sites [2, 9, 10].

From a clinical perspective, the giant cell fibroma lesion appears as an asymptomatic pedunculated nodule with a papillary-like surface. The examined lesions were small, measuring less than 1 cm in diameter [1, 4, 11], frequently less than 0.5 cm [2–4, 10], which may cause them to be mistaken for a papilloma or gingival hyperplasia [11]. The consistency can vary from soft to firm [12]. It is a slow-growing lesion [10]. Histologically, the giant cell fibroma is an uncapsulated mass of loose fibrous connective tissue, noninflammatory, and covered with stratified squamous hyperplastic epithelium [1, 4, 11]. The conclusive diagnostic features of these lesions

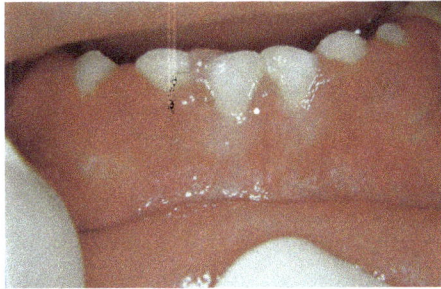

FIGURE 1: Frontal view of a tissue growth in the lingual gingiva next to the primary incisors in a 2-year-old girl. Note that gingivitis is present.

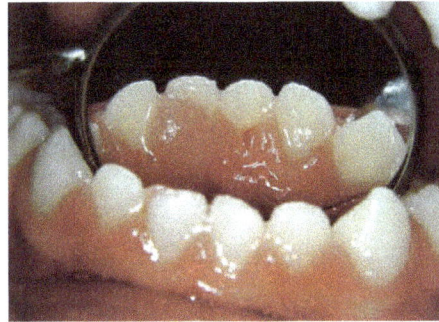

FIGURE 2: Lingual view of the gingival lesion. This image was shot six months after Figure 1.

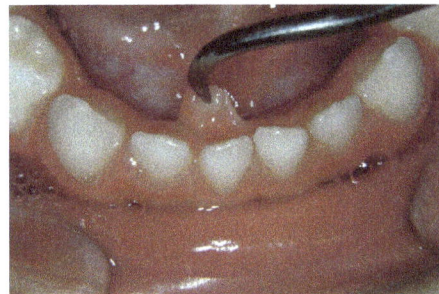

FIGURE 3: Pedunculated lesion in the lingual gingival mucosa, next to primary incisors.

are the presence of large spindle-shaped, stellate-shaped, and mononuclear and multinucleated fibroblasts. The stellate cells showed large vesicular nuclei with prominent nucleoli. The cytoplasm of these cells was well demarcated and occasionally dendritic processes were observed. The cellular boundaries appeared to be separated from the surrounding collagen fibers in some areas and some of these cells contained melanin granules [1, 4, 11]. A prominent vascular element composed mainly of capillaries was also noticed [1, 4, 11]. Inflammatory processes rarely occur, unless the surface epithelium is ulcerated. When present, the inflammatory infiltrate is mono- and polimorfonuclear [1, 10, 11]. Giant cell fibroma could be diagnosed only on histopathological examination [5, 13].

The cause of giant cell fibroma is not well determined; however, some studies show that giant cell fibroma was considered as a response to trauma or recurrent chronic irritation and is characterized by functional changes in fibroblastic cells [14]. The treatment is surgical removal [4, 10, 12–15], and recurrence is rare [13].

This study reports a case of giant cell fibroma, located in the lingual gingival mucosa of the lower right primary incisors in a 2-year-old girl, and describes the main clinical and histologic findings, as well as the treatment.

2. Case Report

A 2-year-old Caucasian girl was brought for treatment at the Research and Clinical Center of Dental Trauma in Primary Teeth, where practice for the Discipline of Pediatric Dentistry (Faculty of Dentistry, University of São Paulo, Brazil) takes place. She presented total intrusion of the central lower right primary incisors. During clinical examination, tissue growth was detected on the lingual gingival mucosa of the lower right primary incisors teeth (Figure 1). According to the mother, the lesion was asymptomatic and she had not noticed it before. The child did not have any medical complications.

The patient was referred for treatment of traumatized primary tooth, as well oral preventive measures, since oral biofilm and gingivitis were present. The patient failed to attend the following session and returned only 6 months later.

On clinical examination, a pedunculated fibrous lesion was observed. This lesion was nonhemorrhagic of firm consistency and covered by intact white mucosa of approximately 5 mm × 5 mm × 3 mm in size. The primary teeth adjacent to the lesion maintained their original position. The lesion partially covered the lingual surface of the central and lateral lower right primary incisors. No other alteration was present in the oral cavity (Figures 2 and 3).

Based on the clinical appearance of the lesion, the differential diagnosis included primarily reactive and benign neoplastic lesions, such as fibroma, fibrous hyperplasia, peripheral ossifying fibroma, peripheral odontogenic fibroma, giant cell fibroma, and odontogenic hamartoma. As the procedure was simple, the lesion was excised under local anesthesia. The parents favoured less physical constraint; therefore, local anesthesia was used instead of general anesthesia. The young patient was sat on the dental chair. Her mother bent over her, holding her hands, whilst the assistant supported the child's head.

A mouth prop was used to maintain adequate mouth opening. After topical anesthesia, local anesthesia was administered to the region of the incisors. Surgical removal was limited to the margins of the lesion in the gingival tissue. The excision was carried out using surgical scalpel blade number 15. Bleeding was very slight and was controlled using gaze compression. No suture was required (Figure 4).

Excised tissue was stored in 10% formaldehyde solution and submitted to the Oral Pathology Department of the Faculty of Dentistry, University of São Paulo, for histological

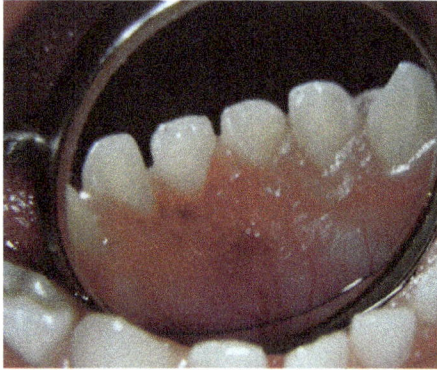

FIGURE 4: Appearance after surgical removal of the lesion.

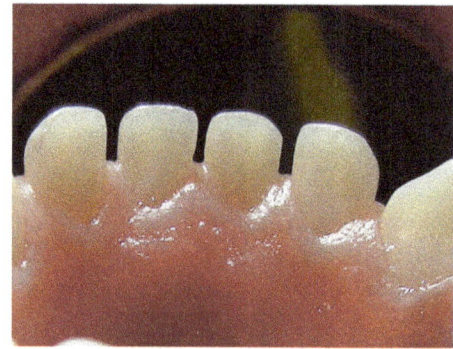

FIGURE 7: Clinical appearance after a 20-month follow-up.

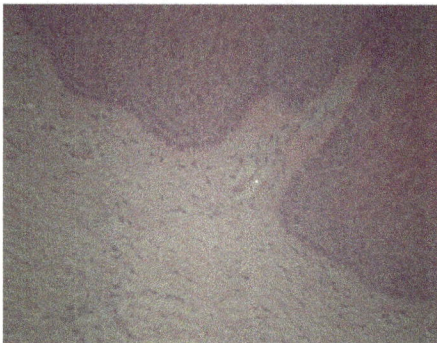

FIGURE 5: Scattered fibroblasts located just beneath the epithelium are enlarged and angular but are not hyperchromatic. Some cells have multiple nuclei. (H&E, original magnification 200x).

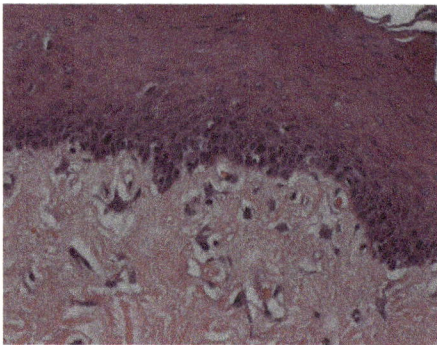

FIGURE 6: Slightly stellate multinucleated fibroblasts. (H&E, original magnification 400x).

analysis. The histological diagnosis revealed giant cell fibroma consisting of mucous tissue. This, in turn, was composed of parakeratinized stratified epithelium, which sent projections into the adjacent conjunctive tissue. Acanthosis, spongiosis, and exocytosis were also present. The lamina propria consisted of dense hyalinized connective tissue. Next to the juxta-epithelial hyalinization area, giant fibroblasts were found; they had two nuclei and stellate-form cells. In addition to the histological findings (Figures 5 and 6), extravasated red blood cells and often congested vascular spaces were found, which completed the findings.

No recurrence of the lesion was observed after a 20-month follow-up (Figure 7). The patient maintained good oral hygiene throughout this period.

3. Discussion

The clinical and histological features of the case we described were similar to the ones reported in the literature regarding giant cell fibroma. The giant cell fibroma is a benign fibrous tumor and it is most prevalent amongst the second and third decade of life [5–7], representing an average of 5% of all biopsied fibrous lesions [4, 9, 15] and around 1% of the total accessions in biopsy services [4, 9].

The differential diagnosis includes papilloma, fibroma, fibrous hyperplasia, and peripheral ossifying fibroma. The clinical aspects of these lesions are similar to those of the giant cell fibroma, such as the pedunculated nodule, the fibrous-looking papillary surface, and the ordinary colouration [1, 4, 11]. Despite this fact, the giant cell fibroma has its own particularities, that is, its own histological features and the prevalence of occurrence in certain (i) age groups, (ii) sex, and (iii) races, which makes it distinct from other lesions [1, 4, 5, 8, 11]. Last but not least, it should be noted that conducting a histopathological examination is essential to confirm the giant cell fibroma diagnosis [1, 5, 9, 11, 13].

Mono-, bi-, or multinucleated giant cells are not exclusive features of the giant cell fibroma, and they are detected in other lesions as well, such as ungual fibromas, acral angiofibroma, fibrous hyperplasia, and fibroma of the oral cavity [1, 7, 11].

The histopathological features found in this investigation are in agreement with the findings in the literature: benign fibroma showing mucous tissue, which are covered by parakeratinized stratified epithelium, projecting into a richly dense hyalinized connective tissue; such tissue is presenting many giant binucleated stellate-form fibroblasts [2–4, 10, 12, 16, 17].

The origin of the multinucleated and stellate cells in the giant cell fibroma is still unknown [18, 19]. It has been suggested that the mononuclear and multinucleated cells of giant cell fibroma may come from melanocytes or Langerhans cells [2, 4]. Histochemical studies have shown that these cells cannot be derived from the lineage of macrophages, monocytes, as they presented a negative reaction to CD68,

LCA, and HLA-DR reagents [18, 19]. Other investigations have shown the fibroblastic origin of these cells. Campos and Gomez [18] suggested that the stellate and multinucleated cells of the giant cell fibroma are of fibroblastic origin and that there is certain difficulty in determining whether these cells undergo functional or degenerative changes [18].

Some authors reported that giant cell fibroma showed no predilection for gender [2–4], but other authors have indicated a preference for females [5, 6, 10, 12]. In this case report, the patient was a girl. Regarding race, literature has reported a marked predominance in Caucasians [2, 10], such as in this case report.

The giant cell fibroma usually occurs in young adults [10, 12, 14, 16, 20]. However, 5 to 15.5% of the evaluated giant cell fibroma was found in children from birth to 10 years of age [5, 8, 20]. Therefore, the case of a giant cell fibroma in a 2-year-old girl, as reported in this article, is a rare finding.

Regarding location, the lesion was found in the lingual gingival mucosa next to the lower right primary incisors, which confirms the information provided in the literature [2, 4, 8, 13, 20]. It is more commonly found in the mandible gingiva than in the maxilla (2 : 1) [2, 8, 13].

The clinical aspects of the lesion in this 2-year-old girl are similar to the ones reported by other authors [2, 4, 5, 10, 12, 13], as it presented a fibrous pedunculated asymptomatic characteristic; it was small, precisely less than 1 centimeter in size.

Recommendation was the complete surgical removal of the lesion, which is procedure that has commonly been suggested in other investigations [4, 5, 13, 15]. Total surgical removal was recommended in this case, as the lesion was very small. Furthermore, the lesion was detrimental to the child's oral hygiene. There was no recurrence of the lesion after a 20-month follow-up. Literature reports that recurrence is rare [4, 10, 12]. Houston only found 2 cases of recurrence in a total of 464 cases [4].

Children of very young age usually show resistance to dental treatment and, therefore, this is why diagnosis and treatment of oral lesions are not always made and offered at such an early age. In this case, the parents did not know their child had a lesion in her oral mucosa. This is probably due to the difficulty in examining baby's mouth and in identifying the exact time of eruption of the primary teeth, as well as others issues such as poor oral hygiene and presence of gingivitis. Oral and dental care should start at a very young age in order to enable dentists to provide effective guidelines for prevention and precocious diagnosis and enable them to offer adequate treatment of diseases of the oral cavity, thereby improving the chances of a correct prognosis and avoiding future problems.

4. Conclusion

It is very important that both oral and dental care begin at the very first months of life in order to promote oral health and enable doctors to make precocious diagnosis and offer more appropriate treatments for diseases of the oral cavity. In short, the clinical diagnosis of a giant cell fibroma in a 2-year-old girl was possible due to a thorough clinical examination. The lesion was asymptomatic and located in the lingual gingiva mucosa. The giant cell fibroma was successfully removed under local anesthesia. No recurrence was observed after a period of 20-months of monitoring.

Consent

The patient's parents have signed an informed consent, authorizing the treatment and the use of images for scientific purposes.

Competing Interests

The authors hereby represent and warrant that there are no competing interests in producing this academic piece of work and that they are capable of identifying a situation that constitutes a potential conflict of interest. The authors further declare that they have refrained and will refrain from engaging in activities that may create or appear to create a conflict of interest.

Acknowledgments

Special thanks are due to Professor Paulo Henrique Braz da Silva, Department of Stomatology, School of Dentistry, University of São Paulo, São Paulo, Brazil, in acknowledgment of his review to the histological chapter of this study.

References

[1] D. R. Gnepp, *Diagnostic Surgical Pathology of the Head and Neck*, Saunder Elsevier, Philadelphia, Pa, USA, 2nd edition, 2009.

[2] D. R. Weathers and M. D. Callihan, "Giant-cell fibroma," *Oral Surgery, Oral Medicine, Oral Pathology*, vol. 37, no. 3, pp. 374–384, 1974.

[3] D. R. Weathers and W. G. Campbell, "Ultrastructure of the giant-cell fibroma of the oral mucosa," *Oral Surgery, Oral Medicine, Oral Pathology*, vol. 38, no. 4, pp. 550–561, 1974.

[4] G. D. Houston, "The giant cell fibroma. A review of 464 cases," *Oral Surgery, Oral Medicine, Oral Pathology*, vol. 53, no. 6, pp. 582–587, 1982.

[5] R. J. Vergotine, "A giant cell fibroma and focal fibrous hyperplasia in a young child: a case report," *Case Reports in Dentistry*, vol. 2012, Article ID 370242, 5 pages, 2012.

[6] S. Torres-Domingo, J. V. Bagán, Y. Jiménez et al., "Benign tumors of the oral mucosa: a study of 300 patients," *Medicina Oral, Patología Oral y Cirugía Bucal*, vol. 13, no. 3, pp. E161–E166, 2008.

[7] N. W. Savage and P. A. Monsour, "Oral fibrous hyperplasias and the giant cell fibroma," *Australian Dental Journal*, vol. 30, no. 6, pp. 405–409, 1985.

[8] L. H. Bakos, "The giant cell fibroma: a review of 116 cases," *Annals of Dentistry*, vol. 51, no. 1, pp. 32–35, 1992.

[9] N. G. Nikitakis, D. Emmanouil, M. P. Maroulakos, and M. V. Angelopoulou, "Giant cell fibroma in children: report of two cases and literature review," *Journal of Oral & Maxillofacial Research*, vol. 4, no. 1, 2013.

[10] R. H. Swan, "Giant cell fibroma: a case presentation and review," *Journal of Periodontology*, vol. 59, no. 5, pp. 338–340, 1988.

[11] W. Shafer, M. Hine, and B. Levy, "Odontogenic tumors," in *A Textbook of Oral Pathology*, pp. 287–290, Elsevier, Philadelphia, Pa, USA, 6th edition, 2009.

[12] S. Fadavi and I. Punwani, "Oral fibromas in children: reports of two cases," *ASDC Journal of Dentistry for Children*, vol. 54, no. 2, pp. 126–128, 1987.

[13] V. K. K. Reddy, N. Kumar, P. Battepati, L. Samyuktha, and S. P. Nanga, "Giant cell fibroma in a paediatric patient: a rare case report," *Case Reports in Dentistry*, vol. 2015, Article ID 240374, 3 pages, 2015.

[14] M. M. Braga, A. L. G. Carvalho, M. C. P. Vasconcelos, P. H. Braz-Silva, and S. L. Pinheiro, "Giant cell fibroma: a case report," *The Journal of Clinical Pediatric Dentistry*, vol. 30, no. 3, pp. 261–264, 2006.

[15] A. J. Mighell, P. A. Robinson, and W. J. Hume, "Immunolocalisation of tenascin-C in focal reactive overgrowths of oral mucosa," *Journal of Oral Pathology & Medicine*, vol. 25, no. 4, pp. 163–169, 1996.

[16] Y. Takeda, R. Kaneko, A. Suzuki, and J. Niitsu, "Giant cell fibroma of the oral mucosa: report of a case with ultrastructural study," *Pathology International*, vol. 36, no. 10, pp. 1571–1576, 1986.

[17] J. A. Regezi, R. M. Courtney, and D. A. Kerr, "Fibrous lesions of the skin and mucous membranes which contain stellate and multinucleated cells," *Oral Surgery, Oral Medicine, Oral Pathology*, vol. 39, no. 4, pp. 605–614, 1975.

[18] E. Campos and R. S. Gomez, "Immunocytochemical study of giant cell fibroma," *Brazilian Dental Journal*, vol. 10, no. 2, pp. 89–92, 1999.

[19] E. W. Odell, C. Lock, and T. L. Lombardi, "Phenotypic characterisation of stellate and giant cells in giant cell fibroma by immunocytochemistry," *Journal of Oral Pathology & Medicine*, vol. 23, no. 6, pp. 284–287, 1994.

[20] B. C. Magnusson and L. G. Rasmusson, "The giant cell fibroma A review of 103 cases with immunohistochemical findings," *Acta Odontologica Scandinavica*, vol. 53, no. 5, pp. 293–296, 1995.

32

Congenital Hemifacial Hyperplasia: Clinical Presentation and Literature Review

Karpagavalli Shanmugasundaram,[1] V. K. Vaishnavi Vedam,[2] Sivadas Ganapathy,[3] Sivan Sathish,[4] and Parvathi Satti[5]

[1]Department of Oral Medicine & Radiology, Saveetha Dental College, Saveetha University, Chennai, India
[2]Department of Oral Pathology, Faculty of Dentistry, Asian Institute of Medicine, Science & Technology (AIMST) University, Kedah, Malaysia
[3]Department of Pedodontics and Preventive Dentistry, Faculty of Dentistry, Asian Institute of Medicine, Science & Technology (AIMST) University, Kedah, Malaysia
[4]Department of Oral Medicine and Radiology, Chettinad Dental College & Research Institute, Kancheepuram, India
[5]Chettinad Dental College & Research Institute, Kancheepuram, India

Correspondence should be addressed to V. K. Vaishnavi Vedam; vaishnavivedam@gmail.com

Academic Editor: Daniel Torrés-Lagares

Hemifacial hyperplasia is a rare congenital malformation characterized by noticeable unilateral excess development of hard and soft tissues of the face. Asymmetry in Congenital Hemifacial Hyperplasia (CHH) is usually evident at birth and accentuated at the age of puberty. The affected side grows exponentially as compared to the unaffected side. Multiple tissue involvement has resulted due to etiological heterogeneity like heredity, chromosomal abnormalities, altered intrauterine environment, and endocrine dysfunctions. As this lesion is rarely seen in our routine clinical practice, we present a case of hemifacial hyperplasia with reported orofacial features that supplement existing clinical knowledge. This paper also adds knowledge to the readers regarding detailed investigation procedures which has complemented our diagnosis. Further emphasis has been placed on periodic approach to its diagnosis and multidisciplinary management following correct diagnosis.

1. Introduction

Congenital Hemifacial Hyperplasia (CHH) is a rare developmental malformation exhibited by a unilateral enlargement of hard and soft tissues of the face. This asymmetrical overgrowth traditionally referred to as hypertrophy is more accurately termed as hyperplasia as this pathologic process involves abnormal proliferation of cells (hyperplasia) rather than growth of individual existing cells (hypertrophy) [1]. Synonymously, this condition has been termed as facial hemihyperplasia, partial/unilateral gigantism, hemimacrosomia, and hemifacial hyperplasia [2].

Congenital Hemifacial Hyperplasia was first noted by Meckel JF in 1822 and, later, first case was reported by Wagner in 1839 [3]. Later, Gesell described this lesion as being "essentially a developmental anomaly antedating birth and arising in partial deflection of the normal process of birth" [4].

Hyperplasia presents as an isolated finding or in association with several syndromes like Beckwith Wiedemann syndrome, Proteus syndrome, Russell silver syndrome, and Sotos syndrome. Rowe [5] proposed a classification of hemihyperplasia based on its anatomic location as (1) simple hemihyperplasia (single limb), (2) complex hemihyperplasia (one-half of the body), and (3) facial hemihyperplasia (one side of the face). Depending on the soft tissue involvement, hemifacial hyperplasia can be broadly classified as (1) true hemifacial hyperplasia (increased growth of one or more tissues on one side of the face) and (2) partial hemifacial hyperplasia (increased growth limited to one structure only) [6].

We present an interesting case of true congenital hemifacial hyperplasia (true CHH) in a 39-year-old male with

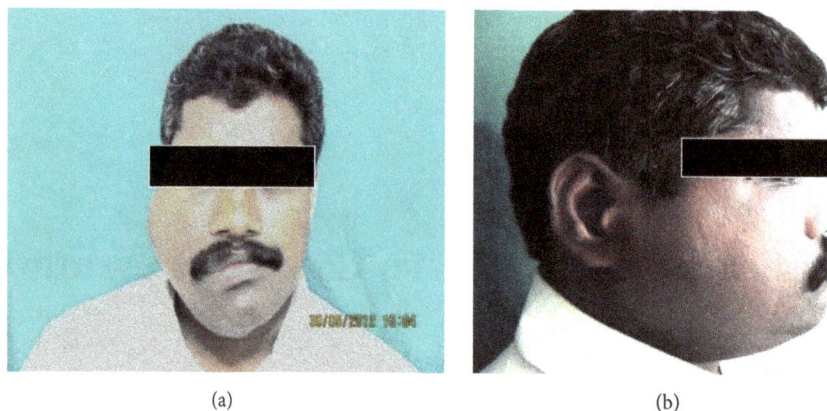

(a)   (b)

FIGURE 1: ((a) and (b)) Extraoral examination of the patient exhibiting a diffuse swelling pertaining to hard and soft tissues of right side of the face.

unique orofacial manifestations, radiographic findings, and differential diagnosis with treatment in detail to supplement the existing knowledge.

2. Case Presentation

A thirty-nine-year-old male patient reported to the Department of Oral Medicine and Radiology with a chief complaint of asymptomatic swelling in his right cheek region since birth. The swelling gradually progressed to the present size and ceased to grow after 18 yrs of age. Family history was noncontributory. The patient was well oriented with stable vital signs.

On extraoral examination, facial asymmetry with diffuse swelling was evident on the right side of the face measuring about 5×6 cm. The swelling extended superiorly to upper canthus of right eye, inferiorly up to 1 cm below the lower border of mandible, anteriorly until nasolabial fold, and posteriorly till the tragus of the ear [Figures 1(a) and 1(b)]. Nose and chin were deviated with an observable arc shaped facial midlines (nasion-gnathion). Enlarged soft tissue mass was observed involving maxilla, mandible, and zygoma on the affected side. On palpation swelling was nontender, hard in consistency, and noncompressible. Skin over the swelling was normal with no evidence of secondary changes. Patient showed mild tenderness on the right condylar region. Restricted temporomandibular joint (TMJ) movements and incompetent lips with marked enlargement of both upper and lower lips on the right side were evident. There was no evidence of regional lymphadenopathy.

On intraoral examination, there was restricted mouth opening with a maximum interincisal distance measuring about 1 cm only. Enlarged right maxillary and mandibular alveolar arches, upper and lower labial mucosa, and buccal mucosa were observed. Dorsum surface of the tongue appeared engorged with polypoid excrescences ("multiple pebbly" appearance) representing enlargement of fungiform papillae [Figure 2]. Distinct tooth size discrepancy was evident between right and left sides. Maxillary and mandibular right teeth increased in labiolingual, mesiodistal, and buccopalatal dimensions [Figures 3(a) and 3(b)]. Midline

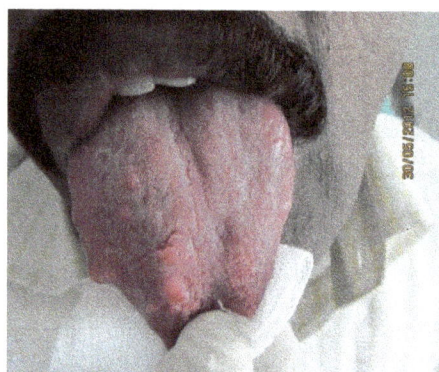

FIGURE 2: Intraoral examination of dorsum surface of the tongue showing multiple nodular structures exhibiting "pebbly" appearance on the right side only.

shift and a downward canting of the occlusal plane were noted.

Orthopantomogram (OPG) [Figure 4] revealed an obvious diffuse enlargement of right side coronoid, condylar processes, lower border of mandible, inferior alveolar canal, jaws, and teeth (macrodontia). Computerized tomography (CT) [Figure 5] scan of the face revealed enlarged right petrous part of temporal bone, pituitary fossa, maxilla, mandible, condyle, zygoma, and cranial bones. Deviation of nasal bone and chin was observed towards left side due to an obvious enlargement of overlying soft tissues on right side of the face. Bone scintigraphy [Figure 6] revealed hyperactivity and excess bone growth on right side maxilla and mandible. A physician consultation was arranged and no systemic abnormality was noted. Routine blood investigations were also under normal limits.

Based on the clinicopathological findings, a final diagnosis of Congenital Hemifacial Hyperplasia (CHH) was made. The patient refused to undergo extensive surgical procedures as the lesion was asymptomatic. Follow-up with this patient exhibited good prognosis and no evidence of malignant changes.

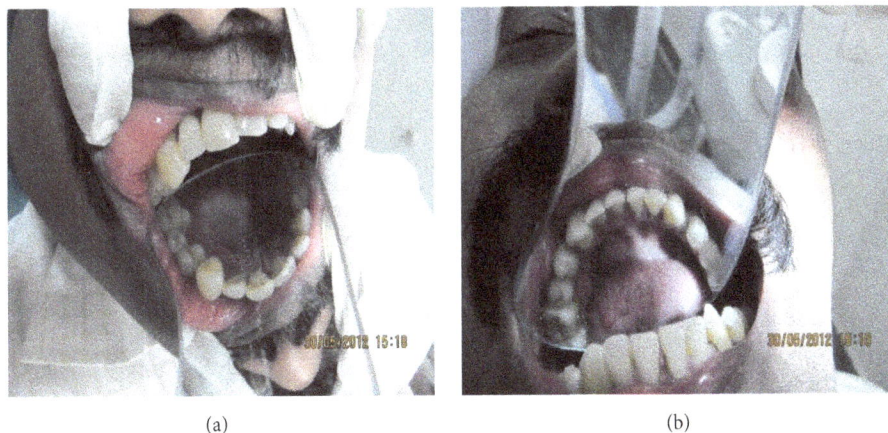

(a)   (b)

FIGURE 3: ((a) and (b)) Intraoral examination showing right sided enlargement of maxillary and mandibular arches with corresponding macrodontia.

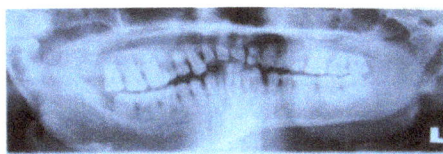

FIGURE 4: OPG reveals diffuse enlargement of skeletal and dental hard tissue enlargement on right side of the face.

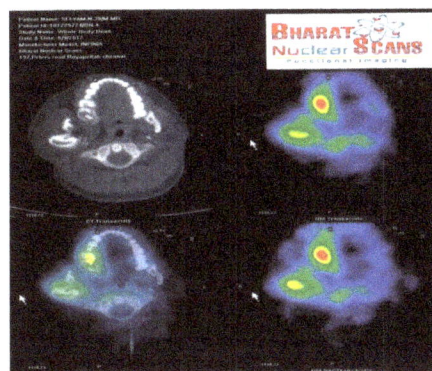

FIGURE 6: Bone scintigraphy shows increased uptake and hyperactivity in right sided maxilla and mandible of the face.

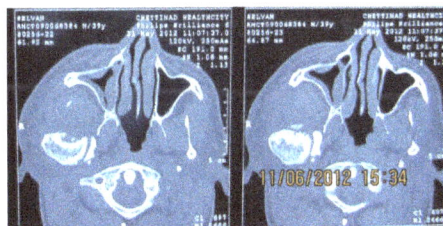

FIGURE 5: CT scan exhibits enlarged petrous part of temporal bone, pituitary fossa, maxilla, and mandible.

3. Discussion

Hemifacial hyperplasia (HFH) is a rare developmental anomaly exhibiting asymmetric facial growth by unilateral localized enlargement of all tissues in the affected area that is facial bones, teeth, and soft tissues [5]. The degree of anatomical variations appears variable from mild to most severe cases. Hence limited cases of hemifacial hyperplasia are documented.

The prevalence of hemifacial hyperplasia is approximately 1 in 86,000 live births [1, 3]. Women are commonly affected compared to men with right side predominantly affected as in the present case. The affected side tissue growth occurs in an exponential manner in comparison to the uninvolved side resulting in facial asymmetry following a skeletal arrest. This results in a relative asymmetry that is taken forward throughout the growth until adulthood [7].

Various etiological factors like heredity, chromosomal abnormalities, altered intrauterine development, endocrine dysfunction, and vascular and lymphatic abnormalities remain implicated in this lesion. However, no single factor is directly related to the occurrence of this disorder [8].

Of importance, Gesell suggested this condition due to the process of twinning mechanism. According to Noe and Bergman, mitochondrial damage overripened one-half of the fertilized egg resulting in excess generation of cells [9]. Recently, literature suggests that hemifacial hyperplasia may be more aptly attributed to defect in neural crest cell differentiation and migration. In this theory, Pollock and colleagues stated that neural fold appears to be larger on one side compared to the other part of structure. This enlarged neural fold produces increased number of neural crest cells throughout prenatal and postnatal periods of life owing to unilateral overgrowth of crest cell derived bone, teeth, and soft tissue on affected side of the face. Based on the current knowledge, Yoshimoto et al. stated that basic fibroblast growth factor (bFGF) along with its receptor stimulated osteoblastic differentiation on the affected side as compared to the uninvolved part of the face [10].

Limited cases of hemifacial hyperplasia have been documented. These patients present with dental, skeletal, and soft tissues of the affected portion of the face [11]. Dental abnormalities of deciduous teeth are less common and often overlooked. Variations in size, shape of crowns and root of teeth, rate of development (precocious development), and number of teeth are seen. Tooth crown and root size/shape appear distorted. Permanent canines, bicuspids, and first molars are involved most frequently [12, 13]. Of note, our case presented with marked dental abnormalities like precocious tooth development and macrodontia.

Skeletal development of cranial bones (*frontal, parietal, temporal, and skull base*), zygoma, maxilla, and mandible is accentuated. Midline shift and altered occlusion with deviated occlusal plane are noticed. Accelerated jaw growth frequently results in exostoses with malocclusion [14, 15]. Soft tissue abnormalities include gingival and labial mucosal thickening. Large soft tissue excrescences are evident predominantly on the dorsum of tongue ("pebbly") and buccal mucosa ("lipoma-like growth"). Tongue exhibits enlargement of fungiform papillae unilaterally. Lower lip is twice commonly affected than upper lip. Involvement of upper lip causes displacement of philtrum to the uninvolved side of the face. Palate also shows an arch shaped deformity ipsilaterally [16, 17]. All these skeletal features and soft tissue abnormalities were evident in the above case.

Radiographically, this lesion presents with hard tissue and soft tissue enlargement on the affected side. These patients exhibit premature development and altered crown and root size/shape discrepancy along with a downward slant of the occlusal plane [18, 19]. Our case is consistent with the previous findings.

Differential diagnosis of facial hemihyperplasia includes fibrous dysplasia, dyschondroplasia, congenital lymph edema, arteriovenous aneurysm, hemangioma, lymphangioma, neurofibromatosis, and malignant lesions (osteosarcoma and chondrosarcoma). These clinical conditions can be clearly differentiated from CHH based on specific radiographs and laboratory and clinical findings that supplemented our case diagnosis [20].

Treatment ideally is not indicated for Congenital Hemifacial Hyperplasia (CHH) unless cosmetic considerations are involved. Procedures are deferred until physiological growth ceases. An integrated multidisciplinary approach in the field of dentistry is essential in providing an asymptomatic treatment. Treatment options may include soft tissue debulking of masticatory and subcutaneous tissues, preservation of neuromuscular functions, and reconstructive procedures (osteotomy/orthognathic surgical procedure with/without orthodontic treatment) postoperatively. Till date, previous literature survey indicated no evidence of malignant transformation.

4. Conclusion

A true case of Congenital Hemifacial Hyperplasia (CHH) is rare and unfamiliar to a clinician due to underreported number of cases in literature. This article presents a unique case report of a typical case of CHH with a detailed emphasis on diagnostic criteria (clinical and radiographic appearance) thus emphasizing to all the readers its importance. Treatment planning in such patients is tremendously difficult due to the involvement of multiple major surgeries for the removal of excessively grown hard and soft tissues. Further cases need to be brought into documentation so as to have a clear understanding regarding various aspects of this disease.

Competing Interests

The authors declare that they have no competing interests.

References

[1] K. Mutafoglu, E. Cecen, and H. Cakmakci, "Isolated hemihyperplasia in an infant: an overlooked sign for wilms tumor development," *Iranian Journal of Pediatrics*, vol. 20, no. 1, pp. 113–117, 2010.

[2] R. A. Pollock, M. H. Newmann, A. R. Burdi, and D. P. Condit, "Congenital hemifacial hyperplasia: an embryological hypothesis and Case Report," *Cleft Palate Journal*, vol. 22, no. 3, pp. 173–184, 1985.

[3] S. Mark, O. H. Clark, and R. A. Kaplan, "A virilized patient with congenital hemihypertrophy," *Postgraduate Medical Journal*, vol. 70, no. 828, pp. 752–755, 1994.

[4] A. Gesell, "Hemihypertrophy and twinning," *The American Journal of the Medical Sciences*, vol. 173, pp. 542–555, 1927.

[5] N. H. Rowe, "Hemifacial hypertrophy: review of the literature and addition of four cases," *Oral Surgery, Oral Medicine, Oral Pathology*, vol. 15, no. 5, pp. 572–587, 1962.

[6] B. A. Bhuta, A. Yadav, R. S. Desai, S. P. Bansal, V. V. Chemburkar, and P. V. Dev, "Clinical and imaging findings of true hemifacial hyperplasia," *Case Reports in Dentistry*, vol. 2013, Article ID 152528, 7 pages, 2013.

[7] R. Nayak and M. S. Baliga, "Crossed hemifacial hyperplasia: a diagnostic dilemma," *Journal of Indian Society of Pedodontics and Preventive Dentistry*, vol. 25, no. 1, pp. 39–42, 2007.

[8] C. E. Rudolph and R. W. Norvold, "Congenital partial hemihypertrophy involving marked malocclusion," *Journal of Dental Research*, vol. 23, no. 2, pp. 133–139, 1944.

[9] O. Noe and J. A. Bergman, "The etiology of congenital hemifacial hypertrophy and one case report," *Archives of Pediatrics*, vol. 79, pp. 278–288, 1962.

[10] H. Yoshimoto, H. Yano, K. Kobayashi et al., "Increased proliferative activity of osteoblasts in congenital hemifacial hypertrophy," *Plastic and Reconstructive Surgery*, vol. 102, no. 5, pp. 1605–1610, 1998.

[11] R. J. Gorlin and L. Meskin, "Congenital hemihypertrophy," *Journal of Pediatrics*, vol. 61, no. 6, pp. 870–879, 1962.

[12] P. H. Burke, "True hemihypertrophy of the face," *British Dental Journal*, vol. 91, no. 8, pp. 213–215, 1951.

[13] F. J. Hanley, C. E. Floyd, and D. Parker, "Congenital partial hypertrophy of face: report of three cases," *Journal of Oral Surgery*, vol. 26, no. 2, pp. 136–141, 1968.

[14] H. S. Lo, "Congenital hemifacial hypertrophy," *British Dental Journal*, vol. 153, pp. 111–112, 1982.

[15] P. Verma, K. Gupta, S. Rishi, A. Triwedi, and S. Kailasam, "Hemifacial hypertrophy: a rare case report," *Journal of Indian Academy of Oral Medicine and Radiology*, vol. 24, pp. 334–337, 2012.

[16] M. N. Islam, I. Bhattacharyya, and J. Ojha, "Comparison between true and partial hemifacial hypertrophy," *Oral Surgery Oral Medicine Oral Pathology Oral Radiology Endodontics*, vol. 104, no. 4, pp. 501–509, 2007.

[17] J. O. Lawoyin, J. O. Daramola, and D. O. Lawoyin, "Congenital hemifacial hypertrophy. Report of two cases," *Oral Surgery, Oral Medicine, Oral Pathology*, vol. 68, no. 1, pp. 27–30, 1989.

[18] S. Hayashi, T. Tomioka, H. Aoki, K. Nakakuki, and K. Mekaru, "Hemifacial hypertrophy. Report of two cases," *Oral Surgery, Oral Medicine, Oral Pathology*, vol. 35, no. 6, pp. 750–761, 1973.

[19] S. Lee, R. Sze, C. Murakami, J. Gruss, and M. Cunningham, "Hemifacial myohyperplasia: description of a new syndrome," *American Journal of Medical Genetics*, vol. 103, no. 4, pp. 326–333, 2001.

[20] S. Deshingkar, S. Barpande, and J. Bhavthankar, "Congenital hemifacial hyperplasia," *Contemporary Clinical Dentistry*, vol. 2, no. 3, pp. 261–264, 2011.

33

A Case of Bisphosphonate-Related Osteonecrosis of the Jaw in a Patient with Subpontic Osseous Hyperplasia

Chiaki Tsuji, Hiroshi Watanabe, Hidenori Nakayama, Mitsuo Goto, and Kenichi Kurita

Department of Oral and Maxillofacial Surgery, School of Dentistry, Aichi Gakuin University, Nagoya, Japan

Correspondence should be addressed to Chiaki Tsuji; chiatsuji@hotmail.com

Academic Editor: Asja Celebić

Subpontic osseous hyperplasia (SOH) is a growth of bone occurring on the edentulous ridge beneath the pontics of fixed partial dentures (FPDs). This report describes a case of bisphosphonate- (BP-) related osteonecrosis of the jaw (BRONJ) in a SOH patient followed by deciduation of the bony lesion. A 73-year-old woman visited a dental clinic after experiencing pain and swelling beneath the pontics of a FPD that had been inserted 15 years ago. The pontics were removed, but the symptoms persisted and she was referred to our hospital. There was an osseous bulge and gum swelling around the edentulous ridge of teeth 18 and 19, as well as bone exposure. As she had been taking an oral BP for 6 years, we diagnosed this case as stage 2 BRONJ. Following BP withdrawal, the bony lesion detached from the mandible. The tissue was diagnosed as sequestrum based on the histopathological findings. Two months after deciduation, epithelialization over the area of exposed bone was achieved and no recurrence has been observed.

1. Introduction

Fixed partial dentures (FPDs) with pontics are commonly used to replace missing molars. Osteoblastic deformation occurring under pontics was first introduced as subpontic osseous hyperplasia (SOH) by Calman et al. in 1971 [1]. Since then, many studies have investigated SOH. The condition is normally discovered when individuals wearing FPDs for several years undergo simple radiography because of discomfort and pain at FPD sites. Many patients with SOH undergo surgical resection because the spontaneous detachment of hyperplastic bone has not been reported previously. Here, we report a rare case of detachment of hyperplastic bone in a patient with SOH leading to bisphosphonate-related osteonecrosis of the jaw (BRONJ).

2. Case

2.1. Patient. The patient was a 73-year-old woman.

2.2. First Examination. The first examination was carried out in June 2012.

2.3. Chief Complaints. The patient complained of dull pain in the left mandible.

2.4. Past Medical History. Past medical history included hypertension, paroxysmal atrial fibrillation, cerebral infarction, and osteoporosis.

2.5. Present Medication. The present medication included aspirin, amlodipine besylate, cimetidine, gloriamin, and alendronate sodium hydrate (ASH), which had been taken for 6 years since May 2006.

2.6. Current Medical History. In May 2012, she felt pain and noticed gingival swelling under the pontic in the mandibular FPD that had been placed in another dental clinic 15 years earlier. Serial radiographic images taken by the former dentist revealed subpontic bone formation (Figure 1).

The pontic was removed by the dentist in early June 2012, and the patient was followed up. However, the patient was referred to our department for a comprehensive examination in late June 2012 because of the lack of improvement in pain and swelling.

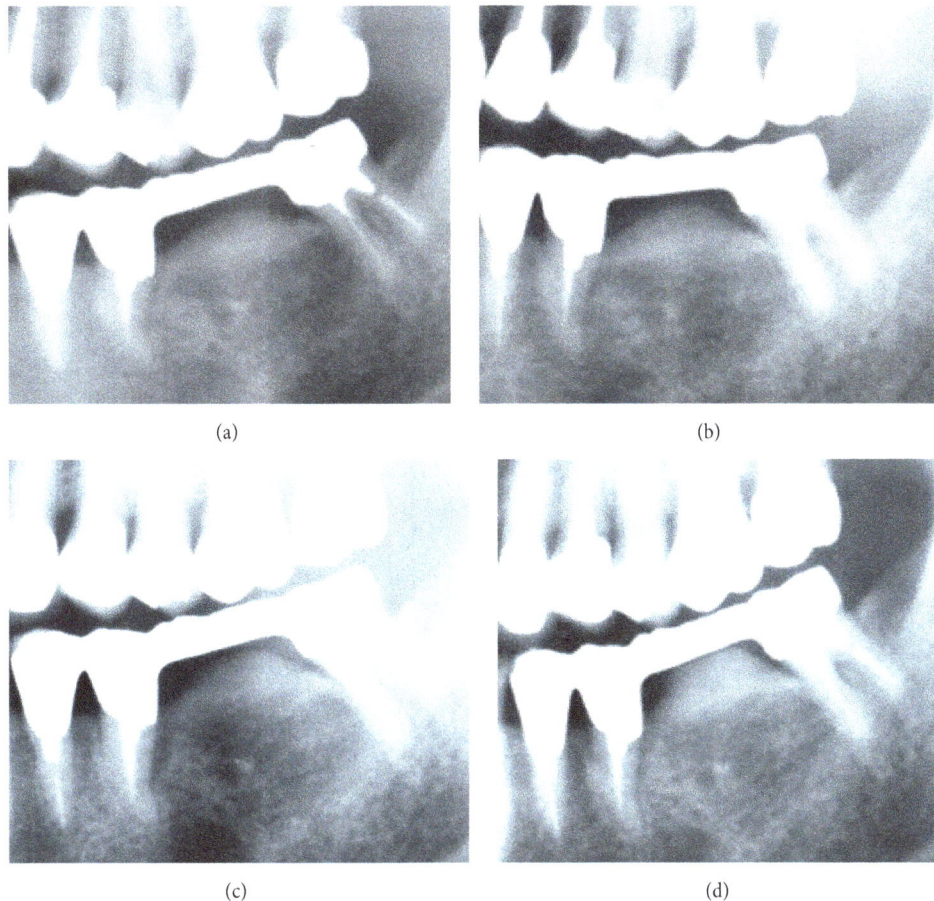

FIGURE 1: Panoramic radiographic images. (a) Image taken in October 2002 (before starting the oral bisphosphonate [BP]). (b) Image taken in February 2005 (before starting the oral BP). (c) Image taken in September 2008 (1 year and 4 months after starting the oral BP). (d) Image taken in September 2011 (5 years and 4 months after starting the oral BP). These images show chronological changes in the subpontic bone formation.

3. Present Symptoms

3.1. Extraoral Findings. Extraoral findings were unremarkable.

3.2. Intraoral Findings. In the alveolar crest of the lower left teeth 18 and 19, a 10 × 11 mm protrusion was accompanied by the exposure of bone approximately 3 mm in diameter, gingival swelling, and discharge of pus (Figure 2).

3.3. Imaging Findings. Panoramic radiographic images taken in the first examination revealed a radiopaque area, resembling cortical bone, with moderately demarcated but distinct borders in the alveolar crest of the lower left teeth 18 and 19 (Figure 3).

Computed tomography revealed similar findings indicative of osteosclerosis (Figure 4).

3.4. Clinical Diagnosis. Hyperostosis and BRONJ of the alveolar bone at lower left teeth 18 and 19 were suspected.

3.5. Treatment and Disease Course. The bone was exposed for 9 weeks. Because the patient had taken oral ASH for 6 years

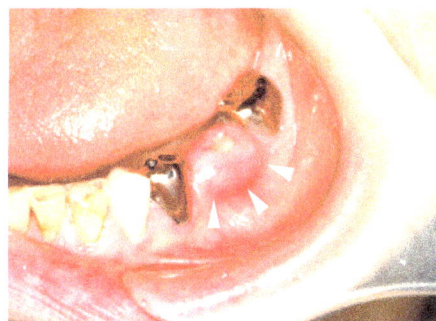

FIGURE 2: Intraoral photographic image taken in the first examination. The bone is exposed from the alveolar crest of the lower left teeth 6 and 7, with swelling and redness in the surrounding gingiva.

with no history of radiotherapy to the mandible, we made a diagnosis of stage 2 BRONJ. To treat inflammation, the patient was prescribed the antibiotic clarithromycin for 7 days and was instructed to continuously gargle 0.2% benzethonium chloride mouthwash solution (Neostelin Green 0.2%, Nishika). ASH was discontinued because the patient had a

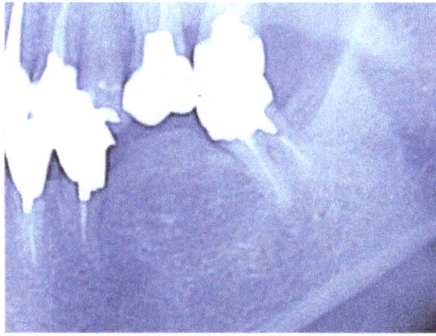

FIGURE 3: Panoramic radiographic image taken in the first examination. Radiopaque area in the alveolar crest of lower left teeth 6 and 7, showing osteosclerosis and formation of bone resembling cortical bone.

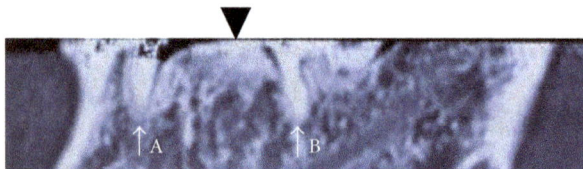

FIGURE 4: Sagittal computed tomographic image. Arrows: (A) the root of the lower left tooth #4 and (B) the root of the lower left tooth #8. Arrowhead: bone formation.

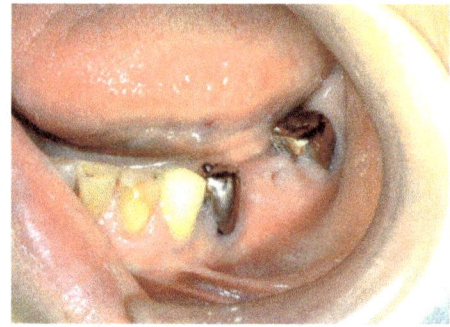

FIGURE 5: Intraoral photographic image after detachment of the sequestrum. Epithelialization was underway with no exposed bone.

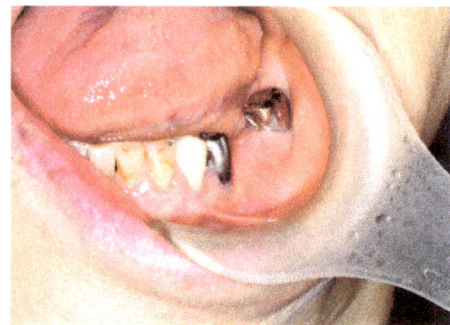

FIGURE 6: Intraoral photographic image taken 2 months after exfoliation. Epithelialization was observed, with no signs of inflammation in the surrounding mucosa.

low risk of bone fracture from osteoporosis according to a plastic surgeon who we consulted, and the patient was scheduled to undergo plastic surgery to resect the bone 3 months later. However, she visited our department in November 2012 and brought in bone tissue that had spontaneously detached. Examination revealed that the area from which the tissue had detached was almost completely covered by the gum and had no discharge of pus (Figure 5).

Two months later, the original area of bone exposure was completely covered by the epithelium (Figures 6 and 7).

3.6. Histopathological Findings. The bone tissue had a compact laminated structure and did not contain the cellular components of bone, but, instead, a bacterial mass was observed inside the tissue (Figures 8 and 9).

3.7. Histopathological Diagnosis. The histopathological diagnosis was sequestrum.

4. Discussion

Since its first report by Calman et al. [1] in 1971, 62 studies have investigated SOH, revealing that it commonly occurs unilaterally in the mandibular area that is missing molars and that only two maxillary cases have been reported previously [2, 3]. FPDs often develop in patients who have been wearing dentures for over 3 years, but it can occur in those wearing the denture for less than 1 year [4], with a mean duration of 13 years [5]. The mean age of onset is 56.6 (range: 29–81) years, with no differences by age group or sex [5]. Although a previous study by Islam et al. [6] investigated SOH among

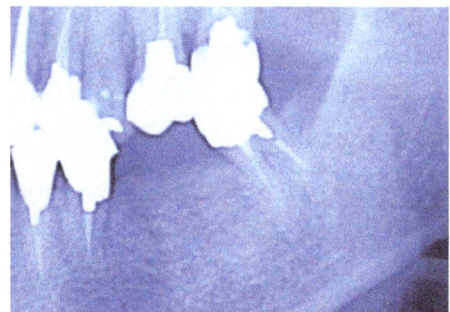

FIGURE 7: Panoramic radiographic image taken 2 months after exfoliation. No recurrence of bone formation was observed.

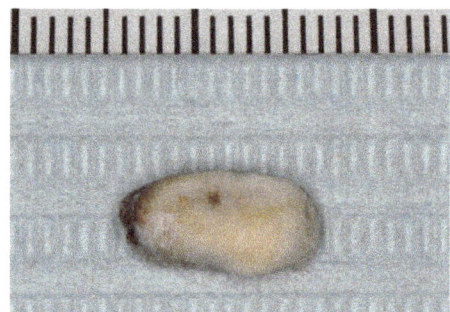

FIGURE 8: Spontaneously detached sequestrum.

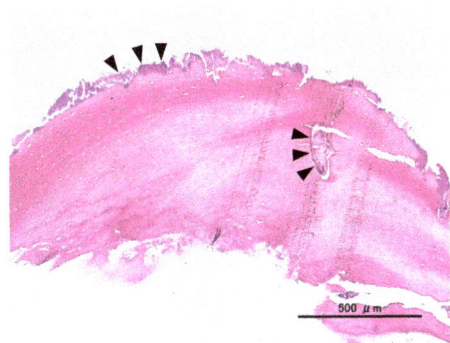

FIGURE 9: Histopathological findings (hematoxylin and eosin stain, slight magnification). Bone tissue, consisting of compact laminated structures, is void of cellular components but contains bacterial masses (arrow).

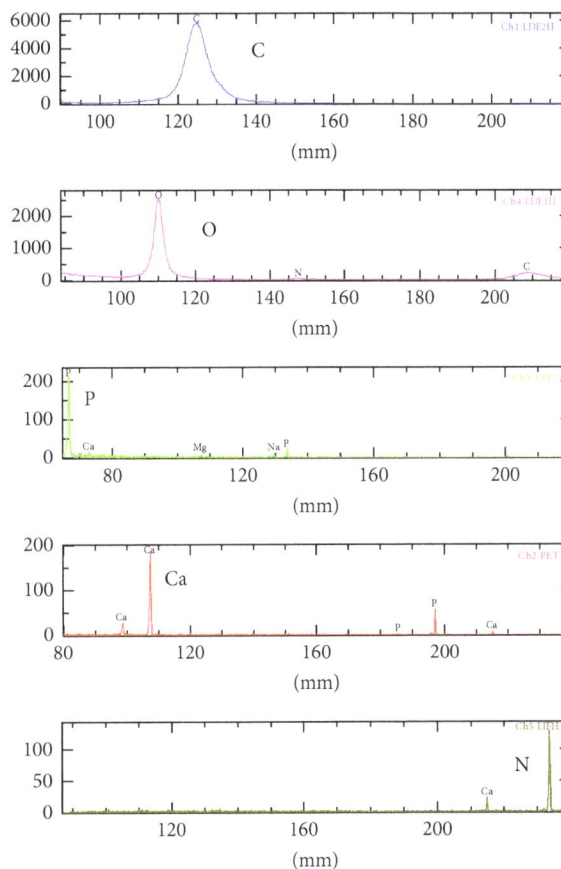

FIGURE 10: Analysis of bone composition. Cellular compositions were similar to those observed in normal bone tissue.

patients taking oral BP, the details of the disease course are currently unclear. Our patient developed SOH and had taken BP for 6 years before the bone became exposed for 9 weeks, as shown in Figures 1(a) and 1(b). In addition, the patient had not received radiotherapy to the mandible. Therefore, this appears to be a rare case of SOH accompanied by BRONJ.

The possible causes of SOH include generic components, chronic stimuli, or mechanical stresses. In patients wearing FPDs, the loading of occlusal force onto abutment teeth and surrounding bone tissue is thought to induce bone formation [6], and this hypothesis is supported by the fact that the removal of FPDs sometimes leads to the reduction of SOH [3, 6]. Similar mechanisms may be involved in this study. It is interesting to observe the progression of bone formation even after commencement of the oral BP, as shown in Figures 1(c) and 1(d), but the involvement of the BP in bone formation in this case is currently unclear.

The mechanism of BRONJ is unclear in the present SOH case, but in the areas where the tori and mylohyoidean line are present, the mucosa is thin and susceptible to development of a decubitus ulcer and is a common site for BRONJ. Similarly, in our patient, the exposure of bone and the development of BRONJ appeared to have been caused by the pontic repeatedly stimulating the mucosa that had been thinned by the SOH. Considering that previous studies of SOH did not reveal the spontaneous exposure of bones, it is possible that BRONJ occurred with SOH in the present case. The mechanism may also have involved the suppression of osteoclasts and osteoblasts by the BP, exacerbation of oral infection, suppression of neovascularization, vascular obstruction, lowered blood flow, proliferation of epithelial cells, inhibition of leukocyte migratory ability, osteosclerosis, or immune compromise [7].

The spontaneous detachment of sequestrum has not been observed in SOH but occurs often in BRONJ [8]. Therefore, it appears that bone formation in SOH progressed into BRONJ because the pressure to the mucosa exerted by the pontic caused circulation impairment and then necrosis of the mucosa. The natural detachment of sequestrum was thought to be caused by a reduction in the effect of the BP after its discontinuation, causing the sequestrum to

separate from the laminated bone. Although we analyzed the separated sequestrum, the compositions were similar to those in normal bone tissue, revealing no relationship with the BP (Figure 10).

In simple radiography, the specific features of SOH are an increase in subpontic radiopacity, osteosclerosis of cortical bone, and a mixture of radiopacity and radiotransparency [3, 5]. Although the radiographic findings of BRONJ vary by stage, they are characterized by radiolucent, radiopaque, or mixed poorly demarcated patches. In the advanced stages, osteosclerosis, irregular bone surface, and the separation of sequestrum are observed [7]. In this study, simple radiographic images taken 10 years earlier at the former clinic revealed an increase in the radiopacity of the subpontic cortical bone in the alveolar crest. Although radiolucent patches were absent, the osteosclerosis continued to grow with time, resulting in imaging findings consistent with those of either SOH or BRONJ.

The histopathological findings of resected SOH specimens include mature laminated bone layers with osteocytes and exostosis-like proliferation resulting in Haversian canals [6, 9–11], similar to those observed in this study. On the other hand, the histopathological findings of BRONJ are characterized by sequestrum, agglomeration of microorganisms, and necrotic tissue filled with neutrophils and other cells, with no specific histopathological findings. As a result, BRONJ is often reported as osteomyelitis or sequestrum [12]. In this study, the sequestrum had laminated bone tissue containing bacterial aggregations, and, based on the histopathological findings, we thought that this was a case of SOH that turned into BRONJ.

5. Conclusion

Here, we reported a rare case of BRONJ where the formed bone in a patient with SOH spontaneously detached.

Competing Interests

No competing interests are declared in this study.

References

[1] H. I. Calman, M. Eisenberg, J. E. Grodjesk, and L. Szerlip, "Shades of white. Interpretation of radiopacities," *Dental Radiography and Photography*, vol. 44, pp. 3–10, 1971.

[2] K. B. Frazier, P. S. Baker, R. Abdelsayed, and B. Potter, "A case report of subpontic osseous hyperplasia in the maxillary arch," *Oral Surgery, Oral Medicine, Oral Pathology, Oral Radiology, and Endodontics*, vol. 89, no. 1, pp. 73–76, 2000.

[3] U. Aydin, D. Yildirim, and E. Bozdemir, "Subpontic osseous hyperplasia: three case reports and literature review," *European Journal of Dentistry*, vol. 7, no. 3, pp. 363–367, 2013.

[4] E. J. Burkes, D. L. Marbry, and R. E. Brooks, "Subpontic osseous proliferation," *The Journal of Prosthetic Dentistry*, vol. 53, no. 6, pp. 780–785, 1985.

[5] C. A. Lee, M. B. Lee, C. R. Matthews, and D. N. Takakis, "Subpontic osseous hyperplasia: a case series and literature review," *General Dentistry*, vol. 62, pp. 46–52, 2014.

[6] M. N. Islam, D. M. Cohen, M. T. Waite, and I. Bhattacharyya, "Three cases of subpontic osseous hyperplasia of the mandible: a report," *Quintessence International*, vol. 41, pp. 299–302, 2010.

[7] Y. Imai, "Osteonecrosis of the jaw that cannot be overlooked in prosthodontic treatment—new findings of BRONJ/ARONJ relevant to bone resorption inhibitors—," *Annals of Japan Prosthodontic Society*, vol. 6, pp. 233–241, 2014.

[8] S. L. Ruggiero, T. B. Dodson, J. Fantasia et al., "American association of oral and maxillofacial surgeons position paper on medication-related osteonecrosis of the jaw - 2014 update," *Journal of Oral and Maxillofacial Surgery*, vol. 72, no. 10, pp. 1938–1956, 2014.

[9] E. R. Lorenzana and W. W. Hallmon, "Subpontic osseous hyperplasia: a case report," *Quintessence International*, vol. 31, no. 1, pp. 57–61, 2000.

[10] W. C. Daniels, "Subpontic osseous hyperplasia: a five-patient report," *Journal of Prosthodontics*, vol. 6, no. 2, pp. 137–143, 1997.

[11] E. Nagahama, Y. Hamada, T. Kondoh, K. Murakami, T. Nakajima, and K. Seto, "A case of subpontic osseous hyperplasia of the mandible," *Japanese Journal of Oral and Maxillofacial Surgery*, vol. 47, no. 10, pp. 627–629, 2001.

[12] T. Ikeda and A. Yamaguchi, "Bisphosphonate-related osteonecrosis of the jaw: review from pathological observation," *Japanese Journal of Oral and Maxillofacial Surgery*, vol. 56, no. 6, pp. 352–356, 2010.

34

Natural Tooth Pontic: An Instant Esthetic Option for Periodontally Compromised Teeth

Rishi Raj, Kriti Mehrotra, Ipshita Narayan, Triveni Mavinakote Gowda, and D. S. Mehta

Department of Periodontics, Bapuji Dental College & Hospital, Davangere, Karnataka 577004, India

Correspondence should be addressed to Kriti Mehrotra; kriti1004@gmail.com

Academic Editor: Sukumaran Anil

Sudden tooth loss in the esthetic zone of the maxillary or mandibular anterior region can be due to trauma, periodontal disease, or endodontic failure. The treatment options for replacing the missing tooth can vary between removable prosthesis, tooth-supported prosthesis, and implant-supported prosthesis. Irrespective of the final treatment, the first line of management would be to provisionally restore the patient's esthetic appearance at the earliest, while functionally stabilizing the compromised arch. Using the patient's own natural tooth as a pontic offers the benefits of being the right size, shape, and color and provides exact repositioning in its original intraoral three-dimensional position. Additionally, using the patient's platelet concentrate (platelet rich fibrin) facilitates early wound healing and preservation of alveolar ridge shape following tooth extraction. The abutment teeth can also be preserved with minimal or no preparation, thus keeping the technique reversible, and can be completed at the chair side thereby avoiding laboratory costs. This helps the patient better tolerate the effect of tooth loss psychologically. The article describes a successful, immediate, and viable technique for rehabilitation of three different patients requiring replacement of a single periodontally compromised tooth in an esthetic region.

1. Introduction

Esthetics and function of the orofacial region are very important aspects of human life, which are affected by anterior tooth loss regardless of personal factors such as age, gender, and level of education, eventually impacting the quality of life [1]. As dentists, we occasionally face daunting conditions that warrant removal of teeth from a high esthetic zone due to trauma, periodontal disease, root resorption, or failed endodontic treatment [2]. Extraction of these teeth mainly leads to esthetic and phonetic difficulties and a functional disability to some extent with pathologic migration. Mostly, such patients either strongly desire to postpone the extraction of their natural teeth or demand immediate management of the esthetic crisis which could adversely affect their social life.

Conventional treatment options available include the removable temporary acrylic prosthesis, resin bonded bridges, and traditional metal and ceramic fixed partial denture (FPD) and amongst the relatively newer options is osseointegrated implant-supported prosthesis [3]. Understanding the

patients' cosmetic demands, functional needs, and affordability becomes imperative in delivering the best possible dental service.

In certain clinical scenarios, using an intact natural tooth which is in good clinical condition as pontic for interim duration could offer a plethora of benefits like excellent color, shape, and size match, positive psychological value, minimal cost, and minimum chairside time with no laboratory procedure involved [4]. With recent advancements in adhesive technology and the advent of newer and stronger composite resin materials, it is possible to create a conservative, highly esthetic prosthesis that is bonded directly to teeth adjacent to the missing tooth.

Socket preservation, as a tool for optimizing the preservation of the hard and soft tissue components of the alveolar ridge immediately following tooth extraction, has been accepted as a clinical protocol for more than a decade now [5]. Autologous platelet concentrates are claimed to enhance hard and soft tissue healing due to the considerable amount of growth factors that are released after application in the

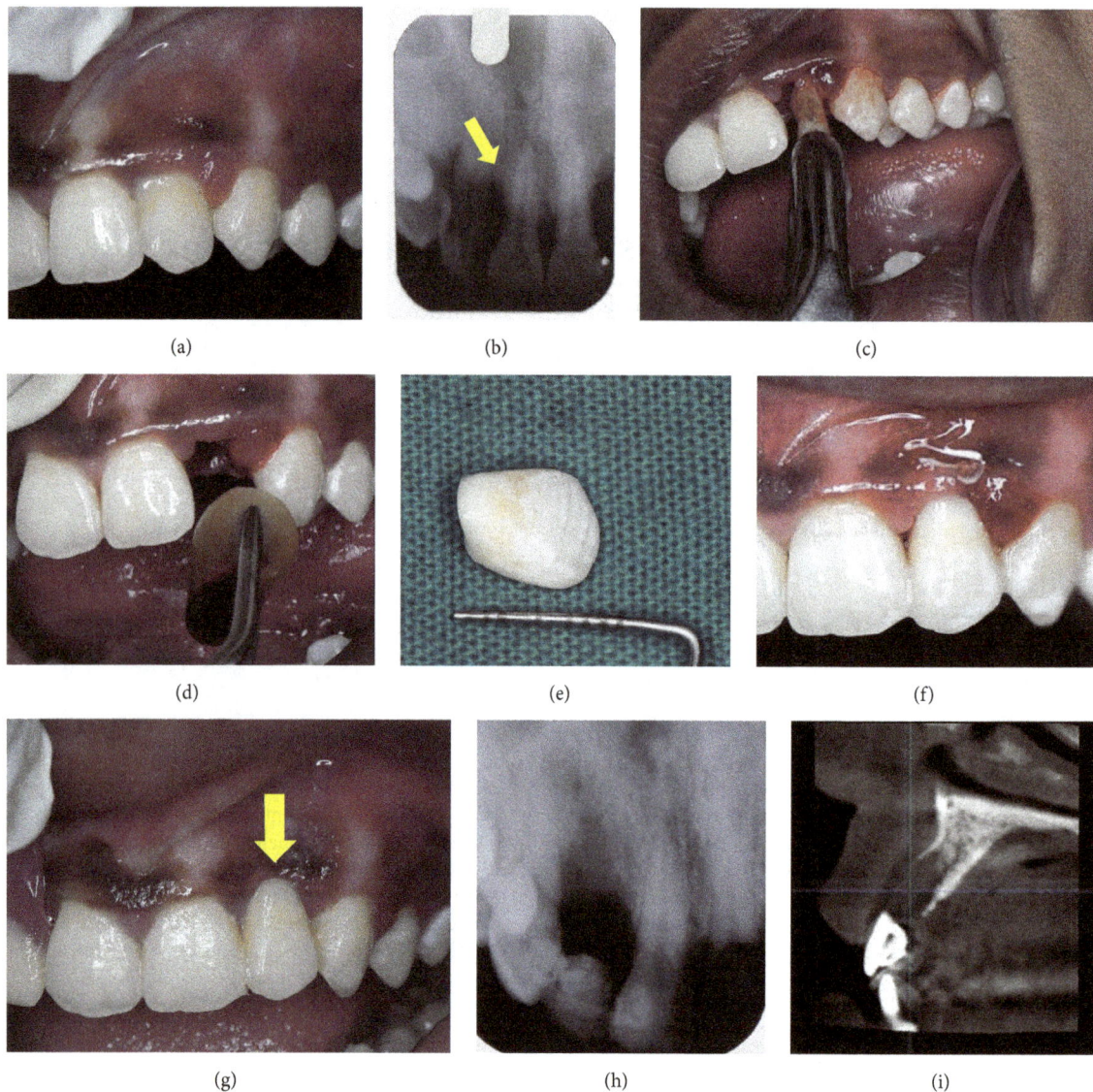

FIGURE 1: (a) Preoperative. (b) Preoperative radiograph. (c) Extraction of 22. (d) Insertion of PRF. (e) Customized NTP. (f) Immediate postoperative. (g) 1 week postoperatively. (h) 1 week postoperatively. (i) CBCT NTP with respect to 22.

surgical site [6]. This article describes the clinically replicable technique of socket preservation using platelet rich fibrin (PRF) followed by immediate tooth replacement utilizing the extracted natural tooth as pontic (NTP) to assist the clinicians in providing an esthetically acceptable treatment option.

2. Case Series

The case selection criteria for NTP include patient desiring an immediate replacement, patient's unwillingness for any kind of invasive procedure, for example, implant-supported prosthesis, areas with high esthetic demand, and need for a cost-effective treatment protocol.

2.1. Case 1. A 22-year-old healthy female patient reported to our department with the chief complaint of mobility in the upper front tooth region along with pus discharge and pain and requested that we provide her with the best treatment possible. Oral and radiographic examination revealed moderate generalized bone loss except for #22 which showed grade III mobility (Figures 1(a) and 1(b)). As the prognosis of #22 was hopeless, different treatment options available to the patient were explained and she chose to use the clinical crown as natural pontic. Extraction of #22 was performed atraumatically under local anaesthesia (Figure 1(c)) and the socket was curetted thoroughly. Then, 5 mL of venous blood was collected from the antecubital fossa of the patient and was immediately transferred to a sterile *(Choukroun's A-PRF)* test tube. The blood was centrifuged at 2700 rpm for 12 minutes, following which PRF obtained was placed in the extraction socket (Figure 1(d)) and stabilized using figure-of-eight suture using 5–0 polyamide *(Ethicon)*.

Thereafter, the length of the natural tooth pontic was determined using periodontal probe and an additional 2 mm was added to compensate for the gingival shrinkage during the healing phase of the extraction site. The natural crown was sectioned from the root using diamond disc to achieve modified ridge-lap shape (Figure 1(e)). Its position was ascertained before bonding, to exclude any occlusal interferences. The pulp chamber was then cleaned, sealed with composite resin *(3M ESPE, Filtek™ Z350)*, and stored in normal saline till replacement. By using floss as template, adequate length of bondable reinforcement ribbon *(Ribbond)* was determined to be inclusive of adjacent teeth. The abutment teeth and the pontic were then etched with 35% phosphoric acid *(3M ESPE)* for 30 seconds, washed, and dried. Thereafter, bonding agent *(Dentsply)* was applied to the etched enamel and cured. A thin layer of composite resin (flowable composite 3M ESPE, Filtek) was placed across the abutment teeth and the pontic. The precut Ribbond fiber was thoroughly wetted by using the bonding agent and placed over the composite and cured. A further layer of composite was placed over the fiber, ensuring that the whole tape was covered by the composite. The excess composite resin was removed and the occlusal interferences were rechecked in protrusion and lateral excursions. Finishing and polishing procedures were carried out by using composite finishing discs and stones. The treatment outcome has been monitored over the last six months and there has been no evidence of any esthetic or functional problems. As the patient desired to undergo implant therapy, CBCT was advised (Figure 1(i)).

2.2. Case 2. A 35-year-old healthy female patient reported to the department with the chief complaint of mobility of teeth. She was diagnosed with generalized chronic periodontitis with grade III mobility of #12 (Figure 2(a)) which was unsalvageable. Extraction of #12 was performed atraumatically (Figure 2(b)). On inspection, the extraction socket revealed presence of intact bony plate. Hence, we decided to proceed with graft placement. PRF was prepared as described above and mixed with β-TCP *(Virchow Co.)* graft material to form a sticky mixture (Figure 2(c)) which was thereafter placed in the extraction site to facilitate socket preservation (Figure 2(d)). PRF plug was used to seal the site and the wound was closed using figure-of-eight ("8") suture with 5–0 polyamide *(Ethicon)*. The natural crown was used as a pontic in a similar fashion, as has been discussed above (Figures 2(e)-2(f)).

Thereafter, the patient was treated for full mouth periodontal therapy. Posttreatment follow-up was done over the last 9 months and the patient was found to be greatly enthused by the final esthetics and function.

2.3. Case 3. A 50-year-old healthy female reported to our department with the chief complaint of mobility in the lower front tooth region. Clinical examination revealed grade III mobility in #42. After extraction of #42 (Figure 3(a)), the extraction socket was preserved using PRF and the natural crown was used as pontic (Figure 3(b)).

General oral hygiene instructions were given to all three patients.

3. Discussion

The restoration of a smile is one of the most appreciative and gratifying services that a dentist can render. Patients with lost anterior teeth require immediate attention for the restoration of esthetics and function and also the prevention of social trauma. Each of the treatment modalities available has its own benefits and detriments.

Removable temporary partial dentures placed in the immediate postextraction phase are unesthetic due to the presence of clasps that inadequately preserve extraction socket while impeding the healing process and are bulky, hence causing discomfort to the patient and jeopardizing oral hygiene maintenance. For many years, metal-ceramic fixed partial dentures (FPDs) have been the treatment of choice. However, the display of metallic framework is less than esthetically pleasing and also entails aggressive tooth of abutment teeth which increases risk of pulp exposure [7]. Resin retained bridges could provide an alternative owing to limited tooth preparation of the adjacent teeth. However, high frequency of debonding and substantial modification to achieve an acceptable color, size, and shape of the prefabricated acrylic poses a challenge [8].

Postextraction healing and maturation of the bone occur with three-dimensional remodeling even after three months of healing [9]. The clinically growing demand for adequate alveolar housing for implant placement necessitates performing guided bone regeneration (GBR) procedures which would prolong the treatment duration. Immediate implant placement on the other hand is a very case specific protocol. However, some patients reject this therapeutic option, because of either the higher cost or the fear of surgery. Systemic problems may also contraindicate the surgery.

The natural tooth pontic (NTP) technique could be a suitable alternative in such clinical scenario because it is commonly opted for and highly appreciated by the patients for being a single visit technique, not involving any waiting period and temporization. Moreover, cutting of the neighboring teeth can be avoided and is highly cost-effective. Another major advantage of retaining the patient's natural crown is that the patient can better tolerate the effect of tooth loss psychologically [10].

There have been a number of different techniques described in the literature related to restorative dentistry, for splinting teeth using adhesive composite resins, wire, metal mesh, nylon, and so forth bonded to adjacent teeth and adding a natural tooth pontic, denture tooth, or composite resin tooth pontic [7]. The inherent problem with these materials was their inability to be chemically incorporated in composite resin and thus clinical failures were more prevalent due to repeated loading stresses placed on the bridge during normal and paranormal functions. Also, owing to the low fracture strength of the bonded composite resin, pontic might debond unexpectedly and results in an unpleasant social situation. Hence, the challenge was to place a thin but strong bonded composite resin-based single visit bridge using natural tooth as pontic. This was achieved using high-strength polyethylene, bondable, biocompatible, esthetic, easily manipulatable fiber ribbons (Ribbond) that could be

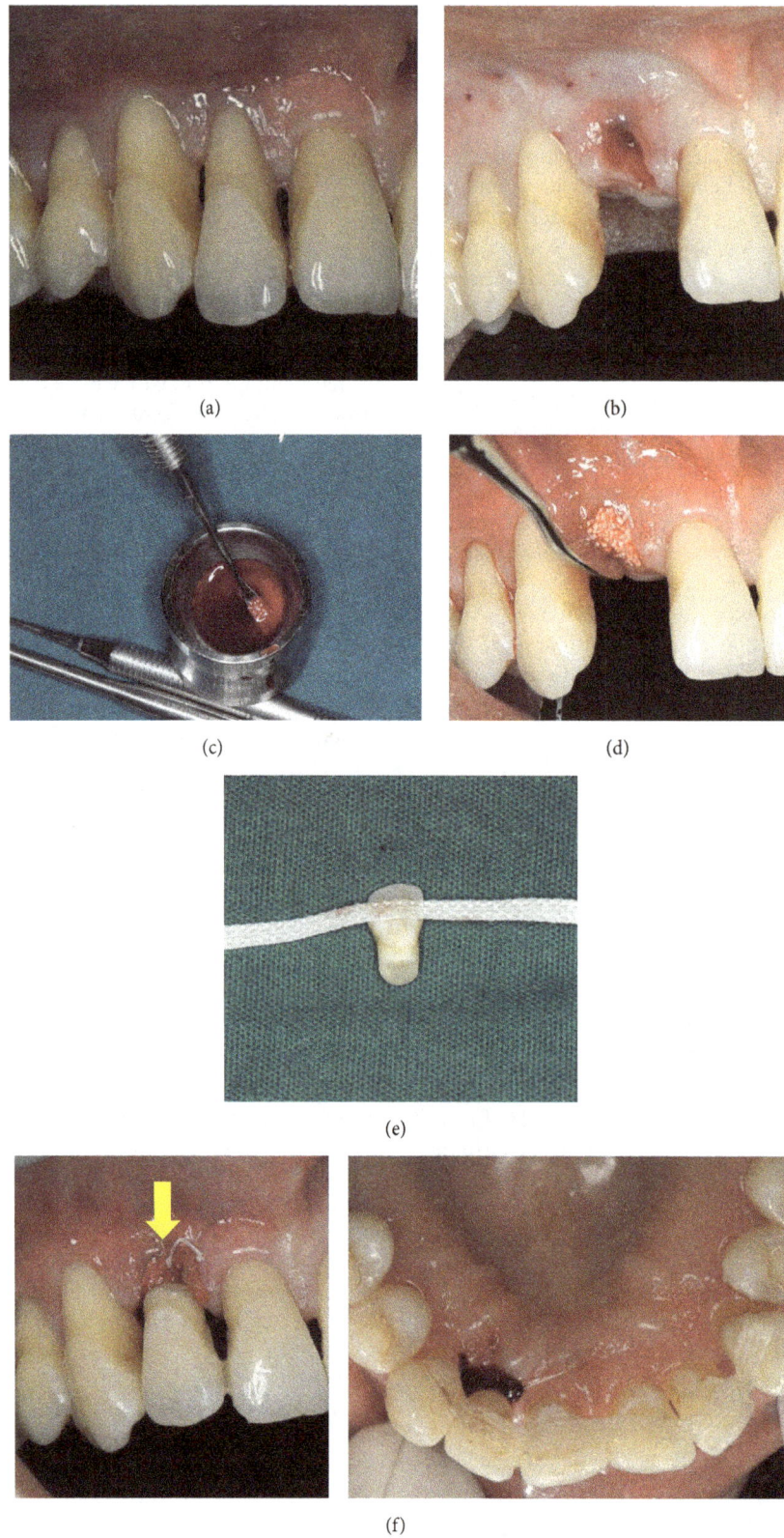

FIGURE 2: (a) Preoperative. (b) Atraumatic extraction. (c) Preparation of sticky bone. (d) Socket preservation. (e) Ribbond attached to natural crown. (f) Immediate postoperative NTP with respect to 12.

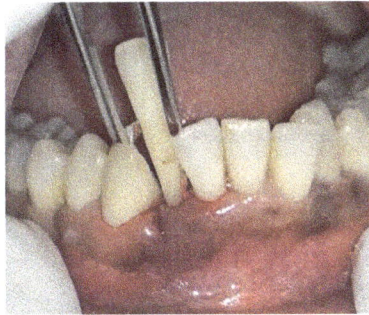

(a)

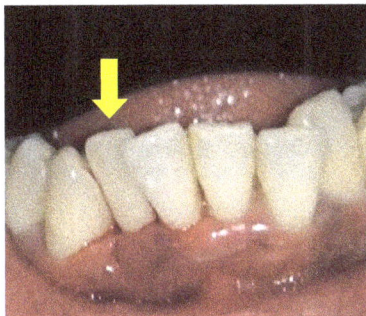

(b)

FIGURE 3: (a) Extraction of 42. (b) NTP with respect to 42.

embedded into a resin structure [11]. Although reinforced composite materials seem to provide excellent esthetics, some authors do not recommend its use for permanent restoration because of unstable esthetics, increased wear, and liability to plaque accumulation [12]. Clinical studies have shown substantial clinical performance of the fiber reinforced composite (FRC) prosthesis with an overall survival rate of 75% after about 5 years, which is higher than that of the FPDs with metal frameworks [13].

In this case, shape of natural tooth pontic was given as modified ridge-lap pontic with a well-polished and smooth, convex surface that results in pressure-free or mild contact with the alveolar ridge over a very small area for better preservation of the soft tissue health. This particular shape of pontic also helps to give the illusion of the replaced tooth emerging from the gingiva like a natural tooth [4]. Also, the ease of usage and almost no adaptability period as it is with the removable partial denture make it a patient-friendly modality. As with any other treatment modality, this procedure is also associated with a number of limitations like relying on patient's motivation and manual dexterity to maintain oral hygiene around the pontic, limited functional efficiency, irritation to the tongue, and chances of splint breakage. Despite these, studies have shown successful long-term follow-ups of such natural tooth pontics [14, 15].

The use of PRF in the oral cavity has been implicated in different procedures such as extraction socket preservation, intrabony defects, sinus augmentation, and sinus lift procedures for implant placement, bone augmentation, root

coverage procedures, and healing in donor site with successful results [16]. The biomaterial acts by releasing high-concentration growth factors to the wound site, thereby stimulating healing and new bone formation [17]. Unlike other socket preservation procedures, the use of PRF is a simple method that requires minimal cost and reduces the need for grafting material. Because it is a completely autologous product, there is absolutely no risk of disease transmission and graft rejection. In the second case, containment of extraction socket allowed socket preservation using PRF and bone graft material.

4. Conclusion

All the three patients were satisfied with the esthetic outcome and functioning of this treatment modality, reinforcing its utility as a routine viable option for cases, indicated for extraction of anterior tooth. Natural tooth pontic (NTP) can be placed as interim restoration until an extraction site heals which later if the patient so desires can be replaced by a conventional bridge or an implant. However, appropriate patient selection, their motivation levels, plaque control, and precision during placement of NTP are imperative for its success.

Competing Interests

The authors declare that there are no competing interests.

References

[1] M. K. Al-Omiri, J. A. Karasneh, E. Lynch, P.-J. Lamey, and T. J. Clifford, "Impacts of missing upper anterior teeth on daily living," *International Dental Journal*, vol. 59, no. 3, pp. 127–132, 2009.

[2] S. Avinash and S. Jagadish, "Natural tooth pontic—a case report," *Endodontology*, vol. 19, pp. 17–18, 2007.

[3] A. R. Purra and M. Mushtaq, "Aesthetic replacement of an anterior tooth using the natural tooth as a pontic; an innovative technique," *Saudi Dental Journal*, vol. 25, no. 3, pp. 125–128, 2013.

[4] A. T. Ulusoy and Z. C. Cehreli, "Provisional use of a natural tooth crown following failure of replantation: a case report," *Dental Traumatology*, vol. 24, no. 1, pp. 96–99, 2008.

[5] C. J. Landsberg and N. Bichacho, "A modified surgical/prosthetic approach for optimal single implant supported crown. Part I. The socket seal surgery," *Practical Periodontics and Aesthetic Dentistry*, vol. 6, no. 2, pp. 11–17, 1994.

[6] A. Khetarpal, S. Talwar, and M. Verma, "Creating a single-visit, fibre-reinforced, composite resin bridge by using a natural tooth pontic: a viable alternative to a PFM bridge," *Journal of Clinical and Diagnostic Research*, vol. 7, no. 4, pp. 772–775, 2013.

[7] K. P. Kumar, S. K. Nujella, S. S. Gopal, and K. K. Roy, "Immediate esthetic rehabilitation of periodontally compromised anterior tooth using natural tooth as pontic," *Case Reports in Dentistry*, vol. 2016, Article ID 8130352, 4 pages, 2016.

[8] K. Hebel, R. Gajjar, and T. Hofstede, "Single-tooth replacement: bridge vs. implant-supported restoration," *Journal of the Canadian Dental Association*, vol. 66, no. 8, pp. 435–438, 2000.

[9] M. G. Araújo, F. Sukekava, J. L. Wennström, and J. Lindhe, "Ridge alterations following implant placement in fresh extraction sockets: an experimental study in the dog," *Journal of Clinical Periodontology*, vol. 32, no. 6, pp. 645–652, 2005.

[10] M. Ashley and V. Holden, "An immediate adhesive bridge using the natural tooth," *British Dental Journal*, vol. 184, no. 1, pp. 18–20, 1998.

[11] C. J. Goodacre, G. Bernal, K. Rungcharassaeng, and J. Y. K. Kan, "Clinical complications in fixed prosthodontics," *Journal of Prosthetic Dentistry*, vol. 90, no. 1, pp. 31–41, 2003.

[12] H. E. Strassler, D. Taler, and L. Sensi, *Single Visit Natural Tooth Pontic Bridge with Fiber Reinforcement Ribbon*, Oral Health, North York, Canada, 2007.

[13] A. Chafaie and R. Portier, "Anterior fiber-reinforced composite resin bridge: a case report," *Pediatric Dentistry*, vol. 26, no. 6, pp. 530–534, 2004.

[14] S. Belli, F. K. Cobankara, O. Eraslan, G. Eskitascioglu, and V. Karbhari, "The effect of fiber insertion on fracture resistance of endodontically treated molars with MOD cavity and reattached fractured lingual cusps," *Journal of Biomedical Materials Research-part B Applied Biomaterials*, vol. 79, no. 1, pp. 35–41, 2006.

[15] M. Behr, M. Rosentritt, D. Latzel, and G. Handel, "Fracture resistance of fiber-reinforced vs. non-fiber-reinforced composite molar crowns," *Clinical Oral Investigations*, vol. 7, no. 3, pp. 135–139, 2003.

[16] J. Choukroun, A. Diss, A. Simonpieri et al., "Platelet-rich fibrin (PRF): a second-generation platelet concentrate. Part IV: clinical effects on tissue healing," *Oral Surgery, Oral Medicine, Oral Pathology, Oral Radiology and Endodontology*, vol. 101, no. 3, pp. E56–E60, 2006.

[17] M. T. Peck, J. Marnewick, and L. Stephen, "Alveolar ridge preservation using leukocyte and platelet-rich fibrin: a report of a case," *Case Reports in Dentistry*, vol. 2011, Article ID 345048, 5 pages, 2011.

Permissions

List of Contributors

Fernando Pedrin Carvalho Ferreira
CORA Vilhena, Vilhena, RO, Brazil

Anderson Paulo Barbosa Lima, Eliana de CássiaMolina de Paula, Ana Claudia de Castro Ferreira Conti, Danilo Pinelli Valarelli and Renata Rodrigues de Almeida-Pedrin
Department of Orthodontics, Universidade do Sagrado Coração, Bauru, SP, Brazil

Afshin Teymoortash and Stephan Hoch
Department of Otolaryngology, Head and Neck Surgery, Philipp University, Marburg, Germany

Yusuke Hamada, Srividya Prabhu and Vanchit John
Department of Periodontics and Allied Dental Program, Indiana University School of Dentistry, Indianapolis, IN 46204, USA

Deepika Pai and Saurabh Kumar
1Department of Pedodontics & Preventive Dentistry,Manipal College of Dental Sciences,Manipal,Manipal University,Manipal, India

Abhay T. Kamath
Department of Oral and Maxillofacial Surgery, Manipal College of Dental Sciences, Manipal, Manipal University, Manipal, India

Vipin Bhaskar
Department of Pedodontics & Preventive Dentistry, Mahe Institute of Dental Sciences, Mahe, Kerala, India

Ayush Goyal and Vineeta Nikhil
Department of Conservative Dentistry & Endodontics, Subharti Dental College, Meerut, Uttar Pradesh, India

Ritu Singh
Department of Paediatric and Preventive Dentistry, Subharti Dental College, Meerut, Uttar Pradesh, India

Arthur Furtado deMendonça and Mario Furtado de Mendonça
Department of Prosthodontics, Fluminense Federal University, Niterói, RJ, Brazil

George Shelby White and Georges Sara
Department of Prosthodontics, Columbia University College of Dental Medicine, New York, NY, USA

Darren Littlefair
University of Manchester (Formerly UMIST), Manchester, UK

Luna Salinas Tatiana and Del Valle Lovato Juan
Central University of Ecuador Dental School, Quito, Ecuador

Vanchit John, Daniel Shin, Allison Marlow and Yusuke Hamada
Department of Periodontics and Allied Dental Program, Indiana University School of Dentistry, Indianapolis, IN 46202, USA

Manar A. Abdul Aziz
1Oral Pathology Department, Faculty of Oral & Dental Medicine, Cairo University, Cairo, Egypt

Nermin M. Yussif
2National Institute of Laser Enhanced Sciences (NILES), Cairo University, Cairo, Egypt

Ramalingam Suganya, Narasimhan Malathi and Harikrishnan Thamizhchelvan
Department of Oral Pathology and Microbiology, Faculty of Dental Sciences, Sri Ramachandra University, Tamil Nadu, India

Subramaniam Ramkumar and G. V. V. Giri
Department of Oral and Maxillofacial Surgery, Faculty of Dental Sciences, Sri Ramachandra University, Tamil Nadu, India

Corina Marilena Cristache
Faculty of Midwifery and Medical Assisting, "Carol Davila" University of Medicine and Pharmacy, 8 Blvd Eroilor Sanitari, 050474 Bucharest, Romania

Maysa Nogueira de BarrosMelo, Viviane Almeida Sarmento and Christiano Sampaio Queiroz
Federal University of Bahia, Salvador, BA, Brazil

Lidyane Nunes Pantoja and Sara Juliana de Abreu de Vasconcellos
Department of Diagnostics and Therapeutics, Dentistry School,The Federal University of Bahia, Araújo Pinho Avenue, No. 62, 40110-150 Canela, Salvador, BA, Brazil

Priscilla Santana Pinto Gonçalves, Daniela Alejandra Cusicanqui Mendez, Daniela Rios and Thiago Cruvinel
Department of Pediatric Dentistry, Orthodontics and Public Health, Bauru School of Dentistry, University of São Paulo, Bauru, SP, Brazil

Paulo Sérgio da Silva Santos and José Humberto Damante
Department of Surgery, Stomatology, Pathology and Radiology, Bauru School of Dentistry, University of São Paulo, Bauru, SP, Brazil

Debopriya Chatterjee and Setu Mathur
Department of Periodontics, Government Dental College, Jaipur, India

Aishwarya Chatterjee
SMS Dental Department, SMS Medical College, Jaipur, India

Manoj Agarwal
Department of Endodontics, Government Dental College, Jaipur, India

Meetu Mathur
Department of Endodontics, Rajasthan Dental College, Jaipur, India

R. Mallikarjun
Department of Prosthodontics, AB Shetty Dental College, Karnataka, India

Subrata Banerjee
Department of Medicine, SMS Medical College, Jaipur, India

Luca Landi, Stefano Piccinelli and Roberto Raia
Studio di Odontoiatria Ricostruttiva, Rome, Italy

Fabio Marinotti
Dental Laboratory Technician, Studio di Odontoiatria Ricostruttiva, Rome, Italy

Paolo Francesco Manicone
Institute of Clinical Dentistry, Department of Prosthodontics, Catholic University of the Sacred Heart, Rome, Italy

Subramaniam Ramkumar
1Department of Oral & Maxillofacial Surgery, Faculty of Dental Sciences, Sri Ramachandra University, Chennai, India

Lakshmi Ramkumar
Dr. Ram'sDental Care & Maxillofacial Center, Chennai, India

Narasimhan Malathi and Ramalingam Suganya
Department of Oral Pathology and Microbiology, Faculty of Dental Sciences, Sri Ramachandra University, Chennai, India

Pradnya S. Nagmode, Archana B. Satpute, Ankit V. Patel and Pushpak L. Ladhe
Department of Conservative Dentistry and Endodontics, SMBT Dental College & Hospital, Sangamner, India

Sarah K. Y. Lee
Department of Prosthodontics, School of Dentistry, University of North Carolina at Chapel Hill, Chapel Hill, NC, USA

Rocio B. Quinonez
Department of Pediatric Dentistry and Pediatrics, Schools of Dentistry and Medicine, University of North Carolina at Chapel Hill, Chapel Hill, NC, USA

Alice Chuang
Department of Obstetrics and Gynecology, School of Medicine, University of North Carolina at Chapel Hill, Chapel Hill, NC, USA

Stephanie M.Munz and Darya Dabiri
Department ofOral and Maxillofacial Surgery/Hospital Dentistry, School of Dentistry, University of Michigan, Ann Arbor, MI,USA

Fernanda Faot
School of Dentistry, Federal University of Pelotas (UFPEL), Pelotas, RS, Brazil

Geninho Thomé, Caio Hermann, Ana Cláudia Moreira Melo, Luis Eduardo Marques Padovan and Ivete Aparecida de Mattias Sartori
Implantology Team, Latin American Institute of Dental Research and Education (ILAPEO), Curitiba, PR, Brazil

Amália Machado Bielemann
Graduate Program in Dentistry, School of Dentistry, Federal University of Pelotas, Pelotas, RS, Brazil

Paulo de CamargoMoraes
Department of Oral Surgery, School of Dentistry, SLMandic, Campinas, SP, Brazil

Luiz Alexandre Thomaz, José Luiz Cintra Junqueira and Luciana Butini Oliveira
Department of Oral Radiology, School of Dentistry, SLMandic, Campinas, SP, Brazil

Victor Angelo Martins Montalli
Department of Oral Pathology, School of Dentistry, SLMandic, Campinas, SP, Brazil

Camila Maria Beder Ribeiro
Department of Oral Pathology and Stomatology, FOP-UNICAMP, Piracicaba, SP, Brazil

Anand Deep Shukla, Abhay T. Kamath, Adarsh Kudva and Nilesh Patel
Department of Oral and Maxillofacial Surgery, Manipal College of Dental Sciences, Manipal, India

Deepika Pai
Department of Pedodontics, Manipal College of Dental Sciences, Manipal, India

Pravinkumar G. Patil
Division of Clinical Dentistry, School of Dentistry, International Medical University, Kuala Lumpur, Malaysia

Smita Nimbalkar-Patil
Department of Orthodontics, Faculty of Dentistry, MAHSA University, Kuala Lumpur, Malaysia

Terry Zaniol and Alex Zaniol
Studio Dentistico Zaniol, Crocetta del Montello, Italy

Luiz Evaristo Ricci Volpato and Álvaro Henrique Borges
Master's Program in Integrated Dental Sciences, University of Cuiabá, Cuiabá, MT, Brazil

Cristhiane Almeida Leite
Department of Oral Pathology, University of Cuiabá, Cuiabá, MT, Brazi

Brunna Haddad Anhesini
Master's Program in Restorative Dentistry,University of São Paulo, São Paulo, SP, Brazil

Jéssica Marques Gomes da Silva Aguilera
University of Cuiabá, Cuiabá, MT, Brazil

Carolina Cortez-Ortega, José Arturo Garrocho-Rangel, Joselín Flores-Velázquez, Socorro Ruiz-Rodríguez, Miguel Ángel Noyola-Frías, Miguel Ángel Santos-Díaz and Amaury Pozos-Guillén
Pediatric Dentistry Postgraduate Program, Faculty of Dentistry, San Luis Potosi University, 78290 San Luis Potosí, SLP, Mexico

O. Marouane and N. Douki
Restorative Dentistry, Dental Surgery Department, University Hospital Sahloul, Sousse, Tunisia

M. Ghorbel
Department of Removable Prosthodontics, Faculty of Dental Medicine of Monastir, Monastir, Tunisia

M. Nahdi and A. Necibi
Orthodontic Department, Faculty of Dental Medicine of Monastir, Monastir, Tunisia

Ayush Goyal, Vineeta Nikhil and Padmanabh Jha
Department of Conservative Dentistry & Endodontics, Subharti Dental College, Meerut, Uttar Pradesh, India

Luciana Munhoz and Felipe Pereira Marcos Marsan
Department of Stomatology, School of Dentistry, University of São Paulo, 2227 Lineu Prestes Avenue, 05508-000 São Paulo, SP, Brazil

Emiko Saito Arita
Department of Odontology, University of São Paulo, 448-475 Cesário Galeno Street, 03071-000 São Paulo, SP, Brazil

Sathish Muthukumar Ramalingam, Sandhya ArunKumar and Sriram Kaliamoorthy
Department of Oral and Maxillofacial Pathology, Chettinad Dental College & Research Institute, Tamil Nadu, India

Daya Srinivasa and Joe Louis ChiriyanKandath
Department of Pedodontia and Preventive Dentistry, Chettinad Dental College & Research Institute, Tamil Nadu, India

Yehoshua Shapira, Tamar Finkelstein, Rana Kadry, Shirley Schonberger and Nir Shpack
Department of Orthodontics, The Maurice and Gabriela Goldschleger School of Dental Medicine, Tel Aviv University, Tel Aviv, Israel

Karpagavalli Shanmugasundaram
Department of Oral Medicine & Radiology, Saveetha Dental College, Saveetha University, Chennai, India

V. K. Vaishnavi Vedam
Department of Oral Pathology, Faculty of Dentistry, Asian Institute of Medicine, Science & Technology (AIMST) University, Kedah, Malaysia

Sivadas Ganapathy
Department of Pedodontics and Preventive Dentistry, Faculty of Dentistry, Asian Institute of Medicine, Science & Technology (AIMST) University, Kedah, Malaysia

Sivan Sathish
Department of Oral Medicine and Radiology, Chettinad Dental College & Research Institute, Kancheepuram, India

Parvathi Satti
Chettinad Dental College & Research Institute, Kancheepuram, India